The Trusted Doctor

The Trusted Doctor

Medical Ethics and Professionalism

ROSAMOND RHODES

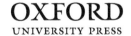

OXFORD
UNIVERSITY PRESS

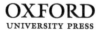

OXFORD
UNIVERSITY PRESS

Oxford University Press is a department of the University of Oxford. It furthers the University's objective of excellence in research, scholarship, and education by publishing worldwide. Oxford is a registered trade mark of Oxford University Press in the UK and certain other countries.

Published in the United States of America by Oxford University Press
198 Madison Avenue, New York, NY 10016, United States of America.

CIP data is on file at the Library of Congress
ISBN 978–0–19–085990–9

1 3 5 7 9 8 6 4 2

Printed by Integrated Books International, United States of America

To my husband, Joe Fitschen,
for your love and support, all the way.

And in memory of my parents, Michael and Helen Rhodes, and my
grandparents, Morris and Anna Gendelman.

When my grandfather attended my Masters graduation he asked what they
all had been thinking, "When you graduate from medical school you work as a
doctor. When you graduate from law school you work as an attorney. What do
you do when you graduate in philosophy?"

Contents

Illustrations

Figure

Tables

Acknowledgments

As I explored the issues in medical ethics that I encountered, I developed my thoughts incrementally over a number of years. Along the way, I presented my evolving ideas at various meetings and published them in chapters and articles (see the list that follows). I am grateful to co-authors, audience members, reviewers, and editors for their comments and questions. This work has surely benefitted from their attention and thoughtful remarks.

Chapter 1

Rhodes, R. (2001). Understanding the Trusted Doctor and Constructing a Theory of Bioethics, *Theoretical Medicine and Bioethics*, 22(6): 493–504.

Rhodes R. (2006). The Ethical Standard of Care, *American Journal of Bioethics*, 6(2): 76–78.

Rhodes R. (2007). The Professional Responsibilities of Medicine, in Rhodes R, Francis L, and Silvers A, editors, *The Blackwell Guide to Medical Ethics*, Hoboken, NJ: Blackwell: 71–87.

Rhodes R. (2013). The Ethics of Medicine: UnCommon Morality, *APA Newsletter on Philosophy and Medicine*, 12(2): 16–20. A version of this article was originally presented at the Bernard Gert Applied Ethics Conference, Dartmouth College, April 4, 2009. On that occasion, Gert offered comments in reply along the lines that I suggest in this chapter. http://c.ymcdn.com/sites/www.apaonline.org/resource/collection/250A3149-F981-47C2-9379-618149806E75/V12n2Medicine.pdf

Rhodes R. (2018). Hobbesian Medical Ethics, in Courtland S, editor, *Hobbesian Applied Ethics*, New York: Routledge: 69–90.

Rhodes R. (2019). Why Not Common Morality? *Journal of Medical Ethics*, 45: 770–777.

Rhodes R. (2019). A Defence of Medical Ethics as Uncommon Morality, *Journal of Medical Ethics*, 45: 792–793.

Chapter 2

Rhodes R and Strain JJ. (2000). Trust and Transforming Medical Institutions, *Cambridge Quarterly of Healthcare Ethics*, 9(2): 205–217.

Rhodes R. (2001) Understanding the Trusted Doctor and Constructing a Theory of Bioethics, *Theoretical Medicine and Bioethics*, 22(6): 493–504.

Rhodes R. (2003) Trust and Trustworthiness in Organ Transplantation: Good Samaritan and Emotionally Related Living Donors, *The Mount Sinai Journal of Medicine*, 70(3): 174–177.

Rhodes R. (2006) The Ethical Standard of Care, *American Journal of Bioethics*, 6(2): 76–78.

Rhodes R. (2006) The Professional Obligation of Physicians in Times of Hazard and Need: A Response to the Opinion of the AMA Council on Ethical and Judicial Affairs, *Cambridge Quarterly of Healthcare Ethics*, 15(4): 424–428.

Rhodes R. (2007) The Professional Responsibilities of Medicine, in Rhodes R, Francis L, and Silvers A, editors, *The Blackwell Guide to Medical Ethics*, Hoboken, NJ: Blackwell: 71–87.

Chapter 3

Capozzi JD and Rhodes R. (2001). Ethics in Practice: Poor Clinical Results, *The Journal of Bone and Joint Surgery*, 83A(10): 1595–1597.

Rhodes R and Schiano T. (2010). Moral Complexity and the Delusion of Moral Purity, *American Journal of Bioethics*, 10(2): W1–W3.

Schiano T and Rhodes R. (2010). The Dilemma and Reality of Transplant Tourism: An Ethical Perspective for Liver Transplant Programs, *Liver Transplantation*, 16(2): 113–117.

Chapter 4

Rhodes R. (2002). UnSafe Presumptions in Clinical Research, *American Journal of Bioethics*, 2(2): 49–51.

Rhodes R. (2003). An Innovative Paradigm for Clinical Research, *American Journal of Bioethics*, 3(4): 59–61.

Rhodes R. (2005). Rethinking Research Ethics [Target article], *American Journal of Bioethics*, 5(1): 7–28. Reprinted (2010) as the "Most Controversial Article" in the journal's 10-year history. *American Journal of Bioethics*, 10(10): 19–36.

Rhodes R. (2008). In Defense of the Duty to Participate in Biomedical Research, *American Journal of Bioethics*, 8(10): 37–38.

Rhodes R. (2008). Response to de Melo-Martin: On a Putative Duty to Participate in Biomedical Research, *American Philosophical Association Newsletter on Philosophy and Medicine*, 7(2): 12–13.

Rhodes R, Azzouni J, Baumin SB, et al. (2011). De Minimis Risk: A Proposal for a New Category of Research Risk, *American Journal of Bioethics*, 11(11): 1–7.

Capozzi JD and Rhodes R. (2013). Ethical Considerations in Clinical Research, in Einhorn T, editor, *Orthopaedic Basic Science*, 4th edition. Rosemont, IL: American Academy of Orthopaedic Surgeons: 513–520.

Rhodes R. (2015). Love Thy Neighbor: Replacing Paternalistic Protection as the Grounds for Research Ethics, *American Journal of Bioethics*, 15(9): 49–51.

Rhodes R. (2015). A Placebo Controlled Trial for an NMO Relapse Prevention Treatment: Ethical Considerations, *Multiple Sclerosis and Related Disorders*, 4(6): 580–584.

Andreae MH, Rhodes E, Bourgoise T, et al. (2016). An Ethical Exploration of Barriers to Research on Controlled Drugs, *American Journal of Bioethics*, 16(4): 36–47.

Rhodes R and Kolevzon A. (2016). Justice in Selecting Participants for a Study in Phelan-McDermid Syndrome, *American Journal of Bioethics*, 16(4): 74–76.

Chapter 5

Strain JJ and Rhodes R. (2015). Medical-Surgical Psychiatry and Medical Ethics, in Sadler JZ, Fulford W, and Werendly van Staden C, editors, *Oxford Handbook of Psychiatric Ethics*, New York: Oxford University Press: 231–243.

Chapter 6

Rhodes R. (2014). Autonomy, Agency, and Responsibility: Ethical Concerns for Living Donor Advocates, in Steel J, editor, *Living Donor Advocate: An Evolving Role Within Transplantation*, Marlton, NJ: Springer: 301–310.

Chapter 7

Capozzi JD and Rhodes R. (2004). Ethics in Practice: Lying for the Patient's Good, *The Journal of Bone and Joint Surgery*, 86-A(1): 187–188.

Capozzi JD and Rhodes R. (2006). A Family's Request for Deception, *Journal of Bone and Joint Surgery*, 88(4): 906–908.

Rhodes R and Strain JJ. (2008). Affective Forecasting and Its Implications for Medical Ethics, *Cambridge Quarterly of Healthcare Ethics*, 17(1): 54–65.

Capozzi JD and Rhodes R. (2009). Ethics in Practice: Managing Medical Errors, *Journal of Bone and Joint Surgery*, 91: 2520–2521.

Rhodes R. (in press). To Act or Not to Act, That Is the Question, *American Journal of Bioethics*.

Chapter 8

Rhodes R and Schiano T. (2010). Transplant Tourism in China: A Tale of Two Transplants [Target article], *American Journal of Bioethics*, 10(2): 3–11.

Chapter 9

Rhodes R. (2004). Justice in Allocations for Terrorism, Biological Warfare, and Public Health, in Boylan M, editor, *Public Health Ethics*, Dordrecht, Netherlands: Kluwer: 73–90.

Rhodes R. (2005). Justice in Medicine and Public Health, *Cambridge Quarterly of Healthcare Ethics*, 14(1): 13–26.

Rhodes R. (2016). Justice and Resource Allocation in Public Health, in Heggenhougen HK and Quah SR, editors, *International Encyclopedia of Public Health*, 2nd edition, volume 5, Oxford, UK: Elsevier: 544–551.

Rhodes R. (2018). Medicine and Contextual Justice, *Cambridge Quarterly of Healthcare Ethics*, 27(2): 228–249.

Chapter 10

Rhodes R. (1995). Love Thy Patient: Justice and Care in the Doctor-Patient Relationship, *Cambridge Quarterly of Health Care Ethics*, 4(4): 434–447.

Rhodes R and Smith LG. (2006). Molding Professional Character, in Kenny N and Shelton W, editors, *Lost Virtue: Professional Character Development and Medical Education*, New York: Elsevier Press: 99–115.

Chapter 11

Rhodes R and Alfandre D. (2007). A Systematic Approach to Clinical Moral Reasoning, *Clinical Ethics*, 2(2): 66–70.

Alfandre D and Rhodes R. (2009). Improving Ethics Education During Residency Training, *Medical Teacher* 31(6): 513–517.

Chapter 12

Rhodes R and Holzman IR. (2004). The Not Unreasonable Standard for Assessment of Surrogates and Surrogate Decisions, *Theoretical Medicine and Bioethics*, 25(4): 367–385.

Rhodes R and Holzman IR. (2014). Is the Best Interest Standard Good for Pediatrics? *Pediatrics* 134(Suppl 2): S121–S129.

Chapter 13

Rhodes R. (2006). Conscientious Objection in Medicine, The Priority of Professional Ethics Over Personal Morality, Rapid Response to Julian Savulescu, *British Medical Journal*, 332: 294–297. https://doi.org/10.1136/bmj.332.7536.294

Rhodes R and Danziger M. (2018). Being a Doctor and Being a Hospital, *American Journal of Bioethics*, 18(4): 88–90.

Rhodes R. (2019). Conscience, Conscientious Objections, and Medicine, *Theoretical Medicine and Bioethics*, 40(6): 487–506.

Chapter 14

Rhodes R. (2015). Good and Not So Good Medical Ethics, *Journal of Medical Ethics*, 41(1): 71–74.

The Trusted Doctor

Introduction

A medical school is a peculiar place for a philosopher to make a career, and I expect that a philosopher may seem like an unlikely person to propose a new theory of medical ethics. I am a philosopher who has spent the past 30 years as a member of the faculty of Icahn School of Medicine at Mount Sinai, and, perhaps audaciously, in this book I present a novel approach to the ethics of the profession and medical professionalism.

This book is certainly a display of chutzpah in that it aims to inform the medical profession about itself and challenge the reigning views of medical ethics. I regard this work as providing a needed framework that can help doctors understand their professional responsibilities, explain their scope and rationale, and fit them together with the kernels of wisdom, principles, and virtues that are all espoused as elements of medical professionalism. I also see this book as an important corrective to the previously accepted approach that regards the ethics of medicine as an application of common morality to the issues that arise in medicine.

I recognize that I owe readers an explanation for why I consider myself to be up to these tasks. My philosophic training at the Graduate Center, City University of New York (CUNY), focused primarily on the history of moral and political philosophy, but as a graduate student I also had experience in applied ethics. While I was a student at CUNY, a group of faculty members received a grant to develop collaborations with professional schools in the region to incorporate ethics education into their professional training. Their model involved a member of the CUNY philosophy faculty and a graduate student joining with a faculty member at the professional school in leading a class on ethical issues within that profession. First, Virginia Held launched a course at the Hunter School of Social Work, and Marshall Cohen launched a collaboration on military ethics at West Point. Professor Cohen invited me to join his team at West Point, where I participated in his seminars for 2 years. Then Bernard (Stefan) Baumrin began a course on medical ethics with faculty members at Mount Sinai, and invited me to join his Mount Sinai team. Just as the grant funding ended, and as I neared completion of my

The Trusted Doctor. Rosamond Rhodes, Oxford University Press (2020). © Oxford University Press.
DOI: 10.1093/oso/9780190859909.001.0001

dissertation, Mount Sinai's dean, Dr. Nathan Kase, decided to hire a faculty member in bioethics. The search concluded with Dr. Barry Stimmel, Chair of the Department of Medical Ethics, offering me the position.

When I first began my work at Mount Sinai, I was the sole philosopher at the institution, and I certainly felt like a stranger among the hundreds of medical professionals. As the only bioethicist on campus, I was called on by any department that wanted ethics education for their trainees and any team that wanted ethics consultation. I was asked to join the hospital Ethics Committee by its original chair, Dr. Kurt Hirschhorn, then I became the Ethics Committee secretary when Dr. Ian Holzman took over as chair and recently Dr. Ron Shapiro and I became co-chairs of the committee.

Over the years, my position at Mount Sinai exposed me to a broad range of medical environments associated with the full complement of the institution's departments and services, nurses, social workers, patient representatives, and clergy. Some of my most memorable collaborative activities were in teaching rounds that were jointly led by a physician and me. Over the years, these have included weekly rounds with Dr. Richard Gorlin, then chair of medicine, and Dr. James Strain, then director of liaison psychiatry; rounds with Dr. Hirschhorn, then chair of pediatrics; rounds with Dr. Holzman, director of the newborn intensive care unit; rounds with Dr. James Capozzi and the residents in orthopedics; rounds with Dr. Thomas Kalb in the medical intensive care unit and first Dr. Thomas Iberti and then Dr. Ernest Benjamin in the surgical intensive care unit; rounds with Dr. Richard Berkowitz with residents in obstetrics; decades of rounds with the surgeons initiated by then-chair of Surgery, Dr. Arthur Aufses; sessions with Dr. Avi Barbasch and the hematology and oncology fellows; sessions with Dr. Lynne Richardson and the emergency medicine residents; and sessions with Dr. Michael Newton and the ophthalmology residents.

There have also been a host of more formal teaching activities for the medical students, residents, fellows, and graduate students in many of our graduate programs, including years of leading seminars with Dr. James Strain for the psychiatry residents, with Randi Zinberg for the genetic counseling students, and research ethics with Internal Review Board member Karin Meyers, and recently Dr. Daniel Moros for students in the clinical research program. I have also been an active member of the Institutional Animal Care and Use Committee (IACUC) and worked with Dr. Giorgio Martinelli, a participant in kidney transplant meetings led by Dr. Lewis Burrows, and worked closely with Drs. Charlie Miller, Myron Schwartz, Thomas Schiano, and many others in the Transplant Institute. And, for sustained academic analysis, I joined the monthly Faculty Seminars on the Philosophy and History of Medicine, an interdisciplinary journal discussion group led by Dr. Daniel Moros. Those meetings, which provided lively debate over issues in the bioethics literature, have been ongoing since before I started work at Mount Sinai.

Most of my Mount Sinai activities count as education in one way or another, but I have also been involved in research projects, policy development, crafting responses to issues that arise, and planning to address possible future problems. I was involved in these activities because the organizers wanted my bioethics input. At the same time, my exposure allowed me to learn about the conundrums that arise in today's medical practice, the ways that physicians understand their roles, and how medicine is practiced in a tertiary care facility in the middle of New York City. Throughout this 30-year period, I have collaborated with colleagues on writing projects and organizing conferences. All of these interactions were opportunities for me to learn about the environment that was initially so foreign to me and to gain experience in thinking through ethical issues and dilemmas. I had no formal education in medicine, but my engagement in the medical environment provided me with a deep appreciation of the work of physicians, their commitments, and the complicated and difficult ethical matters that they confront.

One annual activity stands out from the rest for expanding my understanding of bioethical issues and providing a venue for testing my ideas and receiving critical feedback from an international group of bioethics scholars. The Oxford–Mount Sinai Consortium on Bioethics has thus far convened 28 annual meetings on both sides of the Atlantic with faculty members from Oxford University, Mount Sinai, King's College London, Vrije University of Amsterdam, and Bar Ilan University in Israel. I have hugely benefitted from the rich conversations that we have shared and the incisive comments on my work as it has progressed. I am especially indebted to the group's long-standing members who have now become dear friends: Tony Hope, Mike Parker, Jonathan Glover, Guy Widershoven, and Noam Zohar.

In addition, I have learned a great deal about explaining the process of clinical moral reasoning from teaching the skill to master's students in the bioethics program that we run jointly with Clarkson University. I have the responsibility for running the program's intensive week-long Clinical Ethics Practicum. Developing this critical part of the curriculum, including the various case analysis activities, standardized patient encounters, and evaluation tools, required me to dissect the thinking process that I developed over decades. Working with Ellen Tobin and Nada Gligorov to constantly improve the course improved my own understanding of the steps involved and enabled me to explain the material in a useful way.

I mention all of these contacts because my debts to each of these colleagues run deep. They have been generous and gracious in allowing me to learn from them, and I am profoundly grateful for the opportunities that they have shared with me. Without their perspectives I would not have been able to adequately appreciate the issues that doctors confront or the multiple facets of relevant considerations that have to be taken into account in medical ethics. Their stories and insights have shaped my understanding of the field and provided me with the perspective for piecing together a theory of medical ethics.

I also note these experiences in order to display the source of my understanding of medicine as a profession and my insight into its ethics. I have come to comprehend the landscape little by little, and I pieced it together one bit at a time. When I began in the field, I accepted the reigning views, and I felt secure that my knowledge of traditional moral philosophy provided me with the theoretical background for addressing the moral problems in medicine. But over the years, I started to notice that the well-accepted views from common morality did not fit with what physicians and nonphysicians considered good clinical practice. For example, after 9/11 I began to realize that many allocations of resources in medical contexts did not adhere with my then-favorite view of what justice required. Similarly, through my work as the living donor advocate for the liver transplant program, I began to notice serious problems in the views on autonomy that were espoused by leading philosophers. One by one the counterexamples began to accumulate until I reached the conclusion that everyday ethics and medical ethics were inconsistent with each other.

That recognition left me with the realization that a new and different account was needed to explain the ethics of medicine. I also developed an appreciation of the fact that even though numerous elements of well-accepted medical practice were radically different from common morality, for the most part those practices were what they should be. I recognized that a new theory of medical ethics would have to cohere with those laudable elements of clinical practice and be able to explain why they were right. It would also have to explain why some accepted behaviors and policies were wrong.

Thus, my first aim in this book is to demonstrate that the ethics of being a doctor is very different from the morality of everyday life. (Throughout the book, I address my remarks to all medical professionals, including doctors, nurses, social workers, patient representatives, physical therapists, genetics counselors, clergy, pharmacists, and so on, but to streamline the text, I refer to "doctors" and "physicians" rather than repeating the more cumbersome "medical professionals.") In that sense, after persuading readers of the distinctiveness of medical ethics and stripping doctors from their mooring in common morality, my next task is to provide a replacement, a new view of the unique ethics of the medical profession.

Thus, my second aim is to develop an account of the source of medical ethics, delineate the core duties of physicians, explain why each one is a necessary element of medical professionalism, and show how the various pieces of required behavior and character fit together and conform to what doctors already recognize as exemplary doctorly behavior and medical professionalism. Along the way, in a manner that is consistent with the tradition of case-based medical education, I provide numerous examples to illustrate the kinds of actions that each duty entails. I also offer a tool to guide clinical moral reasoning and for navigating the inevitable moral dilemmas that arise in clinical practice and provide guidance for avoiding pitfalls in moral analysis that arise from infelicitous and imprecise use of language. In sum, the overview of medical ethics that I propose clarifies the moral dimension of medical practice and serves as a guide to what physicians have to be and do in order to meet the standards set by medical professionalism.

This book does not aim to address all of the issues and questions that involve medicine and society. My focus is on the narrow range of issues that doctors and other medical professionals actually have to decide and actions that physicians and their colleagues actually have to perform. In other words, I deliberately set aside public policy issues such as the legalization of recreational marijuana, the definition of death, and how much of society's resources should be allocated for medical needs. Instead, I turn my efforts to the narrow domain of clinical practice and concentrate on matters that are decided by medical professionals. I see myself as providing doctors with a clear picture of the obligations that they undertake when they put on a white coat so that each physician does not have to start from scratch to decipher the duties that they assume when they join the profession. I also regard this project as clarifying the illusive concept of medical professionalism by explaining it as the standards that are derived from the ethics of medicine. This perspective provides a comprehensive picture of the identity-forming virtues, commitments, and competencies that physicians are expected to embody and exemplify in their professional behavior.

I expect that a good deal of what I expound will feel old hat and sound like mother's milk because it is what thoughtful and noble physicians already know to be their duty and what patients and society already expect of doctors. I fully appreciate that the ways in which I present this material may seem to be nothing new or no more than common sense. Nevertheless, I regard providing an account that unites the ethics of medicine into a comprehensive view by explaining the source of medicine's moral commitments and enumerating and defining its obligations and virtues is a significant and original contribution that advances understanding of medical ethics and professionalism.

At the same time, my challenge to the long-standing and widely accepted view that the ethics of medicine is just common morality applied to the medical field and expressed in the four principles, ten rules, or four topics approaches will seem like heresy to many readers. To that I say that the evidence for concluding that medical ethics is different from everyday ethics is clear and compelling, and it should not be ignored. It's time to set aside bioethics orthodoxy and recognize that traditional convoluted explanations in terms of simplistic concepts fail to explain medicine's distinctive obligations, and that vaguely waving in the direction of professional obligation is jejune and uninformative.

The intended audience for this book includes all varieties of medical professionals, bioethicists, philosophers, and general readers. I mention this because at a few points some of what I say speaks to one audience more than another, so some patience may be in order. I have tried to eschew overly abstract descriptions in philosophic terms, but in some instances a bit of technical philosophical language is necessary. Although I did try to keep the philosophic discussion to a minimum and delegate a few digressions to footnotes rather than include them in the main text, there are points where entering the philosophical debate was necessary. Chapter 1 presents my argument against the reigning common morality view of medical ethics. Those who want to jump into my uncommon morality account of medical ethics may want to skip over that chapter. Later in the book, I also decided that a foray into the history of philosophy or the explication of some moral theory was elucidating and justified. These excursions are especially obvious in

Chapter 9, Why Trustworthy Stewardship Requires Justice, and Chapter 13, Professional Responsibility and Conscientious Objection. Readers should feel free to explore these excursions or avoid my self-indulgence by skipping over those sections.

Throughout the book, I pointedly sidestep engaging in debates that I regarded as tangential to my specific aims to avoid disrupting the flow of the central argument and my account of the duties of a physician. Even though some readers may fault me with dodging philosophic arguments, I considered some issues to be rather settled matters and chose not to engage in a broader discussion of generic issues such as truth-telling and confidentiality. My omissions also justified limiting references to the bioethics literature on those topics: No offense is intended by those exclusions.

As I mentioned, I do provide numerous case examples to illustrate medical duties and the kinds of circumstances in which they arise. Almost all of the cases that I use come from my experience at Mount Sinai, although some details have been changed to protect confidentiality. These examples are cases that I encountered and cases that have been shared by colleagues in various venues, and I have used some of the cases in teaching students in different programs. Aside from their explanatory value, the cases may be useful to those who teach bioethics and others engaged in medical education. In describing the cases, I provide sufficient detail to make the circumstances realistic and clear. I also make the ethical issues accessible to those without a medical background.

In the case descriptions and throughout the book, I alternate the gender of physicians and patients to avoid confusion and avoid the awkward use of "he or she," "him or her." When I present the patient as male, I typically present the doctor as female and vice versa. When I refer to the doctor as a male in one section, in the next section I typically refer to the doctor as a female. Nothing of substance is intended by my random assignment of gender.

The chapters in this book are ordered in a sequence that seems cogent, but each chapter is designed also to stand alone, and I wrote them so that they would be comprehensible when read in any order. Conceptually, Chapter 2, The Distinctive Ethics of Medicine, provides the justification for all of the discussions of duties that follow, but even with that caveat, each chapter should be clear enough without what comes before it. This stand-alone feature is designed to make the entire volume useful in teaching and particularly in medical education. The cost of employing that stand-alone design is a small amount of repetition to flesh out the arguments without relying on what came before. A charitable view of this repetition will be to regard it either as illustrating medicine's typical practice of assessing harms and benefits and balancing them against each other or as useful reminders of what has come before.

Before concluding these introductory remarks, I need to add one more acknowledgment of gratitude. Every complicated well-functioning program is supported by someone working behind the scene who keeps track of the details, follows up on whatever needs attention, overcomes errors and accidents, and makes friends with all of the critical players whose help may be needed at some point. For nearly my entire career at Mount Sinai, Karen Smalls has been that hero for the bioethics program. I am immensely thankful for all that she has done, for her caring and diligent commitment to the program, her intelligence, and most of all, for her friendship. Karen holds the fort and supports everyone who works with us with her resourcefulness, her smiles, and her warmth.

1

Why a New Approach to Medical Ethics Is Needed

The Argument

Although it is commonplace to view medical ethics as the application of traditional moral theory to questions of ethics that arise in medicine, I have a different view. The dominant view was articulated by K. Danner Clouser in his *Encyclopedia of Bioethics* article "Bioethics," where he explained that "bioethics is not a new set of principles or maneuvers, but the same old ethics being applied to a particular realm of concerns."[1] The strategy was further explained by Clouser and colleagues Bernard Gert and Charles Culver in *Bioethics: A Return to Fundamentals*[2] and again in *Bioethics: A Systematic Approach*,[3] where they identified ten moral rules as the crux of ordinary morality. This common morality approach was most prominently expounded by Tom Beauchamp and James Childress in the seven editions of their *Principles of Biomedical Ethics*[4] and adopted by Albert Jonsen, Mark Siegler, and William Winslade in the eight editions of *Clinical Ethics: A Practical Approach to Ethical Decisions in Clinical Medicine*.[5] In their volumes, Beauchamp and Childress argued that the action-guiding norms of traditional ethical theories tend to converge on the acceptance of the norms of common morality "without argumentative support."[6] Drawing on common

---

[1] Clouser KD, "Bioethics," in Reich W, editor, *Encyclopedia of Bioethics* (New York: Free Press, 1978: Volume 1, 115–127, p. 116.
[2] Gert B, Culver CM, and Clouser KD, *Bioethics: A Return to Fundamentals* (New York: Oxford University Press, 1997).
[3] Gert B, Culver CM, and Clouser KD, *Bioethics: A Systematic Approach* (New York: Oxford University Press, 2006).
[4] Beauchamp TL and Childress JF, *Principles of Biomedical Ethics*, 7th edition (New York: Oxford University Press, 2013).
[5] Jonsen AR, Siegler M, and Winslade WJ, *Clinical Ethics: A Practical Approach to Ethical Decisions in Clinical Medicine*, 8th edition (New York: McGraw-Hill Education, 2015). These authors largely accepted the Beauchamp and Childress four principles approach and supplemented it with their four topics method for collecting and organizing the case information that is relevant to making ethical decisions.
[6] Beauchamp and Childress, *Principles*, 2013, 407.

The Trusted Doctor. Rosamond Rhodes, Oxford University Press (2020). © Oxford University Press.
DOI: 10.1093/oso/9780190859909.001.0001

features of prominent moral theories, they identified the four principles of respect for autonomy, beneficence, nonmaleficence, and justice as the "considered judgments that are the most well-established moral beliefs" to "serve as an anchor of moral reflection."[7] They used those principles in their analyses of ethical issues that arise in medicine, and that version of the common morality approach to medical ethics has come to be known as *principlism*.

We also find authors who addressed issues in medical ethics drawing on the historical canon of moral and political philosophy. They discussed autonomy in Kantian terms, and they invoked Aristotle when they discuss professionalism in terms of virtue theory. They cited Bentham and Mill when they debated the allocation of scarce resources in utilitarian terms and numerous early modern and contemporary philosophers when they addressed access to healthcare in terms of rights theory.

As I see it, the well-entrenched approach that regards medical ethics as an extension of common morality, and the vast bioethics literature of the past 50-odd years that largely adopts that view, is simply mistaken. I see the ethics of medicine as being radically different from "the same old ethics" of everyday life. My view of medical ethics as distinct and different from common morality is not entirely original in that others have taken positions along these lines. I count Hippocrates, Thomas Percival, John Gregory, and a few more contemporary authors, including David Thomasma, Edmund Pellegrino, Bernard Baumrin, Benjamin Freedman, Robert Baker, Lance Stell, and Lawrence McCullough as allies in this cause. I also acknowledge that in arguing for the distinctiveness of medical ethics, I am arguing for a position that reflects a point made by John Rawls in *Political Liberalism*. There Rawls noted that "it is the distinct purposes and roles of the parts of the social structure . . . that [explain] there being different principles for distinct kinds of subjects."[8]

Roles and Professions

Moving a step beyond Rawls, I see the need to also distinguish social and institutional roles from professions.[9] For the most part, role morality is

---

[7] Beauchamp and Childress, *Principles*, 2013, 407, 408.

[8] Rawls J, *Political Liberalism* (New York: Columbia University Press, 1993, 262).

[9] In the ethics literature, roles and professions are often lumped together (e.g., Gibson K, "Contrasting Role Morality and Professional Morality: Implications for Practice," *Journal of Applied Ethics* 20, 1 (2003): 17–29. https://doi.org/10.1111/1468-5930.00232

consistent with common morality and special role-related obligations (e.g., being a parent, butcher, baker, or candlestick maker) derive from individuals' voluntarily assuming special responsibilities by making an explicit or implicit promise.[10] The starting point for recognizing that medicine requires its own distinctive ethic, one that is different from common morality and even role morality, lies in appreciating that medicine is a profession and what that means.

Social scientists define professions by describing what they see. For example, sociologist Talcott Parsons observed that professions involve "a cluster of occupational roles, that is, roles in which the incumbents perform certain functions valued in the society," and that they typically provide a livelihood and have their own codes and oaths, their own technical language, and sometimes their own uniforms.[11] All of that is interesting, but then we should ask, why is that so?

Professions are different from roles in that the knowledge, powers, privileges, and immunities that society allows to professions are radically different from what is allowed for ordinary citizens. Because the commissions granted to professionals, and no one outside of those professions, are potentially dangerous,[12] the duties of each profession must be articulated, and the limitations on how their distinctive authority may be employed must be delineated and explained. Table 1.1 enumerates some of the distinctive features of medicine.

Whereas everyone is allowed to take on the duties of parenthood, butcher his own meat, bake her own cakes, and make his own candlesticks, only medical professionals are permitted to perform surgery, only those in the

[10] Role morality and "voluntarism" are discussed by numerous authors, such as Hardimon MO, "Role Obligations," *The Journal of Philosophy* 91, 7 (1974): 333–363. doi:10.2307/2940934; Simmons AJ, "External Justifications and Institutional Roles," *The Journal of Philosophy* 93, 1 (1996): 28–36. doi:10.2307/2941017; Cane P, "Role Responsibility," *The Journal of Ethics* 20, 1–3 (2016): 279–298; Baril A, "The Ethical Importance of Roles," *The Journal of Value Inquiry* 50, 4 (2016): 721–734; MacKay D, "Standard of Care, Institutional Obligations, and Distributive Justice," *Bioethics* 29, 4 (2015): 262–273. https://doi.org/10.1111/bioe.12060; Stern RA. " 'My Station and Its Duties': Social Role Accounts of Obligation in Green and Bradley," in Ameriks K, editor, *The Impact of Idealism: Volume 1, Philosophy and Natural Sciences* (Cambridge: Cambridge University Press, 2013: 299–322).

[11] Parsons T, "The Professions and Social Structure," *Social Forces* 17, 4 (1939): 457–467. Sociologists like Talcott Parson define *profession* by cataloging what they observe about professions. The literature on professions largely follows their lead. See, for example, Latham SR, "Medical Professionalism: A Parsonian View," *Mount Sinai Journal of Medicine* 69, 6 (2002): 363–369 2002.

[12] Alan Tapper and Stephan Millet and also W. P. Metzger take positions that are, in some respects, similar to mine on this issue. Tapper A and Millett S. "Revisiting the Concept of a Profession," *Research in Ethical Issues in Organisations* 13 (2015): 1–18. Metzger WP. "What Is a Profession?" *College & University*, 52, 1 (1976): 42–55.

Table 1.1 Some Distinctive Features of Medicine

Knowledge	Anatomy, physiology, immunology, pathology, pharmacology, genetics, microbiology, genomics, biochemistry, and so on
Powers	Determine lack of decisional capacity Impose treatment over objection Deprive people of freedom (i.e., involuntary commitment)
Privileges	Ask probing questions Examine nakedness Image insides Prescribe and administer medication (i.e., poison) or treatments Perform surgery (i.e., assault with deadly weapons) Inflict pain
Immunities	From prosecution for employing powers and privileges From prosecution for untoward outcomes

military are allowed to explode bombs to kill other humans, and only priests may grant absolution. Because the risks to society of granting professional permissions and exemptions are significant, professions are required to establish explicit and transparent rules and standards of conduct to govern their extraordinary commissions.[13] In order to be trusted with the remarkable freedoms that society allows its members, each profession (e.g., medicine, military, clergy) must articulate its own profession-specific moral rules and describe the distinctive character required from its members.

Why Not Common Morality?

The widely accepted practice of invoking principlism or employing concepts from common morality to explain medical ethics is actually at odds with a longer tradition of understanding professional ethics as distinctly different from the ethics of everyday life. In what follows, I specifically challenge only the views of the most popular of such approaches to medical ethics articulated by Beauchamp and Childress and by Gert, Culver, and Clouser and their followers that medical ethics is just common morality applied to the complex issues that arise in clinical medicine. They see their contribution to

---

[13] Exploring the details of how and why professional identity should be distinguished from roles goes beyond the limited scope of this chapter; it is a project for another day. For the purposes of this chapter, it is enough to enumerate the extraordinary ways in which a license granted to medical professionals exceeds what other individuals may do.

the field as merely specification of common morality, largely as a response to remarkable recent scientific and technological advances in the field.

Initially, I also accepted the common morality view of medical ethics uncritically, and I felt secure that my knowledge of traditional moral and political philosophy provided me with the theoretical background for addressing the moral problems in medicine. But over the years, I started to notice that the well-accepted views did not fit with what physicians and nonphysicians considered good clinical practice. One by one, counterexamples began to accumulate until I reached the conclusion that everyday ethics and medical ethics were incompatible. Over the same period, discussion in academic medicine circles began to shift away from medical ethics and toward medical professionalism. Elements in that discussion rang true, but as critics rightly acknowledged, the accounts of medical professionalism lacked a supporting conceptual framework.[14]

Ultimately, I came to appreciate three facts: (1) that numerous elements of well-accepted medical practice were what they should be, (2) that those practices were not consistent with commonly espoused approaches to medical ethics, and (3) that the most popular approaches to medical ethics were not particularly useful in resolving dilemmas in clinical practice. Those insights led me to recognize that a new theory of medical ethics was needed. A new theory would therefore have to challenge the long-standing and widely accepted common morality approaches and have to cohere with both the laudable elements of clinical practice and explain why some accepted behaviors and policies were wrong. Thus, I realized that developing a new theory of medical ethics would be embarking on a project to contest the common morality approaches to medical ethics, something that was likely to be regarded as bioethics heresy.

In the face of what appears to be clear and compelling evidence for concluding that medical ethics is different from everyday ethics, I am picking up the gauntlet and confronting the challenge head on. Whereas the common morality approach may still be appropriate for guiding public policy related to healthcare,[15] in this chapter I am setting aside bioethics orthodoxy and rejecting the relevance of this common morality approach to the practice of medicine. I recognize that my opposition to this long-standing tradition

---

[14] Wear D and Kuczewski MG, "The Professionalism Movement: Can We Pause?" *American Journal of Bioethics* 4, 2 (2004): 1–10.

[15] For example, Kuczewski MG, "The Common Morality in Communitarian Thought: Reflective Consensus in Public Policy," *Theoretical Medicine and Bioethics* 30, 1 (2009): 45–54.

requires a robust defense. Here, I present my case for distinguishing "medical ethics" from "common morality" and argue that medical professionalism is tied to medicine's distinctive ethics.[16]

The Distinctiveness of the Ethics of Medicine

I begin by demonstrating that the ethics of medicine is distinct and different from common morality. This is critically important because if I can show that the principles or rules of common morality are inadequate guides for the action of medical professionals, and that in some circumstances they direct doctors to do what good doctors should not do, that demonstration would prove that common morality accounts of medical ethics are inadequate. Furthermore, the conclusion would imply that doctors need a different touchstone for their professional behavior, a theory of medical ethics that provides them with clear and reliable moral guidance. Patients' well-being depends on their decisions, so doctors need a moral compass that can point them in the right direction.

The reigning view, that all bioethics is traditional ethics applied in a novel set of circumstances, amounts to a universal claim. It implies that there is nothing distinctive about the moral principles of medicine or the moral virtues of a physician. According to the laws of logic, a single counterexample refutes a universal claim. Although one counterexample should be sufficient repudiation, because the belief that medical ethics is just common morality is so widely accepted and deeply entrenched, to make a compelling argument for the distinctiveness of medical ethics, I offer a week's worth of counterexamples to prove the distinctiveness of medical ethics.

---

[16] The view that the ethics of professions is different in some respects from common morality is implicit in the codes of ethics developed by medical organizations. It has also been defended by a number of authors, such as Freedman B, "A Meta-Ethics for Professional Morality," *Ethics* 89, 1 (1978): 1–19. https://doi.org/10.1086/292100; Freedman B, "What Really Makes Professional Morality Different: Response to Martin," *Ethics* 91, 4 (1981): 626–630. https://doi.org/10.1086/ 292275; Veatch RM, "Professional Medical Ethics: The Grounding of Its Principle," *The Journal of Medicine and Philosophy* 4, 1 (1979): 1–19. https://doi.org/10.1093/jmp/4.1.1; Goldman AH, "The Moral Foundations of Professional Ethics," *Law and Philosophy* 2, 3 (1983): 397–403; Smith J-C, "Strong Separatism in Professional Ethics," *Professional Ethics* 3, 3/4 (1994): 117–140. doi:10.5840/ profethics199433/416. It has also been criticized in the ethics literature, for example, Gewirth A, "Professional Ethics: The Separatist Thesis," *Ethics* 96, 2 (1986): 282–300. https://doi.org/10.1086/ 292747); Martin MW, "Rights and the Meta-Ethics of Professional Morality," *Ethics* 91, 4 (1981): 619– 625. https://doi.org/10.1086/292274). It is beyond the scope of this chapter to discuss the details of similar views or defend against our opponents.

1. Imagine a doctor[17] sitting quietly in a corner. She has not murdered anyone, not stolen anything, and not inflicted any harm on anyone.[18] In the eyes of most observers, her behavior would be judged to be totally acceptable. After all, the bulk of our moral responsibility in ordinary life is negative. We must refrain from harming others by not killing, stealing, injuring, or deceiving. Yet, a doctor who merely sat in a crowded emergency room reading the newspaper and drinking the coffee that she had purchased would not be taken to have acted well. That is because doctors have a positive duty to respond to patient needs and actively promote their patients' good even when it's time for a coffee break.[19]

2. In everyday life, we are free to make decisions any way we like. You can choose to accept guidance from your horoscope, tarot cards, a Magic 8 Ball toy, or your favorite radio personality. You and your friends may decide on a movie by flipping a coin. You might rely on your gut feeling when you select your vacation destination or relocate your family because you decide that it's time for a change. Doctors, however, are expected to rely on scientific evidence when they recommend treatment for their patients. Gut feelings and the like are not acceptable justifications for medical decisions.

3. In the course of ordinary social interactions, we freely share what we learn. We tell one another about what happened in the course of our daily lives, we share our opinions, and we convey information that we discover about others. We speak about who can and cannot be trusted to repay a loan, which restaurants serve bad food, which teachers grade fairly, who is no longer speaking to whom, whose relationships are on the rocks, which doctor was hours late for an appointment, and which dentist has a gentle touch. Such sharing is useful and entertaining, and it is very much a part of the fabric of our lives. We are free to impart

---

[17] For simplicity, in this chapter and throughout this book, I refer to doctors or physicians as my central example. I do, however, take the ethics of medicine to extend broadly and inclusively across the several medical professions and to apply to all medical professionals, such as, for example, nurses, pharmacists, genetics counselors, physical therapists, social workers, and so on. Furthermore, I use *doctor* and *physician* as synonyms and alternate between the terms just for sake of variety.

[18] Here I am explicitly referring to the first five rules that Gert has informally referred to as being "the first tablet."

[19] Medicine's fiduciary duty to act for the benefit of patients and society is discussed in Chapter 2 as the second duty of medical ethics: use medical knowledge, skills, powers, and privileges for the benefit of patients and society. It is further discussed in Chapter 3 as the fourth duty of medical ethics: provide care.

what we learn, and exceptions actually require explicit requests for keeping divulged information in confidence (e.g., making promises, signing nondisclosure agreements) or some special understanding arising from the details of an intimate relationship. In medicine, at least since the time of Hippocrates, however, confidentiality is presumed, although some exceptions can be justified.[20]

4. In ordinary life, we are free to associate with whomever we choose. In fact, we were taught, and we teach our children, to be careful in our choice of friends. We are supposed to attentively distinguish between people based on their character and reputation and avoid the unsavory and those who might have a negative influence on our behavior. We should be discriminating in our judgments about the character of others and associate with people who are likely to be good role models and help us to improve ourselves. But in medicine, doctors are supposed to be nonjudgmental and minister to every patient's medical needs without judgments regarding their character or worth.[21]

5. Most people today consider sexual activity among consenting adults to be both pleasurable and ethically acceptable. Unless force, deception, or indecent exposure is involved, sexual interactions between adults are not immoral. In medicine, however, disclosure and consent do not legitimize a physician's sexual involvement with a patient. We expect that a patient's invitation for a tryst will be declined, and that none would be issued to a patient by a doctor even when all of the parties are adults and no force or deception is involved.[22]

6. In ordinary social situations, asking probing personal questions is regarded as rude. I have heard that in Texas and Oklahoma you should never ask a man how much money or land he has. We shouldn't inquire about the details of other people's sex lives, their constipation, their drug use, or even their weight. Many people don't speak about death, illness, or emotions, and lots of people studiously avoid discussing politics. Yet, taking a complete and detailed patient history can include

[20] Medical confidentiality is discussed in detail in Chapter 5 as the ninth duty of medical ethics.

[21] The duty of nonjudgmental regard is discussed in detail in Chapter 5 as the seventh duty of medical ethics, one of the duties of behavior toward patients.

[22] The duty of nonsexual regard is discussed in Chapter 5 as the eighth duty of medical ethics, a duty of behavior toward patients.

asking about a patient's diet, bowel habits, sexual practices, drug use, previous illnesses, emotions, and fears.[23]

7. The morality of ordinary life requires us to regard others as autonomous beings and to respect their choices. Immanuel Kant instructed us to "cast a veil of philanthropy over the faults of others . . . by silencing our judgments."[24] This injunction amounts to requiring us to regard the acts of others *as if* they were chosen with thoughtful consideration and for good reasons. For the most part, the Kantian attitude of respect commands us to leave others alone and allow them to advance their own conception of the good. Even doctors observe this rule when they are outside of their clinical setting. When they see others smoking cigarettes, they walk by with respectful disregard even though they worry about cancer. They hold their tongues when they observe others sporting multiple tattoos or numerous items of body piercing jewelry, even though they are concerned about hepatitis. They even remain silent as overweight others indulge in decadent deserts although they are aware of the dangers of obesity. Nevertheless, in a visit to the doctor's office, it is hard to imagine that a good doctor would fail to admonish a patient about the risks of cancer, hepatitis, or obesity. Physicians are not allowed to presume that their patients are acting autonomously. Instead, they are responsible for vigilant assessment of patients' decisional capacity, and they are sometimes required to take steps to oppose patients' preferences (e.g., warning patients who'd prefer not to hear it about health risks, overriding the wishes of the patient who refuses surgery for a strangulated hernia or ruptured appendix out of fear that her body will be invaded by aliens through the incision).[25]

All of these examples are presented to make the point that the ethics of medicine is distinct and different from the ethics of everyday life. To summarize the differences that the examples illustrate, I have arranged them in Table 1.2 that makes the dissimilarities glaringly explicit. This graphic depiction of the difference between duties of medical ethics and common morality on

---

[23] Taking a patient's medical history is an element of professional competence. It is discussed in Chapter 3 as a core responsibility, an element of the third duty of medical ethics, professional competence.

[24] Kant I, *Immanuel Kant: Ethical Philosophy (The Metaphysical Principles of Virtue*; Part II of *The Metaphysics of Morals*), translated by JW Ellington (Indianapolis, IN: Hackett, 1993 [§43, 466] 132).

[25] Issues of respect for autonomy and justified paternalism are discussed in Chapter 6, Autonomy and Trust.

Table 1.2 The Distinctiveness of Medical Ethics

Counter-examples	Duties of Medical Ethics	Common Morality Versus Medical Ethics
1. Look after your own interests	Act for the good of patients and society	A moral **ideal** is transformed into a **duty**
2. Make choices your own way	Guide choices with scientific evidence	A moral **ideal** is transformed into a **duty**
3. Share information	Confidentiality	**Permissible** behavior is **impermissible**
4. Judge the worth of others	Nonjudgmental regard	**Permissible** behavior is **impermissible**
5. Enjoy sexual interaction	Nonsexual regard	**Permissible** behavior is **impermissible**
6. Mind your own business	Probe (with examination, tests, and questions)	**Impermissible** behavior is a **duty**
7. Presume others have autonomy	Assess decisional capacity	**Impermissible** behavior is a **duty**

the same issues highlights the fact that our expectations for the behavior of doctors and nonphysicians are different.

If common morality and medical ethics were the same, then the ethically justified behavior for doctors and everyone else would be the same. But, as Table 1.2 illustrates, they're not. If the four principles or ten rules of common morality were doing the explanatory work in medical ethics, logically, the same premises would lead to the same conclusions for everyone. The marked difference in what is optional for ordinary people and required for doctors, and the radical differences in actions that are acceptable and unacceptable for doctors and others, demonstrate that the ethics of everyday life is significantly different from the ethics of medicine in dramatic and important ways.

If any of my examples of the difference between common morality and medical ethics strikes you as persuasive, then common morality and medical ethics are different in an ethically significant way, or the principles involved are different, or both. As I see it, the facts that the actions are performed by medical professionals in a professional context make an ethically significant difference. Those differences go a long way toward explaining the different conclusions and suggest that physician actions should be guided by a distinctive set of moral principles. Doctors should be governed by standards of medical ethics and professionalism and they shouldn't rely on common morality to guide their clinical practice or resolve their ethical dilemmas.

At various points, Beauchamp and Childress did point to professional responsibility as accounting for some of the special responsibilities of medical professionals. Similarly, Gert, Clouser, and Culver expected the rules that require promise keeping and fulfilling one's duty to explain those differences. Nevertheless, both groups persist in maintaining that common morality is doing the explanatory work. In the absence of a robust common morality explanation of how the same premises lead to contradictory conclusions for doctors and others, we should recognize that the ethics of everyday life is not consistent with the ethics of medicine.

Although the four principles or ten rules of common morality explain the morality of nonprofessionals in many circumstances, the only explanation of professional morality that they offer is that performing some required action is a professional duty. For example, everyday ethics can justify sharing information by the benefits that it provides (i.e., usefulness, entertainment [beneficence]) and justify the avoidance of probing questions by respect for autonomy or avoiding harm (i.e., embarrassment [nonmaleficence]). The justification for safeguarding patient information and probing patients with potentially embarrassing questions is that doctors have a professional responsibility to do so. Similarly, the justification for doctors' obligations to provide care and maintain nonjudgmental regard is that such behaviors are necessary elements of medical professionalism. In other words, reasons that are specific to the practice of medicine explain specific physician duties, whereas common morality plays no part in justifying required physician behavior. Neither the four principles nor the ten rules figure directly in the ethical analysis that supports those duties of physicians. Fancy footwork might show that common morality is somewhat applicable in medical practice, but it does not adequately explain why medical ethics requires nonjudgmental regard, nonsexual regard, confidentiality, or the rest. Common morality cannot explain why doctors and others have different obligations. Hand waving may create the impressions that common morality accounts for professional duties, but it offers no explanation for why doctors have their distinctive duties when nonphysicians have no such obligations or even obligations to abstain from doing what physicians must do. This lacuna suggests that medical ethics is derived from a different source, and that different or additional moral factors are involved in the ethics of medicine.

The Gap in Common Morality Accounts

Although most people who teach medical ethics and serve as clinical ethicists explain their ethical reasoning in terms of common morality, they fail to notice that often enough common morality does not help in resolving dilemmas. They overlook the significant gaps in common morality and fill them by importing additional concepts that are neither acknowledged nor defended. That sort of undetected ad hoc backfilling is inconsistent with the common morality approach and it tends to make conclusions unreliable because the basis for resolutions is obscured. And because our medical schools rely on common morality to ground their ethics education, the ethics curricula of today's medical school leave doctors with inadequate guidance for confronting the clinical issues that they are likely to encounter. It is therefore important to highlight what is missing from common morality accounts and show why they are incapable of responding to the actual quandaries that arise in clinical ethics.

Beauchamp and Childress

In their initial discussion of "Professional and Public Moralities" Beauchamp and Childress hold fast to their four principles. They maintain that responsibilities of informed consent and confidentiality "are rooted in the more general moral requirements of respecting the autonomy of persons and protecting them from harm."[26] Later, in their chapter 8 discussion of "Professional-Patient Relationships," they continue to ground their account "of rules of veracity, privacy, confidentiality, and fidelity" in the four principles.[27] Yet, without explaining them or their connection to the four principles, they actually introduce additional moral concepts to explain their positions on various issues, including moral concepts such as promise keeping, liberty, contract, trust, personal and property rights, compassion, fair funding, and many more. It's hard to understand how these additional concepts fit together with the four principles, why they must be added to the analysis, or how they should be used in directing action and resolving ethical dilemmas. If these additional moral concepts have to be incorporated in

---

[26] Beauchamp and Childress 2013, 6.
[27] Beauchamp and Childress 2013, 302–349.

their analysis, then the four principles are not providing the moral compass for medical ethics. Other concepts are doing the work. Furthermore, the way in which Beauchamp and Childress take license to deviate from their own theory by importing additional moral concepts invites their followers to similarly elaborate and embroider at will.

In a recent chapter, Beauchamp expanded his list of conceptual tools from the four principles by adding a list of ten "universal rules of obligation," some "universal virtues," and "universal ideals."[28] These additions support my point that additional concepts have to be invoked to explain the conclusions that Beauchamp and Childress reached in *Principles of Biomedical Ethics*. Nevertheless, Beauchamp still maintained that particular moralities such as those of professions "*share the norms of common morality with all other justified particular moralities*" [italics in the original].[29] In other words, Beauchamp held fast to the view that he and Childress have held for decades—that professional ethics is nothing more than narrowly specified conclusions from common morality.[30] For example, in their Chapter 8 discussion of professional-patient relationships, they continued to ground their account "of rules of veracity, privacy, confidentiality, and fidelity" in the four principles.[31]

Even though the distinction between common morality and the ethics of the medical profession is hardly mentioned in their analyses of particular issues, early on in their book Beauchamp and Childress did suggest that there are "particular moralities" including "professional moralities" that vary from common morality. They also accepted that some ideals of common morality become requirements for people in professions "by their commitment to provide important services to patients, clients, or consumers."[32] While they stated that "professional roles engender obligations that do not bind persons who do not occupy the relevant professional roles,"[33] they said little to explain what that commitment is, how it comes to be, or what the specific obligations are. They did allow that moral ideals can become demands of the moral life and that "special roles and relationships in medicine require rules that other

---

[28] Beauchamp T. "The Compatibility of Universal Morality, Particular Moralities, and Multiculturalism," in Teas W, Gordon J, and Rentln AD, editors, *Global Bioethics and Human Rights* (Plymouth, UK: Rowan & Littlefield, 2014: 34).
[29] Beauchamp, *Compatibility of Universal Morality*, 34.
[30] Beauchamp and Childress, *Principles*, 2013, 6.
[31] Beauchamp and Childress, *Principles*, 2013, 302–349.
[32] Beauchamp and Childress, *Principles*, 2013, 7.
[33] Beauchamp and Childress, *Principles*, 2013, 46.

professions may not need."[34] At the same time, they also followed Jay Katz in rejecting the ethical insights of medical professional societies' codes of ethics by quoting his remark that it has "been all too uncritically assumed that they [ethical issues in medicine] could be resolved by fidelity to such undefined principles as *primum non nocere* ["First do no harm"] or visionary codes of ethics."[35]

In a section on negligence and the standard of due care in their Chapter 5, "Nonmaleficence," Beauchamp and Childress listed four essential elements of negligence that would amount to violations of the responsibility to exercise due care:

1. The professional must have a **duty** to the affected party.
2. The professional must breach that **duty**.
3. The affected party must experience harm.
4. The harm must be caused by the breach of **duty**.[36] [emphasis added]

All of that sounds right, as far as it goes, but the central elements in Beauchamp and Childress's approach are missing. They offered no account of what the duties of medical professionals are and why they are duties for those who join the profession. Without enumerating, justifying, and explaining medical obligations, the requirements of duty are left unspecified. That omission invites disagreements and breaches of duty because physicians can legitimately claim ignorance of being duty bound. For example, Beauchamp and Childress claimed that professions have duties involving self-regulation of the profession and ensuring that medical professionals are competent and trustworthy.[37] Studies have shown, however, that many physicians appear to be unaware of that duty.[38]

Beauchamp and Childress clearly recognized the inconsistency problem associated with their four principles approach because Gert and Clouser raised the issue in several articles that Beauchamp and Childress mentioned in later editions of their work.[39] They actually embraced that inevitable

---

[34] Beauchamp and Childress, *Principles*, 2013, 6.
[35] Katz J, editor. *Experimentation With Human Beings* (New York: Russell Sage Foundation, 1972, ix–x); cf. Beauchamp and Childress, *Principles*, 2013, 8.
[36] Beauchamp and Childress, *Principles*, 2013, 155.
[37] Beauchamp TL and Childress JF, *Principles of Biomedical Ethics*, 6th edition (New York: Oxford University Press, 2009, 7).
[38] Campbell EG, Regan S, Gruen RL, et al. "Professionalism in Medicine: Results of a National Survey of Physicians." *Annals of Internal Medicine* 147, 11 (2007): 795–802.
[39] Beauchamp and Childress, *Principles*, 2013, 393–397.

disagreement, boasting that they remained skeptical of the possibility of providing "a unified foundation for ethics."[40] In the 2009 sixth edition of *Principles of Biomedical Ethics*, Beauchamp and Childress expressed their acceptance of that result unambiguously. There they stated that, "We regard disunity, conflict, and moral ambiguity as pervasive features of the moral life that are unlikely to be eradicated by moral theory."[41] Whereas the resultant variety of views may be a virtue in a liberal pluralistic society, leaving individual medical professionals to interpret, specify, and generalize in order to decide questions of medical ethics can be a serious problem for the medical profession. Whereas the resulting "untidiness, complexity, and conflict"[42] may be well tolerated in philosophy's ivory towers, patients need to know what they may reasonably expect from their doctors, and physicians need clear signposts and guidance for navigating characteristic topographies of medical practice.

Gert, Culver, and Clouser

Similarly, Gert, Culver, and Clouser maintained that their ten rules of common morality adequately account for the differences that I highlight between everyday ethics and medical ethics. They explained that the "moral ideals" of preventing death, pain, disability, loss of pleasure, and loss of freedom go a long way toward explaining my examples.[43] From my point of view, however, the transformation from an ideal of beneficence to a strict duty or, in Kantian terms, from an imperfect to a perfect duty is a very significant difference that is not easy to explain. Also, the application of their common morality rules to the standard medical ethics examples that I offer requires a good deal of unpacking and justification. It is not realistic to expect doctors who are not practiced in the maneuvers of philosophical argument to go through mental gyrations in order to determine what their professional duty is, particularly in each case of responding to a frequently encountered issue. Asking physicians to integrate and analyze the implications of ten rules to figure out what they should do in every situation is burdensome, and it

---

[40] Beauchamp and Childress, *Principles*, 2009, 396.
[41] Beauchamp and Childress, *Principles*, 2013, 374.
[42] Beauchamp and Childress, *Principles*, 2009, 374.
[43] Gert et al., *Bioethics*, 43.

invites computational errors. It is more practical to enumerate and explain the specific duties that doctors should uphold.

Gert, Culver, and Clouser would also argue that their sixth rule, "Keep your promise," and their tenth rule, "Do your duty," explain the different responsibilities of physicians and nonphysicians in my examples. Whereas those two rules might account for a moral ideal becoming a stringent moral requirement for someone who makes a promise to uphold the ideal or takes on a role that involves a stronger commitment to the ideal, I do not see how the sixth and tenth rules could radically change the content of moral responsibility from something to its opposite when the conclusion is supposed to be derived from the same rules.

Gert, Culver, and Clouser did recognize that professions have "particular moral rules and special duties," but they regarded that difference as a matter of "culture."[44] Indeed, their tenth rule requires people to "do your duty,"[45] but they persisted in maintaining that

> many of the duties of a profession are particular applications of the general moral rules (which are **valid for all persons in all times and places**) in the context of the special circumstances, practices, relationships, and purposes of the profession. Thus, the duties are far more precise with respect to the special circumstances characterizing a particular domain or profession.[46] [emphasis added]

In other words, they claimed that the rules of everyday ethics explain the ethics of professions. But aside from granting that those changes are "largely set by the medical profession, though perhaps clarified and modified by law and society,"[47] they said little to explain how the change in moral stringency comes about or how doctors become bound to conform with professional duties that are more demanding than, or diametrically opposed to, what others are required to do.

Deriving medical ethics from the moral rules of everyday life becomes particularly difficult for Gert and colleagues to explain in regard to assessing patients' decisional capacity. Their rules 4 and 5 prohibit the deprivation of freedom or pleasure and express the idea that we should allow others to act

---

[44] Gert et al., *Bioethics*, 88.
[45] Gert et al., *Bioethics*, 36.
[46] Gert et al., *Bioethics*, 89.
[47] Gert et al., *Bioethics*, 92.

as they choose and advance their own conception of the good. Yet, they provided numerous examples to illustrate what I regard as a physician's duty to assess decisional capacity. For example, they described an elderly depressed woman who had lost a great deal of weight. She understood and appreciated her life-threatening situation and acknowledged that an irrational fear kept her from consenting to the electroconvulsive treatment that she knew was likely to cure her of depression.[48] Gert and colleagues therefore concluded that the woman lacked decisional capacity, and that electroconvulsive treatment should be administered over her objection.

Both editions of *Bioethics* devoted significant attention to their astute analysis of competence and medical paternalism. Gert, Culver, and Clouser's careful and insightful attention to the interrelated concepts that are involved demonstrates that they regarded the assessment of competence to be a critical medical responsibility. It is important to notice, however, that acknowledging physicians' moral duty to assess patients' decisional capacity is exactly opposed to the critical duty of common morality, which requires us to go as far as possible in presuming that others have decisional capacity, respecting their choices, and not interfering with their freedom or pursuit of pleasure. Although I fully agree that physicians have the duty that Gert, Culver, and Clouser's discussion suggests they have, the duty to assess capacity is clearly at odds with their commitments to avoid depriving others of freedom or pleasure, and it cannot be derived from common morality.

Maintaining their commitment to the common morality approach also leaves Gert, Culver, and Clouser with the difficult problem of what to say about euthanasia or physician-assisted dying. They saw physicians as obliged by the rules of common morality with at least as much stringency as others are or perhaps with greater stringency because they have made a special promise or taken on a special duty. Then, because they listed "do not kill" as a rule of common morality and because they considered "prolonging life" to be a "moral ideal," they were hard pressed to find a way for physicians to respond to requests from "competent patients who rationally prefer to die."[49]

So, what to do? They opted for dancing a little sidestep and taking a giant leap into specious equivocation. They wrote, "Not treating counts as killing only when there is a duty to treat; in the absence of such a duty, not treating does not count as killing."[50] They went on to maintain that, "if a competent

---

[48] Gert et al., *Bioethics*, 222.
[49] Gert et al., *Bioethics*, 322.
[50] Gert et al., *Bioethics*, 322.

patient rationally refuses treatment, abiding by that refusal is not killing."[51] But in another discussion slightly before that in their book, they held that there is no moral distinction between refusing, withholding, and withdrawing treatment.[52] Nevertheless, they insisted on describing the removal of life-preserving treatment, such as nutrition and hydration, ventilator support, or continuous dialysis, as abiding by a competent patient's current or previous wishes and not as killing.[53]

But if I, a mere philosopher with no duty to treat anyone, walked into a patient's room and disconnected the patient from nutrition and hydration, ventilator support, or continuous dialysis and death resulted, I would be charged with murder because what I did was killing even if I was acting in accordance with the patient's request. And, if a parent simply neglected to feed a very young child who died of starvation, the parent would be charged with negligent homicide because withholding food for a significant period is killing. It is hard to see how the very same act could be both killing and not killing. Such acts are killing because of the link between nutrition and life, because of the implicit responsibilities of the person who withdraws or withholds nutrition, and because of the dependency of the individual who ends up dead. The only way that Gert and colleagues avoided recognizing these incontrovertible facts was by hiding behind the illusion of pretending that people were not doing what they were obviously doing and claiming that they were really only abiding by a competent patient's rational request. Really, they were doing both, abiding by the patient's request and killing the patient.

It is, however, not hard to see that an act that is forbidden for most people may be permitted when performed by people with special social powers, privileges, and immunities. An Army infantryman may be justified in shooting people when others are not. A police officer may be justified in imprisoning people when others are not. And a physician may be justified in administering poisons (e.g., chemotherapy), cutting into another's body with knives, removing a limb or vital organ (i.e., performing surgery), and

---

[51] Gert et al., *Bioethics*, 323.

[52] Gert et al., *Bioethics*, 310–322.

[53] The killing and letting die distinction is discussed in legal decisions, the legal literature, and the philosophic literature, often in the context of arguments related to aid in dying. For example, see the following: Cruzan v. Director, Missouri Department of Health, 497 US; Conroy (486 A. 2d); In re Quinlan, 355 A 2d); Battin MP, Rhodes R, and Silvers A, editors, *Physician Assisted Suicide: Expanding the Debate* (New York: Routledge, 1998). The Battin et al. volume includes Washington et al. v. Glucksburg et al. (378–422), Vacco et al. v. Quill et al. (423–430), "The Philosopher' Brief" (431–441), and an article by Gert, Culver, and Clouser, "An Alternative to Physician-Assisted Suicide" (183–202).

even killing (i.e., performing euthanasia) when others are not. These special powers, privileges, and immunities may be socially and morally allowed to such professionals when society authorizes them to perform those extraordinary acts. There is no obvious reason to presume that the rules that govern the application of extraordinary professional powers and privileges are the same as common morality. In fact, when people in the military kill and when police deprive people of freedom, they are likely to be performing their duty. Similarly, when physicians cause pain (e.g., in an examination), disable (e.g., in an amputation), and kill (e.g., in attempting a high-risk potentially life-saving surgery), they are likely to be performing their duty.

Without recognizing that the moral rules of these professions are radically different from common morality, we end up in the same mess as Gert and his colleagues. They called killing not killing and focused on one intention (to abide by a competent patient's wishes) while pointedly ignoring the other intention (to hasten a patient's death). A simpler and more honest approach involves accepting that professional ethics involve departures from common morality. In the specific case of passive or active euthanasia, medical ethics involves recognizing that the distinctive powers and privileges of physicians allow them to withhold and withdraw life-preserving treatment (which Gert et al. accepted), provide advice on how to hasten death by refusing nutrition and hydration (which Gert et al. endorsed), and administer fatal drugs (which Gert et al. refused to accept).

Gert and colleagues saw no moral difference between acts and omissions, and I agree.[54] The conclusion that they should draw from this point is the one that James Rachels drew decades ago.[55] When it is wrong for a doctor to kill, it is wrong for a doctor to let a patient die. And, when it is morally required for a doctor to allow a patient to die, it may be morally better for a doctor to help a patient die by using humane means that serve the patient's interests.

Gert and colleagues' view holds that the rules of common morality, and particularly the rules that require you to keep your promise and do your duty, fully explain doctors' professional responsibilities. An additional problem with that view is that the approach does not provide an adequate explanatory framework for medical ethics. The reason turns on the old philosophic distinction between act-based ethics, which focuses on the action of a specific

---

[54] The issue of acts and omissions is discussed further in Chapter 7, Medicine's Commitment to Truth; and Chapter 8, Physicians' Commitments to Fellow Professionals.

[55] Rachels J. "Active and Passive Euthanasia," *New England Journal of Medicine* 292 (1975): 78–80.

individual in a unique circumstance, and rule-based ethics, which provides a standard for many common situations.[56] According to the account presented in *Bioethics*, any singular violation of a moral rule requires justification and then an assessment of whether or not the violation could be publicly allowed. Whereas clinicians always have a duty to evaluate and compare the risks and benefits of alternative treatment plans in order to determine options that serve the patient's interests, the *Bioethics* approach requires an additional ethical evaluation at the case level. Before every medical action, Gert and colleagues required clinicians to assess the legitimacy of employing any medical intervention that risks death, pain, disability, loss of pleasure, or loss of freedom, yet these are common features of clinical practice. This means that each and every decision involving risks of death, pain, disability, loss of pleasure, or loss of freedom must be justified with reasons, and then the decision must be tested by their publicity standard, which asks whether the decision would be acceptable to the public if it were to be made known. Clearly, imposing treatments and tests that entail risks and inconveniences without any likelihood of medical benefit violates several moral rules. But employing standard-of-care medical interventions that are justified by a comparison of the risks and benefits should not be regarded as violating moral rules and requiring ethical justification per se; they should be seen as providing "indicated" treatments or tests.

Furthermore, it is hard to understand how Gert and colleagues' publicity standard would work for decisions within medicine. According to them, whether an action is acceptable in common morality turns on being publically allowed. The appropriateness of particular medical interventions, however, turns on medical expertise that is not available to the public and moral standards that are different from what is accepted in everyday life. In medicine, the assessment of the ethical acceptability of an action pointedly disregards public opinion because some of the commitments of common morality are unacceptable considerations for making medical decisions. Rather, professional decisions should reflect whether a consensus of experienced, informed, and respected doctors would accept them as meeting the standard of the profession. Actions that come up to that bar may not follow from principles of common morality: In such circumstances, they may need to be explained to the public and shown to be consistent with society's trust.

---

[56] As I use the terms, standards for action are called principles, rules, or duties without denoting any significant differences.

Although Gert and colleagues may be happy to have each medical decision made in their stepwise fashion, the problem with a case-by-case approach is that it opens medicine to tremendous variability and deprives patients of the ability to rely on clinicians to consistently uphold a set of ethical standards in their practice. Gert and colleagues' approach requires individual clinicians to evaluate the merits of maintaining nonjudgmental regard, a caring attitude, confidentiality, and nonsexual regard and assessing decisional capacity on a case-by-case basis. Case-by-case justification involves particular moral judgments that invite inconsistency and deprive clinicians of the guidance that they need for navigating medicine's fraught moral terrain.

The Incompatibility of Common Morality and Medical Ethics

In considering the applicability of common morality to medical ethics, I identified significant problems with both the Beauchamp and Childress and the Gert, Culver, Clouser approaches. The four principles approach is simpler than the ten rules approach, but to reach ethical conclusions about particular issues, Beauchamp and Childress actually needed more tools than their four principles provide. That makes arriving at moral conclusions complex and less certain than it needs to be because they provided no way to discern when the additional imported concepts are legitimate and relevant ethical concerns. The longer list of considerations and the publicity requirement of the ten rules approach provide a larger set of analytic tools. Gert, Culver, and Clouser were, however, stymied by their insistence that the rules of common morality explained the obligations of professionals. And whereas both approaches acknowledged that ideals can become duties in professions, neither approach offers an adequate account of the genesis, stringency, or content of those duties. In doing so, they failed to acknowledge the priority of professional commitments and eschewed the critical tasks of explicating medicine's distinctive professional duties.

Taken together, these considerations suggest that common morality is significantly different from the ethics of medicine in dramatic and important ways. The examples that I presented show that the ethics of medicine cannot be common morality applied to high-tech medicine, and they reveal that medical ethics requires a different framework to explain its special responsibilities. Although the Beauchamp and Childress and the Gert, Culver, and

Clouser common morality approaches may be useful tools of analysis in everyday ethics, and even in addressing public policy that governs healthcare, neither is useful in the clinical arena of medical ethics.

In the examining room and at the bedside, patients expect their doctors to uphold the standards of medical professionalism and display character traits and attitudes that go beyond the requirements of common morality. Without being able to rely on clinicians cleaving to the standard of care; being non-judgmental, respectful, and caring; upholding confidentiality; maintaining professional competence; and fulfilling the rest of their distinctive responsibilities, patients would have to be guarded and skeptical in their interactions with doctors, and that would undermine much of the good that medicine can provide. And without clearly articulated duties that can be explained in a way that is cogent and convincing, doctors are left without a rudder, to struggle and blunder through issues when better moral guidance could and should be provided.

Why Medicine Needs Its Own Ethics

Returning to our starting point of recognizing that medicine requires its own distinctive ethics, I asked, why is that so? One way to answer the question is by employing a thought experiment and seeing what follows. In this case, we can imagine how medicine came about and see what can be learned from the exercise.[57]

It's easy to imagine that people in early civilizations were aware that over the course of their lives they and their loved ones could suffer disease and injury. They wanted help to be available to avoid those conditions when possible and assistance in addressing their consequences such as pain, disability, and death. They therefore allowed a group, call them doctors,[58] to develop the knowledge of fields that we now call anatomy, physiology, organic chemistry, pharmacology, microbiology, and so on. They also allowed doctors to develop examination and surgical skills. To enable that group to accomplish the goals of using their special knowledge and skill in meeting the needs of the people in their communities, societies granted doctors special powers, privileges, and immunities that are permitted to no one else. Reprising the

---

[57] Philosophers call this strategy the hypotheticodeductive method.
[58] They have also been called priests, shamans, and medicine men.

earlier description, doctors' powers traditionally include the authority to do things like quarantine people to prevent the spread of infectious disease, decide that someone lacks decisional capacity and impose treatment on him over his objections, or determine that someone is no longer alive. Doctors' privileges allow them to ask strangers to undress, concoct and administer treatments, and perform surgery. And doctors' immunities protect them from punishment for exercising their extraordinary powers and privileges or causing harms (e.g., disability, death) that may ensue from their efforts.

Because the powers, privileges, and immunities that are allowed to doctors and no one else are potentially dangerous, society wants clear limits for demarcating how doctors' remarkable licenses may be employed. People who choose to join the profession and become doctors must, therefore relinquish the rights of ordinary citizens to act according to their personal preferences and values and commit themselves to uphold the duties of the profession. Doctors' acceptance of the profession's clearly defined duties protects the public from harms that could be inflicted by the unregulated use of their distinctive liberties and assures society that doctors can be relied upon to provide the medical services that they will require. Doctors recognize that they must publicly declare their commitments to use their special privileges for the benefit of patients and society and observe the proclaimed limitations on their practice so that they can be trusted in wielding their extraordinary freedoms.[59]

Doctors are the ones who define the duties of the profession because they are the only ones who can adequately understand what is involved, appreciate the potential risks and benefits of their services, and distinguish competent practice from unacceptable performance. Therefore, the ethics of medicine is internal to the profession in that it is constructed by the profession for the profession. It is not defined by society, politicians, lawyers, or philosophers.[60] The hallmark of professionalism is, therefore, the commitment to and the internalization of medicine's distinctive ethics. Medical ethics has to be

---

[59] Edmund Pellegrino discussed the importance of doctors publicly proclaiming their commitment to the standards of medical ethics. Pellegrino ED, "Professionalism, Profession and the Virtues of the Good Physician," *The Mount Sinai Journal of Medicine* 69, 6 (2002): 378–384.

[60] Although doctors must, for the most part, abide by the law, there have been instances when legal requirements violate the profession's commitments. Historically, doctors have advocated for changes in the law and even violated legal orders or prohibitions in order to uphold what they regarded as their professional responsibility. Doctors who risked punishment by refusing to violate patient confidentiality and report undocumented immigrants and doctors who acted to promote their patients' interests by providing contraception and abortion have been examples.

inculcated by the profession, and it has to be enforced and policed by the profession because no one else is in a position to do the job.

Medical Professionalism

In the past 20 years, there has been considerable discussion of medical professionalism. Many authors who discuss professionalism recognize that something akin to a social contract is involved in the creation of the profession and that trust is necessary for the practice of medicine. Yet, there has been some disagreement within the medical and medical education communities about what medical professionalism is[61-67] and how it should be incorporated into medical training.[68-72] Some argue that professionalism is about rules[73-76]; others maintain that it is about virtues or

---

[61] Ethics and Professionalism Committee, American Board of Medical Specialties (ABMS) Professionalism Work Group. *ABMS Professionalism Definition.* http://www.abms.org/News_and_Events/Media_Newsroom/features/feature_ABMS_Professionalism_Definition_LongForm_abms.org_040413.aspx.

[62] Birden H, Glass N, Wilson I, et al., "Defining Professionalism in Medical Education: A Systematic Review," *Medical Teacher* 36, 1 (2014): 47–61.

[63] Pavlica P and Barozzi L, "Medical Professionalism in the New Millennium: A Physicians' Charter," *Lancet* 359 (2002): 520–522.

[64] Hafferty F, Papadakis M, Sullivan W, and Wynia MK, *The American Board of Medical Specialties Ethics and Professionalism Committee Definition of Professionalism* (Chicago: American Board of Medical Specialties, 2012).

[65] Swick HM, "Toward a Normative Definition of Medical Professionalism," *Academic Medicine* 75, 6 (2000): 612–616.

[66] Wear D and Kuczewski MG, "The Professionalism Movement: Can We Pause?" *American Journal of Bioethics* 4 (2004): 1–10.

[67] Parsi K and Sheehan MN, "Two Faces of Professionalism," in Parsi K and Sheehan MN, editors, *Healing as Vocation: A Medical Professionalism Primer* (Langham, MD: Rowman & Littlefield, 2006).

[68] Cohen JJ, "Professionalism in Medical Education, an American Perspective: From Evidence to Accountability," *Medical Education,* 40, 7 (2004): 607–617.

[69] Stern DT and Papadakis M, "The Developing Physician—Becoming a Professional," *New England Journal of Medicine* 355, 17 (2006): 1794–1799.

[70] Inui TS, *A Flag in the Wind: Educating for Professionalism in Medicine* (Washington, DC: Association of American Medical Colleges, 2003).

[71] Doukas DJ, McCullough LB, Wear S, et al. "The Challenge of Promoting Professionalism Through Medical Ethics and Humanities Education," *Academic Medicine* 88, 11 (2004): 1624–1629.

[72] Birden H, Glass N, Wilson I, Harrison M, Usherwood T, Nass D, "Defining Professionalism in Medical Education: A Systematic Review," *Medical Teacher* 36, 1 (2014): 47–61.

[73] Irvine D, *The Doctors' Tale: Professionalism and Public Trust* (Oxon, UK: Radcliffe, 2003).

[74] Kao A, editor, *Professing Medicine: Strengthening the Ethics and Professionalism of Tomorrow's Physicians* (Chicago: American Medical Association, 2001).

[75] Cruess SR, Johnston S, Cruess RL, "Professionalism for Medicine: Opportunities and Obligations," *The Medical Journal of Australia* 177, 4 (2002): 208–211.

[76] Cruess RL and Cruess SR, "Expectations and Obligations: Professionalism and Medicine's Social Contract With Society," *Perspectives in Biology and Medicine* 51, 4 (2008): 579–598.

character[77-79] or beliefs[80]; and others hold that it is about achieving (measurable) competencies.[81-84] The disagreement is understandable because all of these elements are involved in medical professionalism.

The critical point that has not been adequately appreciated is that the understanding of professionalism derives from the distinctive ethics of medicine. Professionalism is needed because it involves doctors committing themselves to ethical standards that are different from and more demanding than those of common morality. It requires physicians to understand what the distinctive duties of medicine entail, how they apply to medical practice, and why physicians must uphold those duties. It entails doctors embracing their unique obligations, identifying with them, and accepting the responsibility to fulfill them with a sincere commitment. In that sense, it involves developing a character that takes pleasure in fulfilling professional obligations and committing oneself to moderate desires that might interfere with upholding professional duties. In sum, **professionalism is doctors' personification of medical ethics**. Professionalism involves understanding the obligations of a physician, making oneself into a person who is likely to fulfill those duties, and acting in accordance with the dictates of medical ethics.

Two personal anecdotes illustrate the kind of dedication that marks professionalism. My beloved brother is a doctor, a pediatric cardiologist who lives in Boston. After not having seen each other for a few months, my husband and I drove up to Boston for a weekend visit with him and his family. We arrived on Friday night, but he didn't get home until after we were asleep because he had a very sick patient in the hospital. When we awoke the next

---

[77] Brody H and Doukas D, "Professionalism: A Framework to Guide Medical Education," *Medical Education* 48, 10 (2014): 980–987.

[78] Karches KE and Sulmasy DP, "Justice, Courage, and Truthfulness: Virtues That Medical Trainees Can and Must Learn," *Family Medicine* 48, 7 (2016): 511–516.

[79] Pelligrino ED and Thomasma DC, *The Virtues in Medical Practice* (New York: Oxford University Press, 1993).

[80] Wynia MK, Papadakis MA, Sullivan WM, Hafferty FW, "More Than a List of Values and Desired Behaviors: A Foundational Understanding of Medical Professionalism," *Academic Medicine* 89, 5 (2014): 712–714.

[81] Irby DM, "Constructs of Professionalism," in Byyny RL, Paauw DS, Papadakis M, Pfeil S, editors, *Medical Professionalism Best Practices: Professionalism in the Modern Era* (Aurora, CO: Alpha Omega Alpha Honor Medical Society, 2017: 9–14).

[82] Wilkinson TJ, Wade WB, Knock LD, "A Blueprint to Assess Professionalism: Results of a Systematic Review," *Academic Medicine* 84, 5 (2009): 551–558.

[83] National Board of Medical Examiners, *Embedding Professionalism in Medical Education: Assessment as a Tool for Implementation* (2002). http://www.nbme.org/PDF/NBME AAMC ProfessReport.pdf

[84] Arnold L, "Assessing Professional Behavior: Yesterday, Today, and Tomorrow," *Academic Medicine* 77, 6 (2002): 502–515.

morning, he had already left for the hospital. Again, he returned home late at night and left in the morning before we awoke because he had to attend to his patient's needs. I have no doubt that he wanted to spend time with us, but for him, there was no question and no hesitation in putting his patient's interests before his own.

In a second example, there was a small fire one evening in a storage room on the second floor of our main hospital building. The entire building became engulfed in smoke, forcing the evacuation of all the patients to other buildings. Two mornings later, at 7:00 AM, I met with the orthopedic surgery residents for our regularly scheduled ethics discussion. They shared their stories of gagging on smoke while running up and down staircases to rescue their patients and then racing around all night to locate patients who had been moved in haste so they would not miss any doses of their medications. The residents had been in danger, but to a person, they never hesitated or equivocated about putting their patients' interests before their own. Their zeal and commitment to duty was palpable, and they were all rightly proud of having displayed exemplary professionalism in responding to the emergency.

The Role of a Philosopher in Explaining Medical Ethics and Professionalism

Just as physicians have their distinctive knowledge and skills, philosophers have their own areas of expertise. Philosophers bring to the table their knowledge of moral and political philosophy and philosophy of science. They contribute their understanding of the history of ethics and insights into how the pieces of morality fit together. In particular, philosophers who work closely with doctors over a long period and learn about physicians' practice from them may be in a position to develop an overview of the field. That perspective may also enable a philosopher to recognize the inconsistency between common morality and the ethics of medicine. I found myself in that privileged position.

The task that I set myself is to describe and explain the distinctive morality of the profession and weave together the several elements of medical ethics into an intelligible structure with a rationale that explains why it must be so. Although experienced physicians who are leaders in the field have developed many insightful policies for guiding medical practice and crafted professional codes that are important statements of medicine's professional commitments, the rationale for why those measures are necessary has been lacking and a theory of medical ethics that connects the various pieces of the puzzle into a coherent whole does not exist. Although some leaders of the profession have pointed to a social contract analysis and medicine's need for patient trust in explaining the foundation of the profession, to be compelling that description has to be fleshed out in detail. The theoretical structure that I provide is intended to replace the current four principles and ten rules accounts of bioethics because they employ tools that are unwieldly, often inadequate, and sometimes point doctors in the wrong direction or impose inappropriate restrictions on clinical practice.

Medical Ethics

Like any good moral theory, a clear and coherent theory of medical ethics provides a useful scaffold for reasoning about the issues that arise in clinical practice. The list of the distinctive duties and virtues of medical ethics along with the explanation of why they must be the moral commitments that guide the action of medical professionals comprise the "ethical standard of care" for medicine. Just as the clinical standard of care serves as the touchstone for doctors' treatment decisions, the profession-endorsed duties of medical ethics should be regarded as the criteria for justifying ethical decisions in clinical practice. And just as a doctor has to be prepared to justify to peers deviations from the clinical standard of care with reasons related to the individual patient's health, medical condition, or circumstances, deviations from the ethical standard of care have to be justified to peers in terms of duties of medical ethics. Patients and society expect doctors to act in accordance with clinical and ethical standards of care, and patients rely on physicians to meet those standards.

This means that medical practice and medical ethics are not matters of private judgment. Rather, medical decisions should be what similarly situated experienced and trusted doctors would endorse as matters of professional judgment. Disagreements over different possible treatment choices should be resolved by evidence or by factors related to a particular circumstance. Conflicts over which duties to uphold and which to sacrifice that arise in individual cases have to be resolved in terms of reasons that other medical professionals would also find compelling.

Although the theory of medical ethics that I describe in the rest of this book is innovative in many respects, it conforms to the eight criteria for theory construction delineated by Beauchamp and Childress.[85] In my presentation of the theory of medical ethics, (1) the obligations of medical professionals are **clearly** enumerated as sixteen duties without vagueness or obscurity to make the responsibilities concrete. The theory justifies all the enumerated doctors' duties and explains them in a way that makes clear why physicians must uphold them. (2) The theory is internally **coherent** in that the duties are consistent with each other because they are derived from the same fundamental commitment. It is also coherent in that the prescribed duties and virtues that harmonize with the doctorly behavior that physicians respect. (3) It is **comprehensive** in that it accounts for the moral judgments that doctors typically need to make, and it provides a decision procedure for generating responses to unusual or unforeseen circumstances. (4) It is **simple** in that the theory identifies a sufficient number of duties to cover the common obligations that physicians must fulfill, without being too abstract or too complicated to be useful. (5) By providing a detailed explanation of why each duty is required by medical ethics and how each duty is to be implemented in the clinical arena, the theory has **explanatory power**. (6) By explicating the rationale for why each duty is a necessary element of medical professionalism and why failing to uphold a duty would be a failure of medical professionalism, the theory has **justificatory power**. (7) This theory demonstrates its **output power** by being able to explain and account for medicine's unique duties that cannot be justified by common morality. (8) The theory also meets the standards of **practicability**, in that today's esteemed physicians actually conform to the standards that the theory describes.

Like Beauchamp and Childress and Gert, Culver, and Clouser, in presenting my account of medical ethics I draw on the long history of moral philosophy. Specifically, I take insights from a number of the same moral and political theorists that informed the thinking displayed in their four principles and ten rules accounts of common morality. Although we interpret the positions of important philosophers differently on numerous points, the group of historical exemplars who inform their and my accounts includes Aristotle, Thomas Hobbes, Immanuel Kant, W. D. Ross, John Rawls, and T. M. Scanlon.

---

[85] Beauchamp and Childress, *Principles*, 2009, 334–336.

This particular philosophic tradition acknowledges two important facts: that humans have common needs, desires, and vulnerabilities, and that ethics is not discovered but constructed by giving reasons for moral positions. Because of our common human nature, the principles, rules, and duties that are supported by broadly accepted reasons apply to everyone. Thus, the stated conclusions of moral reasoning are not arbitrary, contingent, or relative to a particular time and place but count as being true for everyone in relevantly similar situations. In philosophic terms, this approach to moral theory is called contractarian constructivism, and it regards ethical conclusions to be rational, propositional, and cognitive.

I also explain the distinctive virtues that doctors must cultivate to enable them to fulfill their professional duties. Professionalism requires doctors to develop the virtues of an exemplary physician. Molding that character requires honing the feelings, attitudes, and inclinations that make meeting professional obligations feel right or even pleasurable, as well as nurturing the dispositions that support duty while moderating excessive desires that could undermine professionalism. In my analysis of doctorly character and virtues, I closely follow Aristotle because I find his insight to be most perspicacious and his template of virtues most relevant to the array of temptations that can lead unwary doctors astray.

Constructing Medical Ethics

In his prescient article, "The Autonomy of Medical Ethics: Medical Science vs. Medical Practice," Bernard H. Baumrin explained what makes a field of knowledge autonomous. He wrote,

> In philosophic circles such a question is usually put this way: is such and such domain or subject matter autonomous? In professional circles the language tends to be more metaphorical: is this or that subject matter merely an offshoot of some more fundamental study? ... To say that such and such a subject is something on its own and not reducible to something else, some other intellectual endeavor, is to say it is an autonomous subject, and that means it is not fully reducible to some other subject, like metallurgy to chemistry, botany to biology, or even chemistry to physics. One domain is reducible to another if, either all of its principal technical terms are expressible in the technical language of the other domain, or if its principles or

theorems are deducible from the other domain. If either of these conditions hold then the domain is not autonomous; but for the independence of some domain to be established there needs to be at a minimum a species of data *sui generis* to it. This, along with principles specific to the domain (i.e., not deducible from any other domain) establishes the autonomy of the discipline.[86]

In this sense, and just as philosopher G. E. Moore argued that ethics is an autonomous field and distinct from fields such as biology and physiology,[87] I argue that it is precisely because the duties of doctors are not derived from the precepts of common morality or any other field, and because they cannot be deduced from the precepts of common morality, that medical ethics is an autonomous field. As an independent domain of ethics, the specific requirements of medical ethics have to be defined and explained.

Starting with the view that the ethics of medicine is distinct and different from common morality, I explicate the ethics of medicine by showing how it is constructed. As Bernard Gert did, I model my account by drawing inspiration from Thomas Hobbes's analysis in his masterpiece, *Leviathan,* where Hobbes identified twenty laws of nature that oblige both rulers and the governed.[88] Gert followed Hobbes's methodology in explaining his ten rules of common morality. My account of medical ethics takes a sharp turn away from Gert's approach by limiting the list to the duties of physicians and other medical professionals.[89]

The list of professional duties that I defend and explain includes sixteen duties that doctors should be committed to uphold. I expect that no informed and experienced physician can reasonably reject the duties of medical ethics that I enumerate. I am not claiming that the list is definitive, that additional duties could not be added, or that some of the duties should not be further subdivided. (For example, doctors may find that a duty to yield to the chain of command may be necessary for the management of medical procedures and in urgent situations.) I do, however, maintain that any additional duties have to be derived from the fundamental commitments to seek and maintain

[86] Baumrin BH, "The Autonomy of Medical Ethics: Medical Science vs. Medical Practice," *Metaphilosophy* 16, 2&3 (1985): 93–102.

[87] Moore GE, *Ethics* (New York: Holt, 1912).

[88] Hobbes T, *Hobbes's Leviathan* (Oxford, UK: Clarendon Press, 1965; reprinted from the 1651 edition).

[89] The Hobbesian roots of my account are detailed in Rhodes R, "Hobbesian Medical Ethics," in Courtland S, editor, *Hobbesian Applied Ethics* (New York: Routledge, 2018): 69–90.

trust and be consistent with the duty to act in the interest of patients and society. Thus, additions to the list would still be in harmony with the rest.

In this presentation I do more than present a list of the core set of distinctive duties prescribed by medical ethics. I explain how medical ethics
should be conceived and argue for the specific duties that must be part of
the distinctive ethics of medicine. In each case, I explain the medically specific and uncommon justification for each duty and describe the structural
features that are necessary for upholding the distinctive commitments of the
field. Following the medical model of case-based learning, I offer examples to
illustrate the importance of each obligation and show its relevance in various
medical contexts.

The conclusions that I reach are consonant with the long-standing
traditions of medical ethics and good medical practice. People from outside
the field, and physicians who have not yet understood the rationale for the
full register of medical duties, may reach different conclusions about some
cases. (For example, people outside of medicine may object to doctors providing excellent medical care to terrorist bombers as well as their victims,
whereas physicians will agree that treatment based on need is required.)
I have found, however, that in the vast majority of situations, experienced
medical professionals arrive at a consensus that is in line with the conclusions
that I have enumerated. That agreement is no accidental coincidence, but
the product of shared moral insights. It amounts to what John Rawls has
termed an "overlapping consensus," a deep and principled agreement as opposed to a modus vivendi, a chance coincidence of different people's personal
priorities.[90]

I suggest that the differences in opinions between those who regard
examples from within medicine and those who regard the same examples
from outside of medicine stem from the contrast between basing decisions
on common morality versus medical ethics. For instance, later I argue that
nonjudgmental regard is a duty for doctors.[91] Medical professionals act on
that duty when they treat patients solely based on their need and pointedly
refuse to discriminate based on social standing, a patient's complicity in the
medical condition that requires attention, or any other nonmedical reason.
Patients with lung cancer, for example, are treated based on their disease and

---

[90] Rawls, *Political Liberalism*.
[91] In Chapter 5, Duties of Behavior Toward Patients, I describe the seventh duty of medical ethics,
nonjudgmental regard.

not according to whether they have the condition because of their genes, because of their smoking history, or because they worked on "the pile" after the collapse of the World Trade Center on 9/11. The consensus of society may support distinguishing between patients whose diseases have different etiologies. But in medical ethics, and in contrast to what Beauchamp and Childress or Gert, Culver, and Clouser held, the standard should not be social consensus or public opinion, but the consensus of experienced and esteemed physicians precisely because of their commitment to the profession's moral perspective. That is to say that medical ethics is internal to the profession, it is constructed by the profession for medical professionals. As the 7th edition of the American College of Physicians Ethics Manual maintains, "The Manual is intended to facilitate the process of making ethical decisions in clinical practice, teaching, and medical research and to describe and explain underlying principles of ethics, about their project . . . [and it] "was written for our colleagues in medicine."[92]

To recapitulate, because no one else may wield the powers, privileges, and immunities that society allows medical professionals, the duties that govern their use cannot come from common morality. Medical ethics cannot be derived from common morality because some of its strict duties are merely optional actions in common morality and others are exactly the opposite of what common morality prescribes for non-physicians. Because such inconsistent conclusions cannot be derived from a shared set of premises, logically the radical distinctness of medical ethics must be acknowledged. Those who crafted codes and oaths of medical ethics for over two thousand years implicitly recognized that doctors relinquish many rights of ordinary people when they take on the distinctive duties of the profession. In this sense, my rejection of common morality as the ethics of medicine is less revolutionary than it may at first appear. The common morality movement arose only in the 1970s. It was well-intentioned, and its simplicity made it attractive. But it should now be seen as a move in the wrong direction that requires correction.

---

[92] American College of Physicians Ethics Manual: Seventh Edition, *Ann Intern Med.* 2019;170(2_ Supplement):S1–S32. DOI: 10.7326/M18-2160. Accessed online 12/13/19 at https://annals.org/aim/ fullarticle/2720883/american-college-physicians-ethics-manual-seventh-edition?_ga=2.138123378 .3519210.1576272473-111550467.1576272473#208345950

Vocabulary

Before moving on to explaining medical ethics, a few remarks on vocabulary are in order. This digression may prevent nit picking quibbles and misinterpretation, what, in the words of Mose Allison, amount to "Your Mind Is on Vacation, and Your Mouth Is Working Overtime"[93].

Many people, and people in fields such as sociology and history, understand *ethics* and *morality* to mean different things. As a philosopher, I take ethics and morality and variations on those terms to be synonymous. Similarly, some people distinguish the terms *doctor, physician,* and *medical professional*. I use them as equivalent for the purpose of presenting this theory. Furthermore, even though I primarily discuss doctors, I intend what I say to apply broadly to people in all medically related professions because I consider them all to be medical professionals, and the duties of medical ethics to apply to doctors, nurses, social workers, physician assistants, pharmacists, genetics counselors, physical therapists, bioethicists, and so on.

Beauchamp and Childress presented their theory of common morality in terms of principles. Gert, Clouser, and Culver presented their theory of common morality in terms of rules. I present my theory of medical ethics in terms of duties. Although Beauchamp and Childress distinguished principles, rules, and obligations[94] as the words are typically used in moral philosophy, all three terms identify what a person should do, what they must do, what is their duty, and what it would be wrong for them not to do. Although the terms may have slightly different meanings in some contexts, when we tell someone to "abide by these principles," "follow these rules," or "uphold your duty," the direction is pretty much the same. In that sense, I use these terms without distinguishing any significant differences. I do appreciate that in some contexts "principles" may suggest direction that is more optional than "rules" or "duties." Perhaps that is why Beauchamp and Childress selected principles as their preferred term. Duties are unambiguous in their dictates, which is the point of professionalism. The actions and attitudes that are required or prohibited by medical ethics are not optional; they are demanded from all medical professionals.

---

[93] From the song, "Your Mind Is on Vacation," by Mose Allison, Atlantic Records, 1976.
[94] Beauchamp and Childress, *Principles*, 2009, 12–14.

The contractarian constructivist tradition that guides my thinking explains human formulation and acceptance of morality as the creation of obligations. When we accept the obligation to observe the rules of common morality (e.g., the first nine rules of Gert, Culver, and Clouser) by agreeing to relinquish our right to do as we please, we commit ourselves to observe the rules for at least so long as others do so as well.[95] Personal commitment under conditions of reciprocity give us the obligations not to kill, injure, or rob others and so forth.

In contrast to the obligations of common morality, special obligations are not based on reciprocity. When a couple decides to become parents, they take on obligations to the offspring they produce, but their children make no commitments to them at all. Similarly, people who choose to become doctors take on the obligations of the profession. Whereas before they undertook their professional role they were free, for example, to be judgmental, once they enter the medical profession they become bound to nonjudgmental regard when acting in their professional role. The obligations of doctors derive solely from their commitments and not from reciprocity because patients do not take on any obligations to them. In fact, physicians have duties to provide care even for patients who refuse to participate in furthering medical education or biomedical research.[96] In that light, I choose to use the word *duty* in presenting this theory of medical ethics. It indicates that doctors are undertaking the obligations imposed by medical ethics when they join the profession. Focusing on duties, rather than principles or rules, also makes it easier to distinguish this account from the four principles and ten rules versions of bioethics.

My Limited Scope

Because my aim in this book is to present and explain a theory of medical ethics, this is not the place for debating all the controversial issues that arise

---

[95] Here I take a position in opposition to Beauchamp and Childress (*Principles*, 2009, 354) and Alan Gewirth in his "Why Rights Are Indispensable," *Mind* 95, 379 (1986): 329–344. Although we all accept the correlativity thesis that duties and rights are linked, these authors maintained that rights create duties in others. I stand with Hobbes (also Rawls and Scanlon) in asserting that undertaking duties creates rights in others. In the case of medical ethics, in accepting the duties of doctors, physicians take on obligations. Their assumption of duties gives patients and society the right to trustworthy medical practice.

[96] Here, again, my position opposes the stand taken by Beauchamp and Childress (*Principles*, 2009, 206) and others who maintained that the physician-patient relationship involves reciprocal duties.

in the broader field of bioethics. There are many contested issues of public policy and common morality that I simply do not address in these pages. Although I agree with Beauchamp and Childress and Gert, Culver, and Clouser on some points and disagree on at least as many, this is not the venue for debating positions that lie outside of my limited scope. Specifically, I do not engage on issues that fall outside of doctors' authority even though in some instances I have argued for particular positions elsewhere. Here I limit my scope to identifying the distinctive duties of medicine, explaining them, and arguing for why they must be professional obligations. Where I do enter into debate, for instance on the issues of best interest and conscientious objection, I do so because these are important and controversial issues within the sphere of medical practice today and because they bear on our understanding of medical professionalism.

2

The Distinctive Ethics of Medicine

Since the ancients, people have recognized their fragility: We are all vulnerable to injury, disease, disability, pain, and death. People have understood their physical limitations and impairments and hoped to overcome them. People have treasured their own health and the health of their loved ones and wished to maintain their fitness.

These natural and widely shared human desires have led people to seek means to avert the feared states of illness, disability, pain, and disease and satisfy their hopes and wishes to overcome poor health and its burdens. These common concerns have also inclined people to try to preserve their good health when possible. Societies therefore have recognized the need for developing and supporting a cadre of individuals who might advance their people's communal goals of creating the means for preventing illness, curing disease, alleviating symptoms, restoring function, easing suffering, and averting death.

To further these collective aims, societies have authorized some individuals to develop the special knowledge and skills that could be effective in advancing those ends. That group practices the profession of medicine, and the members of the profession are our doctors.[1] The profession and institutions of medicine are therefore social creations that provide social goods. This means that medicine has no essential nature. It is not part of the natural world and not governed by any primordial natural necessity or focused on achieving some metaphysical end. Medicine is a human creation that we design, revise, and moderate in order to meet our needs and goals.

At the same time, people are aware of the potential dangers that are associated with creating this particular kind of knowledge and bestowing the

---

[1] Throughout this book, I refer to the profession of medicine and medical professionals with broadly inclusive intent. Often, though not always, when I refer to medical professionals I include physicians, nurses, pharmacists, dentists, genetics counselors, midwives, bioethicists, medical technicians, and so forth. I intend to include all medical specialties as well as all of those who are now described as physician extenders and even those who work in supportive roles in medical offices. I consider all of these individuals to be medical professionals who are bound by the ethics of medicine.

The Trusted Doctor. Rosamond Rhodes, Oxford University Press (2020). © Oxford University Press.
DOI: 10.1093/oso/9780190859909.001.0001

special powers involved in performing medical activities and executing medical decisions. These realizations create a broadly accepted consensus that the distinctive knowledge and skills that society allows doctors to develop must be used for the good of patients and society. Thus, society allows doctors to learn about anatomy, physiology, nutrition, genetics, immunology, pharmacology, the microbiome, environmental toxins, biochemistry, and so on. We want physicians to have all of this knowledge so that they may use it for the good of patients and society. Yet, we are aware that this powerful armamentarium of medical information and understanding is, simultaneously, a potentially dangerous body of knowledge.

Society also permits doctors an extraordinary set of powers, privileges, and immunities.[2] Physicians are allowed to ask probing questions and examine nakedness (i.e., invade privacy), they are given license to prescribe medications (i.e., poisons), they are granted the privilege to perform surgery (i.e., assault with deadly weapons) with immunity from prosecution, and they are also empowered to assess individuals' decisional capacity and sometimes override the expressed wishes of their patients and impose unwanted treatment on them. These remarkable powers, privileges, and immunities amount to an astonishing collection of distinctive rights that create a medical monopoly over a field of employment and a warrant to perform actions that no other group is allowed to execute.

If a mere mortal, a nonphysician such as I, cut into another to remove a vital organ or convinced someone to imbibe a potentially deadly poison, I could be arrested and sent to prison, even if that other had consented to my action. Yet when physicians perform such actions, what they do is accepted as something good. They are typically praised for their activities and paid for their efforts. In other words, physicians are given license and immunity to do what nonphysicians are prohibited from doing.

Societies recognize that the knowledge, powers, and privileges that we allow doctors could also be used for achieving an array of other common human goals that are not directly related to health or life extension. We call on the medical profession to use the tools at their service in relieving the embarrassment and distress caused by blemishes and other conditions that a person might consider unsightly, even though the effective intervention

---

[2] I am following Wesley Newcomb Hohfeld's account of rights. Hohfeld WN, *Rights and Jural Relations in Fundamental Legal Conceptions*, edited by WW Cook (New Haven, CT: Yale University Press, 1919: 35–64). Cf. Feinberg J and Gross H, *Philosophy of Law*, 4th edition (Belmont, CA: Wadsworth, 1991: 357–367).

might impose some risk to life or health. We count on the expertise of doctors to relieve pain and support the dying, even when the required interventions will neither improve health nor extend life and might, in fact, do the opposite. And we want skilled medical professionals to oversee pregnancies and assist in childbirth, even though no illness or disease is involved.

Similarly, in our society today, we call on firefighters to rescue children and cats when they get stuck in tall trees, even when no fires are involved, and we expect the police to deal with pythons and alligators that occasionally show up in cities, even when no laws are violated. We call on these professionals because they have the tools and the skills to address the problems that we need to have resolved.

In the same way, we ask medical professionals to use their special knowledge, tools, and powers to address people's needs and desires. We count requests for medical interventions as medical needs because the people with the knowledge and skills to address them are medical professionals and because we have authorized medical professionals to address human and social concerns. To the extent that only medicine has the tools to address the problems that people experience, medical interventions are appropriate. These needs may involve assisted reproduction, bariatric surgery, aid in dying, and facial reconstructive surgery for transgender people. To the extent that only medical intervention can elevate the experienced distress or contribute to well-being, medical interventions are in order. Such considerations suggest that the boundaries of the medical profession, like other professions, are defined, not by essentialist concepts such as deviations from normalcy or health and disease, but by the scope of knowledge, powers, and privileges that society grants to the profession.

Societies also appreciate that the knowledge, powers, privileges, and immunities that are allowed to doctors could also be hazardous if used carelessly, recklessly, or without goodwill. So, whereas medicine is granted these uncommon commissions, society provides them only on the condition that medicine can be trusted to wield them for the good of patients and society. In a sense, the ethics of medicine is created *as if* in a promise between the profession of medicine and society. Society grants the profession the license to develop its distinctive knowledge and skills; the privileges to pry, examine, prescribe, and administer dangerous drugs; and the powers to execute risky diagnostic interventions, treatments, and therapies with impunity. At the same time, the profession, and every individual who joins the profession, publicly pledges to be trustworthy and competent and use the profession's special knowledge, skills, privileges, powers, and immunities to help society and the individuals in it.[3]

Because society's trust is essential to the practice of medicine, society and the medical profession itself have developed explicit and implicit conventions, laws, and penalties to constrain physician behavior and ensure the trustworthiness of the profession.[4] The clearly articulated statutes and codes of ethics that are drafted and publicly displayed online by medical associations and medical specialty groups around the world, as well as numerous unspoken implied understandings, express the conditions that must be observed in order for doctors and the profession to be trusted and trustworthy. Although all of the duties of physicians have not previously been fully defined and explained, at least not in the way that I believe they need to be, a general understanding of many of them has been assimilated into the practice of medicine since at least the time of Hippocrates. They have been accepted by physicians as the duties that they must fulfill, and they are articulated in short and lengthy lists posted in the codes of ethics on the websites of medical societies. To illustrate the sort of consensus that I have observed in clinical environments, as well as the remarkable silence on some issues, I refer to a sample list of codes of ethics prominently posted on the websites of the World Medical Association and national medical associations in the world's largest English speaking countries[5]:

American Medical Association Code of Medical Ethics (2001)[6]
Australian Medical Association Code of Ethics (2016)[7]

---

[3] I regard my account of medical ethics to be consistent with the views of H.L.A. Hart and Edna Ullmann-Margalit on the generation of the "rules of obligation" or "specific norms" that are necessary for maintaining essential features of a functioning human society. In this case, I am providing the derivation of the obligations or morally binding norms of the medical profession. The game-theoretical conclusion, "seek trust and be deserving of it" provides the security for society granting the profession its distinctive liberties. The contextual details of medical practice (not game theory) then guide the derivation of medicine's fiduciary duty and the subsequent deduction of 14 additional duties of the profession. Hart, HLA, *The Concept of Law*. Oxford: Oxford University Press, 1961. Ullmann-Margalit, E, *The Emergence of Norms* Oxford: Oxford at the Clarendon Press, 1977.

[4] I am suggesting that genesis of the medical profession is similar to the genesis of other professions. Each profession is granted its own domain of knowledge, powers, privileges, and immunities, and that their use is constrained by that profession's own socially generated distinctive ethics.

[5] The codes that I mention here and elsewhere in the book are reproduced in the Appendix. Some other English-speaking national medical associations, such as the South African Medical Association, subscribe to the World Medical Association Declaration of Geneva.

[6] American Medical Association. *AMA Code of Medical Ethics: AMA Principles of Medical Ethics* (2001). Accessed October 28, 2018, at https://www.ama-assn.org/sites/default/files/media-browser/principles-of-medical-ethics.pdf

[7] Australian Medical Association. *AMA Code of Ethics 2004. Editorially Revised 2006. Revised 2016* (2016). Accessed October 28, 2018, at https://ama.com.au/system/tdf/documents/AMA%20Code%20of%20Ethics%202004.%20Editorially%20Revised%202006.%20Revised%202016.pdf?file=1&type=node&id=46014

Canadian Medical Association Code of Ethics (2004)[8]
Medical Council of India, Code of Medical Ethics (2002)[9]
New Zealand Medical Association Code of Ethics (2014)[10]
UK General Medical Council, Good Medical Practice (2014)[11]
World Medical Association Declaration of Geneva (2017)[12]
World Medical Association International Code of Medical Ethics (2006)[13]

These codes differ in their scope and amount of generality and detail, and at various points take opposing positions on the same issue. The areas of consensus are especially instructive. The shared commitments that these and other similar codes enshrine have become the duties that patients rely on their doctors to uphold. When individuals join the profession and take on the trappings that publicly proclaim them to be doctors, they publicly proclaim their commitments by declaring an oath,[14] using the letters MD after their names, and wearing the white coat. In doing so, doctors give patients and society reason to expect that they are committed to upholding their distinctive professional obligations.

A Thought Experiment

To more vividly illustrate medicine's ongoing need for trust, consider the kind of situation that could happen to almost anyone anywhere. Imagine a young pregnant woman visiting a city that is far from her home. In the airport terminal, shortly after her arrival, she is overcome with vomiting and

---

[8] Canadian Medical Association. *CMA Code of Ethics (Update 2004)* (2004). Accessed July 30, 2019 at https://www.cma.ca/cma-code-ethics-and-professionalism
[9] Medical Counsel of India. *Indian Medical Council (Professional Conduct, Etiquette and Ethics) Regulations 2002* (2002; amended up to October 8, 2016). Accessed October 28, 2018, https://www.mciindia.org/documents/rulesAndRegulations/Ethics%20Regulations-2002.pdf
[10] New Zealand Medical Association. *Code of Ethics for the New Zealand Medical Profession* (2014). Accessed October 28, 2018, at https://www.nzma.org.nz/publications/code-of-ethics
[11] UK General Medical Council. *Ethical Guidance* (2014). Accessed October 28, 2018, at https://gmc-uk.org/ethical-guidance
[12] World Medical Association. *WMA Declaration of Geneva* (2017). Accessed December 13, 2018, at https://www.wma.net/policies-post/wma-declaration-of-geneva/
[13] World Medical Association. *WMA International Code of Medical Ethics* (2006). Accessed December 13, 2018, at https://www.wma.net/policies-post/wma-international-code-of-medical-ethics/
[14] Edmund Pellegrino discussed the importance of the public proclamation in medicine. Pellegrino ED, "Professionalism, Profession and the Virtues of the Good Physician," *The Mount Sinai Journal of Medicine* 69, 6 (2002): 378–384.

abdominal pain. She is taken by ambulance to a nearby hospital, where she knows no one. A stranger in a white coat plies her with detailed questions about her symptoms, her personal and family history, her sexual and drug history, and her bowel habits. She discloses information that she might not be willing to share with even her most intimate relations. Then the stranger asks her to disrobe and begins to handle and probe her body, even touching sexually sensitive areas and manipulating her body in ways that cause some pain. After a while, the stranger announces that this patient will have to submit to tests that she never would have otherwise sought (e.g., barium enema) or ingest a chemical that is likely to have toxic properties. Imagine further, that the next morning the stranger announces that she will have to permit herself to be made unconscious so that her body can be invaded by knives and allow some body parts to be removed. It is very hard to imagine that she would submit to these bodily intrusions from anyone but a doctor. And for a doctor to be permitted to do any of these things, albeit for her own good, the doctor must, to some degree, be *trusted*.

Furthermore, imagine that this young woman's diagnosis is life threatening and requires surgery within hours. Without surgery, she and her fetus will surely die. If this young woman refuses the urgent surgery and explains that her ancestors on the astral plain 10,000 years ago commanded her to refuse to allow her skin to be punctured, the surgeon, and the psychiatrist who is called for assistance, will assess her decisional capacity. If they determine that their patient lacks decisional capacity, they will override her refusal and proceed with the recommended urgent treatment. Again, it is only because society recognizes that disease, drugs, psychosis, and fear can impair decisional capacity; that the consequences of refusing recommended medical treatment can be serious and enduring; and that medical decisions are often time sensitive, that doctors are trusted to determine that a patient lacks decisional capacity and impose treatment, even surgery, over objection in emergency situations.

This vignette demonstrates that trust is at the core of medicine. Society allows doctors to develop their special knowledge and skills, advantages that could be particularly dangerous to members of society if they were not controlled. Society therefore has a compelling interest in having the uses of medicine's muscle controlled and regulated by clearly delineated professional obligations. Those duties comprise the ethics of medicine, and their constraining force on physician behavior enables patients and society to trust doctors. Individual physicians publicly acknowledge their undertaking of medicine's fiduciary responsibilities and their commitment to abide by the ethics of medicine. The formulation of medical ethics, the enumeration of the duties of physicians, and the enforcement of those standards is what makes the profession trustworthy and allows doctors to be trusted. In other words, the creation of the medical profession is founded on trust. Without that trust the profession would not exist and doctors would not have the wherewithal to conduct their practice.

Misplaced trust can be dangerous to people's health, and a lack of trust impedes medicine's ability to provide services.[15] Yet, frequently patients are not in a position to assess the trustworthiness of their individual physicians, particularly when the patients are ill, incapacitated, fearful, or in the throes of a medical emergency. And often, patients who may have the ability to delve further simply trust the doctor to whom they are assigned, the one they select from an insurance list, the physician recommended by a friend or another doctor, the physician from the needed specialty at a renowned medical institution, or the one identified through an Internet search or a subway advertisement. Most people select their doctors in one of these ways largely because they appreciate that they lack both the ability to discern the relevant characteristics and the access to the relevant information. Thus, whenever people accept someone as their doctor without thoroughly vetting the physician's qualifications, skills, judgment, character, and history, they do not know enough about that individual to be making an informed decision to submit to the doctor's powers and yield to the doctor's recommendations. Instead, they are actually relying on the social trust that is attached to the professional role that the practitioner fills.

To the extent that medicine provides care, patients have to accept the care by investing their doctors with profession-based trust. Combining these insights about trust and medicine makes the point that trust is the fundamental basis of medical practice. It is therefore essential for clinicians and the institutions of medicine to be trustworthy and to seek the trust of patients and society in all of their efforts. No physician who considers the context of medical practice can fail to acknowledge it. No patient who vividly imagines what is being undertaken would want it any other way. Any prospective patient—everyone that is—wants doctors to be trustworthy.

---

[15] Onora O'Neill has the opposite view, that it is unreasonably dangerous to trust doctors. O'Neill O, *Autonomy and Trust in Bioethics* (Cambridge: Cambridge University Press, 2002).

Unfortunately, medical treatment is sometimes delivered without a climate of trust. Some patients have learned to be distrustful because of unfortunate experiences with untrustworthy physicians and our flawed system of healthcare delivery. Distrustful patients sometimes do accept treatment when there is no better option. Nevertheless, examples of distrust do not refute the claims that patients would prefer to be able to trust their doctors, that most doctors would prefer to be trusted by their patients, and that society grants special license to the profession of medicine on the expectation of its trustworthiness.

The Fundamental Commitment of Medical Ethics

The first duty of medical ethics is to seek trust and be deserving of it.
Because people make themselves vulnerable by trusting medical institutions and clinicians based on the institutions' and clinicians' professional standing, the responsibilities of medical ethics require broad endorsement from the profession and the commitment of each practitioner and every medical institution. The distinctive obligations have to be publicly enumerated and professed in codes and oaths, as they have been since at least the time of Hippocrates[16] and up to the present in the Internet-posted statements of the vast majority of medical associations and specialty groups.[17]

The starting point for my explication of the duties of the medical professionals, and the most basic duty that the profession and every doctor must uphold, is **seek trust and be deserving of it.** This is the first and fundamental duty of medical ethics. In deciding what to do and how to do it, doctors must pay attention to promoting trust and not eroding it. And in molding themselves as physicians, they must focus on making themselves trustworthy practitioners.

Patients need to trust their doctors from the first moment of their first visit, even when they know little about their individual physician, medical science, or medical procedures. They need to trust, and actually do trust, doctors who are total strangers to them (e.g., think back to the example of the patient in

---

[16] Hippocrates' oath, translated by H. von Staden, "'In a Pure and Holy Way': Personal and Professional Conduct in the Hippocratic Oath," *The Journal of the History of Medicine and Allied Sciences* 51, 4 (1996): 404–437.
[17] Here I make a similar claim to the position taken by Edmund Pellegrino. Pellegrino ED, "Toward a Reconstruction of Medical Morality," *The Journal of Medical Humanities* 8, 1 (1987): 7–18.

the emergency room setting). To receive the medical benefits that they reasonably hope to secure, they have to yield to the advice of their physicians, at least to some degree. The nature of illness makes patients vulnerable and reliant on trusting their doctors. Physicians also encourage patients to trust them because the practice of medicine requires it. Whereas "buyer beware" is the hallmark of business, medicine is a profession and not a business.

Patients and their families extend their trust to doctors because doctors wear the professional uniform of a white coat or scrubs, because they carry the professional title MD after their name, and often because they encounter the doctor in a medical facility. In sum, patients and society rely on doctors, medical institutions, and the medical profession to be trustworthy. They trust because a history of doctors (for the most part) acting for their patients' good has made medicine trustworthy.

Physicians today are the heirs of the trust that was engendered by those who came before them, and their actions today create the legacy for those who will come after. As beneficiaries of their predecessors' trustworthiness, and as those who create the reputation that the next generation of physicians will inherit, doctors also have the responsibility of acting to ensure that the profession of medicine will be deserving of its necessary trust. As the New Zealand Medical Association Code of Ethics declared in its preliminary statement, "The medical profession has a social contract with its community. In return for the trust patients and the community place in doctors, ethical codes are produced to guide the profession and protect patients."[18] The UK General Medical Council declared much the same commitment in the opening statement of its good medical practice list of duties of a doctor. "Patients must be able to trust doctors with their lives and health. To justify that trust you must show respect for human life and make sure that your practice meets the standards expected of you."[19] And it concludes with the statement, "Never abuse your patients' trust in you or the public's trust in the profession."[20] And as the US physician Jordan J. Cohen has written, "Trust in physicians is the foundation upon which the social contract with society rests. But trust in physicians is not a birthright. Trust is earned, not owed. The only way physicians can earn trust is by being trustworthy as true professionals."[21]

[18] New Zealand Medical Association, *Code of Ethics*.
[19] UK General Medical Council, *Ethical Guidance*.
[20] UK General Medical Council, *Ethical Guidance*.
[21] Cohen JJ, "Tasking the 'Self' in the Self-Governance of Medicine" [Editorial], *JAMA* 313, 18 (2015): 1839–1840.

The fundamental and core guiding *first duty of medical ethics is to seek trust and be deserving of that trust.* It is the source from which all of the other more specific duties are derived.

The command to *seek trust* sets out the basis for defining which kinds of **action** are required and which are forbidden and the source from which the more specific particular duties of the profession are explicated. It directs doctors to do those things that will garner trust for themselves and the profession and to resist the temptation to do anything that is likely to undermine that trust. In other words, *seek trust* directs action.

The command to *be deserving of that trust* means that doctors must mold themselves into being *trustworthy* clinicians because anyone who falls short of that standard does not deserve the tremendous trust that society bestows on doctors. The concept of *trustworthiness* establishes that developing a doctorly **character** is an essential element of the commitment to medicine, and it defines the distinctive virtues that physicians must cultivate.[22] Medical schools carefully select students who are bright and admirable people who show their prospects for becoming good doctors. Then, their knowledge and skills and their doctorly character must be cultivated. Just as medical students do not arrive at medical school knowing all that they need to know, they do not arrive at medical school with a doctorly character. The Canadian Medical Association Code of Ethics acknowledges the need for doctors to be helped to develop the ability to navigate moral conflicts, stating in its introduction that, "Training in ethical analysis and decision-making during undergraduate, postgraduate and continuing medical education is recommended for physicians to develop their knowledge, skills and attitudes needed to deal with these conflicts."[23] The distinctive duties of medical ethics have to be studied and learned, and the virtues that comprise a doctorly character have to be inculcated and honed.

A trustworthy doctor needs to understand each professional duty and the justification for it. In addition, every physician must feel a commitment to upholding each duty of medical ethics. That commitment amounts to an accompanying feeling of identity with the obligation, a powerful inclination to abide by its dictates, and an attitude that supports doing what the duty requires. These feelings of identity with the duties of medicine, the inclinations to abide by professional duties together with a concomitant

---

[22] The importance of developing a doctorly character is explained further in Chapter 10.
[23] Canadian Medical Association, *Code of Ethics.*

aversion to violating them, and the attitude toward upholding professional obligations amount to the virtues of a physician. Taken together, they define what a physician should be and what a doctorly character is.

The command to *seek trust and be deserving of that trust* also serves as the principle for resolving the inevitable conflicts that arise in any system of ethics with more than one single obligation. As the standard for resolving conflicts of duty, the fundamental duty of medical ethics directs doctors to consider which course can be expected to promote trust and which can be expected to undermine trust and resolve the matter in that light. When a circumstance arises in which a doctor cannot satisfy two or more of the duties of medical ethics because they dictate conflicting actions in some particular situation, the dilemma's resolution is likely to require that one or more of the cherished duties must be compromised: One duty may have to be set aside so that another can be upheld.[24]

Aside from the fundamentalduty, there is no hierarchy among the duties of medical ethic: They all have equal standing as inferences from the fundamentalduty. In circumstances that involve dilemmas of incompatible direction, *seek trust and be trustworthy* is the touchstone for resolving the conflict. The decision on how to proceed and which treasured duty to sacrifice should be determined by considering which alternative action is more likely to preserve society's trust and which more likely to erode or undermine the trust. An individual physician confronting a professional dilemma is likely to consider what a trustworthy mentor would do in the situation and follow that course. In today's medical institutions, dilemmas are often hashed out in consultation with peers, at team rounds, or referred to a departmental or institutional committee with jurisdiction over the matter. Broader issues are often referred to professional societies for recommendations. Typically a professional consensus emerges on which path to take, and that agreement expresses the shared view of what is the right thing to do in the situation, what any doctor in such a situation should do, and which course is likely to be accepted by society as what a trusted doctor would do. In other words, the resolution of dilemmas should be decided from the perspective of professional judgment, and not personal preference or a public opinion poll.

---

[24] The resolution of ethical dilemmas is discussed in detail in Chapter 11.

Serve the Interests of Patients and Society

The second duty of medical ethics is promote the interests of patients and society. The second duty of medical ethics is derived from the fundamental first duty that commands physicians to seek trust and be deserving of that trust. As long as a society allows doctors to develop their distinctive knowledge and skills and allows them the powers and privileges to do things that are otherwise forbidden to ordinary citizens, the second duty requires that *doctors relinquish their liberty to pursue only self-interest and commit themselves to using their medical knowledge, skills, powers, privileges, and immunities in the service of patients and society.* This is the core of medicine's *fiduciary responsibility*, and it requires doctors to put their patients' good before their own.[25] Commitment to this obligation means that doctors accept the risks that the profession deems to be reasonable (e.g., exposure to infectious disease), the burdens and inconveniences that are concomitant with providing care to people who require their medical expertise (e.g., assisting in the delivery of a baby at 3:00 AM), and the need to minimize conflicts of interests (e.g., limit opportunities for personal gains or enrichment).

Using similar but somewhat different words, this commitment is asserted by leaders of the profession and in numerous codes and oaths of medical ethics. For example, Jordan J. Cohen has asserted "the hallmark of medical professionalism is a subordination of self-interest to the best interest of patients and the public."[26] The preamble of the American Medical Association's most current version of their "Principles of Medical Ethics" makes a comparable claim. It states that, "A physician must recognize responsibility to patients, first and foremost"; again in Principle VIII, it reiterates that "a physician shall, when caring for a patient, 'regard responsibility to the patient as paramount.' "[27] The UK Medical Council statement of good medical practice requires doctors to "make the care of your patient your first concern."[28] The Canadian Medical Association Code of Ethics instructs doctors to "consider first the well-being of the patient" and "consider the well-being of society in matters affecting health."[29] The Australian Medical Association

---

[25] Edmund Pellegrino actually regarded medicine's fiduciary responsibility as the fundamental principle of medical ethics. Pellegrino ED, "Physician's Duty to Treat: Altruism, Self-Interest and Medical Ethics," *JAMA* 258, 14 (1987): 1939–1940; Pellegrino, ED, "Professionalism, Profession."

[26] Cohen, "Tasking the 'Self,'" 1840.

[27] American Medical Association, *AMA Code of Medical Ethics.*

[28] UK General Medical Council, *Ethical Guidance.*

[29] Canadian Medical Association, *Code of Ethics.*

Code of Ethics declares, "While doctors have a primary duty to individual patients, they also have responsibilities to other patients and the wider community."[30] The Medical Council of India holds that, "The prime object of the medical Profession is to render service to humanity; reward or financial gain is a subordinate consideration."[31] The World Medical Association Declaration of Geneva requires doctors to pledge that "the health and well-being of my patient will be my first consideration."[32]

One important point to note about my articulation of the duty *to serve patients and society* and the versions in numerous professional statements is that this duty encompasses both individual patients and the broader community of patients. Sometimes a single patient is the sole object of attention for a physician, but often enough, there are other patients with claims on the doctor's attention at the very same time, patients who are waiting for their appointments, patients who are in the hospital, patients who are waiting to have their phone call returned. In addition, doctors frequently have to consider the impact on other patients when making a treatment choice for an individual patient. For example, the choice of an antibiotic may reflect growing concerns about antibiotic-resistant bacteria, and a decision about scheduling a patient for surgery will take into account the needs of other patients who have appointments for a procedure and other patients with more urgent needs for surgery. And from time to time, medical decisions may reflect concerns for the entire local or global community. Choices about disease control in the face of a pandemic or the distribution of a vaccine when the supply is limited are relevant examples. Mindful physicians appreciate the moral complexity of this central duty. They also recognize the ethical risks that are inherent in oversimplifying the obligation to focus on the single patient in their present encounter.[33]

The scope of this and the other duties of medical ethics is comprehensive. They not only apply to dramatic matters of life and death, but also apply to choices about the small details of professional action that are frequently neglected, perhaps as seeming too trivial to mention. To illustrate the sweeping implications of this critically important obligation, consider the white coat, a matter that has received very little attention in the medical ethics literature. In

---

[30] Australian Medical Association, *AMA Code of Ethics 2004.*
[31] Medical Counsel of India, *Indian Medical Council.*
[32] World Medical Association, *WMA Declaration of Geneva.*
[33] Pledging that the "health and well-being of my patient will be my first consideration" is an example of what I regard as a dangerous oversimplification. World Medical Association, *WMA Declaration of Geneva.*

Western societies, wearing white has symbolic importance. White represents purity and holiness. Brides, the Pope, and Jewish rabbis on the High Holidays all wear white. Doctors wearing white coats signify the traditional regard of both physicians and society toward the practice of medicine. In the words of the Hippocratic oath, and in the spirit of the oath of Maimonides, the practice of medicine is an activity that must be approached with reverence. The color white also has represented cleanliness and upholding sanitary standards. In that light, when physicians present themselves wearing the white coat, they are taken to be declaring their commitment to medicine as a higher calling and to protecting their patients from harm by possibly transmitting disease.

Questions related to the white coat actually raise subtle but significant ethical issues concerning the color, the length, and the condition of the coat and who gets to wear one. Some institutions reserve long white coats for physicians. They allow medical students to wear short white coats and other medical professionals to wear coats of other colors. Some institutions have moved away from white coats for physicians, adopting, instead, coats of other colors and coats of a single length. Some people argue that reserving white for physicians and distinguishing levels of training by coat length is hierarchical and authoritarian, and that it makes some coat wearers uncomfortable. Others argue that allowing nonphysicians, research assistants for example, to wear long white coats encourages patients to cooperate with them.

That may all be true, but the question that should be asked is whether uniform coats of another color, or white coats worn by nonphysicians, serve the interests of patients. Does it, instead, put the interests of medical professionals before the interests of patients? From the perspective of patients, the symbolic value of whiteness provides the important assurance that their doctor is upholding sanitary practice and treating professional responsibilities "in a pure and holy way."[34] White coats make doctors readily identifiable, and the visible difference in color and coat length allows patients to distinguish doctors from medical students and others on the medical team so that they may use the information in making decisions about how much and what sort of trust to place in each of them. Obliterating those distinctions, or allowing nonphysicians to deceptively masquerade as physicians, does not serve patients' interests and may actually obstruct them.

In addition, at many hospitals the laundry facility that provides clean coats is not conveniently located and has limited hours for distributing clean garments.

---

[34] von Staden, " 'In a Pure and Holy Way.' "

Making access to clean coats inconvenient for staff probably saves money on laundry expenses for the institution, but making it difficult to secure clean coats also leaves physicians feeling excused for changing coats only rarely.

Ignaz Philipp Semmelweis, the nineteenth century Hungarian physician who introduced hand washing at the Vienna General Hospital, described his early clinical experience of being embarrassed by his clean white coat.[35] He explained that the senior physicians at the hospital wore coats that had been dirtied by using them to wipe their hands after examining patients. To Semmelweis, the filth suggested having significant clinical experience and an appropriate lack of concern for mundane matters like washing a coat. But again, the issue should not be what the coat's appearance means to doctors, but what it means to patients. To patients who notice the grimy cuffs, the stains, and slept-in look of the white coat, the slovenly appearance suggests the opposite of cleanliness and sterility. It also shows the doctor's disrespect for patients because we do not present ourselves dirty and disheveled when we care about making a good impression.

Placebo and nocebo effects offer additional reasons for attending to white coats.[36] These are the beneficial or harmful effects that are attributed to patients' beliefs rather than medical treatments per se.[37] Recent studies have shown that the trappings of a medical environment can by themselves promote beneficial effects even when patients are informed that they are only receiving an inert intervention, that is, a placebo.[38–40] The effects are produced by contextual and environmental cues and not by any active ingredients. These findings suggest that by conveying the appearance of professional commitments, a clean white coat can bolster patients' expectations for a good outcome and create a placebo effect. Other studies have shown that a messy desk could have a negative effect on people's experience.[41] Such results imply

---

[35] Carter KC and Carter BR. *Childbed Fever. A Scientific Biography of Ignaz Semmelweis* (Piscataway, NJ: Transaction, February 1, 2005).

[36] Kaptchuk TJ and Miller FG, "Placebo Effects in Medicine," *New England Journal of Medicine* 373, 1 (2015: 8–9.

[37] Finniss DG, Kaptchuk TJ, Miller F, and Benedetti F, "Placebo Effects: Biological, Clinical and Ethical Advances," *Lancet* 375, 9715 (2010): 686–695.

[38] Carvalhoa C, Caetanob JM, Cunhac L, Reboutac P, Kaptchukd TJ, Kirsch I, "Open-Label Placebo Treatment in Chronic Low Back Pain: A Randomized Controlled Trial," *Pain* 157, 12 (2016): 1–7.

[39] Sandler AD and Bodfish JW, "Open-Label Use of Placebos in the Treatment of ADHD: A Pilot Study," *Child: Care, Health and Development* 34, 1 (2008): 104–110.

[40] Kaptchuk TJ, Friedlander E, Kelley JM, et al., "Placebos Without Deception: A Randomized Controlled Trial in Irritable Bowel Syndrome," *PLoS One* 5, 12 (2010): 15591.

[41] Chae B and Zhu R, Why a Messy Workspace Undermines Your Persistence, *Harvard Business Review* (2015, January 28). Accessed April 20, 2017, at https://hbr.org/2015/01/why-a-messy-workspace-undermines-your-persistence

that the aura of a crumpled or dirty white coat could undermine the salutary experience of a medical encounter.[42]

Thus, considering the white coat in light of the commitment to serving the interests of patients leads to important ethical conclusions. Professional garb is not merely something to cover one's outdoor clothing. It means something to the wearer and to those who interact with the wearer. Like the robes worn by judges, white coats are emblematic of the wearers' commitment to fulfilling their professional responsibilities. They remind doctors and their patients of the role that the wearer has taken on. They declare physicians' trustworthiness and thereby serve their patients' interests.[43] Therefore, coats should be white, clean, and well pressed and allow patients to readily identify the name and role of those who contribute to their care.

Associated Duties

Because the ethics of medicine is markedly different from the ethics of everyday life, physicians need to learn what their duties are. A doctor also has to become a person who is likely to fulfill those distinctive duties. Popular culture has had numerous examples of both exemplars of what a good doctor should be (Dr. Kildare, in various incarnations from the 1930s through the 1960s; Marcus Welby, MD, in the 1970s TV series; Dr. Hank Lawson in the 2009–2016 TV series *Royal Pains*) and more controversial examples of how a doctor may be lacking in some doctorly virtues (Dr. Gregory House, 2004–2012). The point is that being a good doctor requires a special character, people want their doctors to have that sort of character, and even when it's not explicitly articulated, for the most part, we can recognize exemplary doctors and distinguish them from those who are flawed.

Drawing on a long tradition in moral philosophy has brought me to appreciate how interconnected behavior is with virtues. Virtues are the habitual inclinations to act and feel as one should with respect to an object or a kind of situation. Virtues dispose a person to choose and behave one way rather than another. Therefore, to achieve the behavior that we want in citizens, civic virtues have to be deliberately cultivated. And to achieve the behavior that we want from our medical doctors, physicians' virtues have to be deliberately cultivated. Because the duties of medical ethics are so markedly different

---

[42] In conversation, Jody Azzouni suggested this point.
[43] Pellegrino ED, "Professionalism, Profession."

from the principles of common morality, the virtues that are needed for complying with the duties of medical ethics must be nurtured. When people accept and endorse the ethical commitments of the medical profession as the duties for guiding their professional actions, they commit themselves to fulfill those obligations. To the extent that professional virtues facilitate professional actions, choosing to become a doctor therefore commits individuals to developing the habitual inclinations and attitudes that will dispose them to fulfill their professional responsibilities. Medical education should aim at developing the professional character that doctors must have. And just as athletes work to form their bodies into the tools that will allow them to succeed in their sport, doctors need to mold themselves into trustworthy individuals who are virtuous.

Because patients are more inclined to trust a doctor who they believe genuinely *cares* about their good, doctors must be caring. Here I use the word *care* to capture the feelings, sentiments, and emotions associated with love, brotherly love, concern for the other's good, empathy, sympathy, compassion, and sensitivity to the other's situation. In Aristotelian terms, I am referring to what Aristotle called "friendship," but I choose to use the term *caring* to denote the particular sense that this virtue has in medical ethics.

Numerous moral theorists in the Western tradition of ethics have recognized that ethical conduct involves an emotional component,[44] but to date, that view has not taken hold, and it has not been widely endorsed in medical ethics.[45] Although I have pointed to an array of codes of medical ethics, I have not found any that mention a duty to care. In fact, the American Nurses Association Code of Ethics for Nurses, the caring profession, did not mention "caring" or anything like it until 2015, when the word *compassion* was inserted into its most recent version.

In response to the profession's predominant silence on the issue, I argue for my anachronistic yet radical position that doctors are obliged to care by presenting an array of medical cases to press my point.

[44] Such theorists include Aristotle, Kant, and Hume.
[45] Some authors in the literature of bioethics and professionalism are identified as virtue theorists in that they see the entire ethics enterprise exclusively in terms of virtue. I am not aligning myself with that approach, but taking a different tack in explaining ethics as a complex matter involving duties to do the right thing along with virtues that incline doctors to abide by their commitment to uphold medical ethics.

Case 1

It was August 1982. A hematologist, Dr. Smith, was aware of a clotting factor therapy that would help his hemophiliac patients live without the painful and crippling crises that have been associated with the disease. He was also aware of some suggestions that there was a risk of contracting hepatitis or an unnamed immune system disorder associated with using the clotting factor that had been killing gay men and intravenous drug users. Should he have encouraged his patients to use the clotting factor?

If this doctor genuinely cared about his patients, would he urge them to use the clotting factor, discourage them from trying it, or choose some other course? Sweeping moral principles of autonomy, beneficence, nonmaleficence, and justice[46] do not tell him what more he needs to consider or what to do. In fact, the different principles seem to give different answers, and there is no obvious way to adjudicate between them.

Respect for autonomy would require him to share what he knows about the risks of using the factor. But he cannot present information on the likelihood of contracting these diseases through the use of clotting factor because, at the time when he had to decide, there were no data. Furthermore, he had no information on how the unnamed immune disorder or the hepatitis virus behaved in the hemophiliac population, where they might be significantly less or more lethal.

By analogy with other diseases that had been spread through the distribution of blood products from pooled donor sources, the doctor might come to believe that the likelihood of contracting and dying from the immune disorder or the hepatitis virus was greater than 1%. He might also believe that plainly sharing this projection with his patients without editorializing might leave them with the view that a 99% chance of having no serious drawback made taking the factor low risk. Would respect for autonomy require him not to share his own sense that a 1% risk represented a significant danger, or should respect for autonomy allow him to present his

[46] Beauchamp TL and Childress JF, *Principles of Biomedical Ethics*, 7th edition (New York: Oxford University Press, 2013).

view colored so vividly to make it hardly possible for his patients to draw a conclusion that was different from his? The directions for applying the principle of autonomy are not clear, precise, or easy to fit to the circumstances.

On the one hand, beneficent considerations could have inclined him to avoid worrying his patients when the connection between the factor and the diseases had not been proven by scientific studies and patients stood to gain a great deal from treatment. If the danger proved insignificant and he had discouraged his patients from using the clotting factor, they would certainly have been harmed by living with pain, the crippling and life-threatening effects of bleeding, and having to limit their freedom of action. On the other hand, nonmaleficence could have persuaded him to avoid using the clotting factor because of the danger of infecting his patients with a fatal, incurable disease. In this situation where the evidence available might not be decisive, invoking a moral principle does not provide the answer.

Case 2

It is now later in 1982, and Dr. Jones, an emergency medicine physician, is having a conversation with an infectious disease expert, a politically cautious official from the Centers for Disease Control and Prevention (CDC). They are discussing the principles at issue in a situation very much like the one that had confronted Dr. Smith earlier that year. Dr. Jones wants the official's advice on whether he should administer clotting factor to bleeding hemophiliac patients in the Emergency Department. The CDC official was a schooled diplomat who had been around the federal agency long enough to choose his words carefully. He offered statements about the absence of proof of a causal link between the clotting factor made from pooled blood and the diseases.

Then, Dr. Jones pressed further, asking, "If your children had hemophilia, would you let them use clotting concentrate?"

The response was unhesitating, "No."[47]

---

[47] This case is based on a report by Michael McLeod, "Bad Blood: Every Day, a Hemophiliac Dies of AIDS. It Didn't Have to Happen," *Orlando Sentinel* December 19, 1993, pp. 10–24, at p. 17. Accessed July 2, 2018, at http://articles.orlandosentinel.com/1993-12-19/news/9312270549_1_hemophilia-foundation-johnny-hemophiliacs

Adding care to the sensitive balance made the weight of the evidence clear to this CDC official. With a megadose of caring for his own children, he was able to resolve the dilemma that appeared to his dispassionate thinking as a choice that could go either way. When this well-meaning but indecisive scientist was moved by feeling the kind of love he has for his sons, he was able to make an assessment of the available evidence and come to a conclusion that he was unable to reach without the emotion.

Psychologists tell us that a great deal of our thinking is unconscious, but efficient and reliable. Some have demonstrated that unconscious thinking is able to integrate and evaluate multiple pieces of information to optimize decisions.[48-51] This anecdote appears to be such an instance. Although relying entirely on feelings and unconscious thinking invites serious hazards, well-tuned emotions can be an aid in resolving dilemmas. In fact, study findings suggest that several strategies can be utilized in deciding among alternatives, and unconscious thinking may be more likely than conscious thinking to assign weight to the various considerations according to their importance.[52]

Beyond the psychological appeal of a caring doctor, physicians, in particular, need to feel caring concern for their patients' well-being in order to be trusted. Caring can be a defense against the ethical danger of making clinical judgments that reflect self-interest rather than patient interest and may also protect against the moral hazard of finding good excuses rather than doing what one should. Furthermore, in order for patients to trust their doctors and accept their medical recommendations, patients need to believe that their doctors are acting from caring rather than selfishness.[53]

If the doctor in this case cares about his patient, he may want to keep her close by so that he can continue to look after her and keep her from feeling abandoned. From beneficence, he would try to do what was best for his patient, and that could involve keeping her in a familiar environment and close to her family and friends so that she would not be uncomfortable and

---

[48] Kahneman D, *Thinking Fast and Slow* (New York: Farrar, Straus and Giroux, 2013).

[49] Dijksterhuis A, Bos MW, Nordgren LF, and Van Baaren RB, "On Making the Right Choice: The Deliberation-Without-Attention Effect," *Science* 311, 5763 (2006): 1005–1007.

[50] Dijksterhuis A & van Olden Z, "On the Benefits of Thinking Unconsciously: Unconscious Thought Can Increase Post-choice Satisfaction," *Journal of Experimental Social Psychology* 42, 5 (2006): 627–631.

[51] Nordgren LF, Bos MW, and Dijksterhuis A, "The Best of Both Worlds: Integrating Conscious and Unconscious Thought Best Solves Complex Decisions," *Journal of Experimental Social Psychology* 47, 2 (2011): 509–511.

[52] Dijksterhuis et al., "On Making the Right Choice."

[53] Medical Counsel of India, *Indian Medical Council.*

Case 3

A patient in the sixth month of her first pregnancy also has a history of Crohn's disease, an inflammatory bowel disorder. She has had no recent Crohn's disease flare-ups and no other complications of the pregnancy until she suddenly started to experience abdominal cramps. She goes to the office of her doctor, which is located within a hospital. Her blood count shows some abnormalities. Should her physician, a competent, experienced surgeon, keep the patient for observation and treatment at the local hospital, have her transferred to an institution with specialists in high-risk pregnancies and inflammatory bowel disease, or devise a plan for periodic reevaluation? Will a transfer reflect the desire to avoid a record of poor outcomes? Will keeping the patient at the local facility express reluctance to forgo the billing?

lonely. Besides the socially significant reasons for keeping the patient close by, there are medical considerations that need to be factored into the equation. Continuity of care is a significant advantage in delivering medical care because knowing the details of a patient's medical history improves the likelihood of proper diagnosis and the selection of the most medically appropriate treatment for the individual patient. Furthermore, a relationship with an involved attending physician who alertly oversees the patient's medical care helps to ensure that the patient will receive the necessary ongoing attention from the staff because the attending physician can draw on his existing relationships with other staff members and advocate for vigilance on behalf of his patient.

An unnecessary transfer to a distant facility or a transfer that would involve a dangerous delay of treatment would be wrong, but it would also be wrong to keep a patient who would be better off getting treatment elsewhere. If the local hospital lacked the needed facilities and experts that could be available to the patient if she were transferred, failing to transfer would be denying the medical needs of the patient.

Acting in bad faith and appreciating that what he was doing was wrong, the doctor could always offer the justification that would make his choice seem right. But, how is a less self-serving doctor to judge whether or not it would be right to transfer his patient in the face of reasons that could be persuasive for going either way?[54] A doctor who cared too much about his patient might keep her close by when she should be transferred. Too much caring (like too little caring) can blind one's view of some crucial moral features of the situation or incline one to undervalue some relevant factors. Caring about the patient's good is helpful in assessing what duty demands, but only when we care the right amount. A good doctor will work to become someone who cares to the right degree. Genuine caring about the well-being of his patient to the right degree could be an effective prophylactic against self-deception and enable the doctor to reach the conclusion that a consensus of his well-informed peers would also endorse.

Case 4

During the 34th week of her third pregnancy, a 30-year-old patient is found to have a serious complication in that the position of the placenta (placenta previa) will prevent a normal delivery. If there is no spontaneous reversal of the condition, a cesarean section and a hysterectomy will be required to save her and her baby, but the surgery will involve blood transfusions. She and her baby will certainly both die without the surgery, and the woman has about an 80% chance of dying because of rapid blood loss if she has the surgery without transfusions.

The patient is a Jehovah's Witness, and she refuses to have any blood or blood products. She has been fully informed of the likely outcomes, and she is willing to cooperate with any treatment that does not involve receiving blood. She wants to live, but she says, "I love my husband and my children, but I love my God more." Should her obstetrician comply with the patient's wishes? Should he refuse to participate in the surgery?

There is no good answer for a caring doctor in this case. He wants to promote her well-being, but does that lead him to do the surgery and let her bleed to death, to give her blood while she is under anesthesia, or to do nothing? Another sort of practitioner, who is not moved by caring but who still wants

---

[54] Bad faith (*mauvaise foi*) is a concept used by French philosophers Jean-Paul Sartre and Simone de Beauvoir. It describes the phenomenon of people inauthentically declaring themselves to be acting from values that are not the ones that actually motivate them. Bad faith may involve both deception of others and self-deception.

to do what is right, might respect cultural diversity and individual choice, the principle of do no harm, or the principle of maximizing life. Again, principles alone are not enough to provide a definitive answer when different principles indicate conflicting action.

Does her obstetrician need to focus on his duties or be guided by caring to make his choice? Should he comply with the patient's wishes? Should he refuse to participate in the surgery? He wants to promote his patient's interests, but what does that direct him to do? An obstetrician who is not moved by caring but who still wants to do what is right might abide by the duty to respect autonomy or the duty to benefit the patient by preserving her life, but which? Again, duty alone is not enough to provide a definitive answer when principles call for conflicting action. At the same time, when there is uncertainty, caring alone does not provide tools for ethical analysis and clarification.

A disinterested doctor could conclude that he was obliged by benevolence to try to save his patient and her baby and, in addition, that he was bound not to provide blood transfusions because of his duty to respect autonomy by complying with a patient's choice. He might accept the consequence that his patient would probably die from blood loss during surgery as an unfortunate, but morally justifiable, outcome. Regardless of the consequences, he would be ensured that he had done the right thing as long as he had made a sincere effort to satisfy his obligations by delivering medical care that conformed to current practice guidelines.

Sympathy with another's predicament can lead a doctor to a more comprehensive assessment of duty than would be made with indifference. A sympathetic physician might be less complacent about accepting this resolution. He would empathize with the seriousness of the conflict for the patient and be pained by the likelihood of her death and leaving three young children without a mother. Moved by complex feelings of care and compassion, fear, doubt, and guilt, he could engage his imagination and energy to vigorously pursue treatment options that were not part of the standard vocabulary for patient management.

The physician who was actually involved in this case engaged expert hematologists to explore innovative alternatives for using artificial blood and diminishing the effect of blood loss. He enlisted the participation of vascular surgeons to apply their skill in preparing for embolization of vessels that could start to bleed during the surgery. And he recruited the creativity of an anesthesiologist to develop a management plan that would meet the special requirements of this case. Because these special efforts are not normally regarded as a physician's duty in such cases, it is hard to imagine that a physician who cared less would have gone to these extraordinary lengths.

An uncaring physician who might make a similar effort because of the intellectual challenge presented by this case and the publication opportunities it offered would not be heroically attentive in a scenario that did not offer the challenge of a cerebral puzzle or the possibility of fame. We can also imagine that an uncaring physician would minimize his assessment of what his duty to the patient entailed if the Jehovah's Witness was fat, in need of a bath, and had malodorous collections under every fold of skin.

The treating physician who I described saw all of his extra efforts as part of the job. To him, all of the time, energy, and creativity he devoted to trying to save this patient were merely required by his professional obligation.

The disinterested physician and the deeply caring physician would both be required to do their duty, but the scope of what they identified as required by duty would be vastly different because of the lack or presence of caring. The absence of sympathetic caring can lead to narrowly circumscribing the extent of obligation. Excessive compassion can similarly mislead someone into taking an overextended view of what duty requires. Caring only promotes right action when the feeling has appropriate strength. Only well-moderated caring facilitates ethical judgment.[55]

Even when people are committed to fulfilling their moral obligations, emotions play a role in what we identify as being required by duty. This epistemological factor makes the problems of identifying and categorizing what we see into problems of morality. The purely dispassionate stance that has been idealized in some theoretical discussions should be dismissed because appropriate emotions are essential moral apparatus for beings whose vision, imagination, and will are hindered or aided by their feelings. Achieving the right amount of emotion is a self-adjusting process of moral self-education. It begins with the existential doubt of recognizing that what we feel may be insufficient or excessive and that emotions can and sometimes should be modified. Cultivating emotions from the desire to fulfill one's professional responsibilities and acting with the aid of those fostered emotions is the

---

[55] Curzer HJ, "Is Care a Virtue for Health Care Professionals?" *The Journal of Medicine and Philosophy* 18, 1 (1993): 51–70. Curzer has argued that care is a vice. He focused on what I see as an excess of caring, and I agree that such an extreme of feeling is vice. In this discussion, I am focused on the mean, not the extreme, and I advocate for well-regulated feelings of goodwill.

opposite of being dragged around by our feelings. Rather, it is taking responsibility for our feelings just as we take responsibility for our actions.

On to the Other Duties of Medical Ethics

I explain my remaining list of physician duties and virtues in the chapters that follow. Aside from the first fundamental duty, *to seek trust and be deserving of it,* and the second broadly inclusive duty, *to use medical knowledge, skills, powers, and privileges for the benefit of patients and society,* none of the duties I will list have any priority over others, and I do not mean to suggest any hierarchy by the order of my presentation .

Most of the professional duties that I explain are neither novel nor new, although the way that I explain them may illuminate their meaning and implications. Some dating back to Hippocrates have at least a 2,000-year tradition, so I expect that very little of what I have to say will be regarded as a dramatic change in medical practice or call for any radical change in what is required for medical professionalism. For the most part, the duties that I enumerate and explicate have been implicitly incorporated into the practice of medicine over centuries. For the most part, societies and the medical profession have reached harmonious conclusions on what the duties must be and have incorporated them into their legitimate expectations and medical practice. Some standards that have been developed were not clearly articulated, but over time professionals arrived at an understanding of expected behaviors that were consistent with the needs and goals of medical activity.

There are instances, however, where what I have to say calls for immediate changes in behavior (e.g., my discussion of white coats in this chapter) and other circumstances in which my explorations and conclusions will spur critical reanalysis of how medical practice should be implemented. Occasionally incompatible directions became popular and stood out like false notes; most of those deviations from medical ethics have been identified and corrected. Without guidance from my theoretical approach, they were noted in the way that people who know nothing about music theory recognize a segment of a musical performance being out of tune when they hear it.

Because having a map makes it easier to navigate the terrain, my aim in what follows is to provide what I take to be a clear picture of the underlying theory of medical ethics and provide some clear and readily discernible guideposts. I am not creating new duties for doctors to follow in their practice, but providing new and coherent explanations of the duties that have already been espoused, accepted, and used to direct the behavior of physicians. I also explain just why these duties oblige physicians so that doctors can appreciate their moral responsibilities. In one sense, these goals are modest because my presentation largely endorses the long-standing ideals of the profession. In another sense, my goals are immodest in that I present what I take to be a full-blown theory of medical ethics that provides useful guidance for traversing the complex and perplexing ethical dilemmas that arise in the work of medical professionals.

3

Medicine's Core Responsibilities

Several further specific duties of medical ethics follow from the first two foundational duties. Each one is justified as a necessary means to achieve or maintain trust, either as deriving from an understanding of medicine's need for trust or as a feature of medicine's fiduciary responsibility. The profession's fundamental commitments to trustworthiness and fiduciary responsibility generate the moral force of the additional ethical duties of physicians.

Professional competence, the duty to provide care, and the duty of mindfulness are core duties of a physician. These particular duties are also tied to distinct elements of a medical professional's character. They define both how a physician is obliged to behave and the virtues that are necessary in a trustworthy physician. These duties and virtues are commonly recognized as professional responsibilities, and without anything being said, patients rely on their doctors to uphold them. Competence and the duty to provide care are both specifically acknowledged as essential duties by most statements of medical ethics. Mindfulness, another core responsibility, is also something we expect from doctors even though it is seldom stated. All of this is to say that, in addition to acting for the good of patients and society, maintaining professional competence, providing care to those in need, and being mindful of what needs to be done, doctors need to identify with these commitments and pride themselves as being committed to their patients' welfare and being caring, competent, and mindful professionals.

Professional Competence

The third duty of medical ethics is professional competence.
In ordinary life, developing some expertise or skill may be a source of satisfaction and personal esteem. People pride themselves on the outstanding abilities they have nurtured (e.g., skiing, music, cooking, language mastery), but these excellences are all personal options.

The Trusted Doctor. Rosamond Rhodes, Oxford University Press (2020). © Oxford University Press.
DOI: 10.1093/oso/9780190859909.001.0001

For doctors, competence is more than a matter of competitive pride, personal curiosity, ambition, or prudence. Knowledge and skill are essential to trustworthiness and therefore they are moral obligations for physicians. To be a trustworthy doctor, a person must be fully informed of the most recent clinical studies relevant to her practice, capable of performing the tasks and maneuvers that are required, and able to assess personal strengths, weaknesses, and their implications. Without professional competence, the physician is not deserving of trust. Expressing this awareness, the Canadian Medical Association Code of Ethics identifies "engaging in lifelong learning to maintain and improve your professional knowledge, skills and attitudes" as a core responsibility of doctors.[1] The American Medical Association (AMA) lists competence as its first principle, declaring that, "A physician shall be dedicated to providing competent medical care, with compassion and respect for human dignity and rights," and also as its fifth principle, "A physician shall continue to study, apply and advance scientific knowledge, maintain a commitment to medical education, make relevant information available patients and colleagues, and the public, obtain consultation, and use the talents of other health professionals when indicated."[2] The UK General Medical Council good medical practice list of duties of a doctor expresses similar thoughts. The council declares that a doctor has the duty to "provide a good standard of practice and care, keep your professional knowledge and skills up to date, and recognize and work within the limits of your competence."[3] These and other similar professional statements suggest that competence is a well-recognized, broadly encompassing core duty of medicine. Anyone who assumes the title *doctor* and pretends to practice medicine without competence is a charlatan and a quack.

The duty of competence involves a commitment to lifelong learning that must be incorporated into the character of a physician. Such an attitude toward learning is necessary because it enables doctors to deliver care in accordance with advances in knowledge. Someone who fails to keep up with the literature on treatment advances or keep up with technological advances

---

[1] Canadian Medical Association. *CMA Code of Ethics* (updated 2004), item 8 and also items 3 and 5. https://www.cma.ca/cma-code-ethics-and-professionalism
http://www.cpsa.ca/wp-content/uploads/2019/01/CMA_Policy_Code_of_ethics_of_the_Canadian_Medical_Association_Update_2004_PD04-06-e.pdf

[2] American Medical Association. *American Medical Association Code of Medical Ethics: AMA Principles of Medical Ethics* (2001), principles 1 and 5. Accessed October 28, 2018, at https://www.ama-assn.org/sites/default/files/media-browser/principles-of-medical-ethics.pdf

[3] UK General Medical Council. *Ethical Guidance* (2014). Accessed October 28, 2018, at https://gmc-uk.org/ethical-guidance

that may require the development of new skills may fail in the duty to deliver competent care. Lacking important knowledge or skills, a physician may be unable to offer patients treatment with minimal risks, diminished symptoms, or quicker recovery. This is not to say that every physician must be equipped to provide the latest modes of treatment, but it does mean that doctors should be informed about them so that they may make their patients aware of new treatment options and their advantages and disadvantages and offer referrals to physicians who can competently provide those services. Competence is an obligation for the profession, and a variety of different professionals and structures of healthcare delivery can be employed in concert to fulfill the duty.

Competence and Medical Education

Because the need for medical care will persist, and because a society's competent physicians cannot continue to practice indefinitely, the profession and its members have to shoulder the responsibility of educating future doctors and ensuring their future competence. For the most part, educational and training activities as well as setting standards and assessing performance must be performed by doctors. They are typically the only ones with the relevant knowledge and experience to teach the material and evaluate the competence of trainees. As the Australian Medical Association Code of Ethics notes, a doctor is required to "honour your obligation to pass on your professional knowledge and skills to colleagues and students, where appropriate."[4] And as the Canadian Medical Association Code of Ethics declares, every doctor has the responsibility to "contribute to the development of the medical profession, whether through clinical practice, research, teaching, administration or advocating on behalf of the profession or public."[5]

Medical training itself is a lengthy process that is designed, implemented, and overseen by the profession. Since at least the time of Hippocrates, the profession has accepted its responsibility for training future doctors and ensuring their competence. In modern medicine, training future doctors is

---

[4] Australian Medical Association. *AMA Code of Ethics 2004* (editorially revised 2006; revised 2016), item 2.6.1. Accessed October 28, 2018, at https://ama.com.au/system/tdf/documents/AMA%20Code%20of%20Ethics%202004.%20Editorially%20Revised%202006.%20Revised%202016.pdf?file=1&type=node&id=46014

[5] Canadian Medical Association, *Code of Ethics*, item 8.

accomplished by medical schools, with residency and fellowship programs selecting trainees who have the potential for becoming trustworthy physicians and then educating them through didactics, skills training, and mentorship. In the United States today, medical training includes undergraduate medical education (UME), provided in medical school, and graduate medical education (GME), provided through residency and fellowship programs in the major specialty fields. The system involves national accreditation of training programs, requiring their structure and content to conform to rigorous standards. It also requires trainees to pass national board examinations and the periodic reevaluation of practicing clinicians to ensure their continued competence.

Medical training must also include a robust element of medical ethics education. To be competent, physicians have to recognize, understand, and appreciate their distinctive professional responsibilities, and their training must mold them into doctors who are committed to fulfilling those duties by acting with exemplary professionalism. To accomplish that goal, trainees have to be helped to develop the characteristic attitudes of physicians. They and their patients will need to rely on those feelings and attitudes to incline them toward fulfilling their professional responsibilities and honing the skills to accomplish their distinctive responsibilities.

Beyond the formal preparatory training that doctors receive, medical institutions typically grant doctors privileges to perform only specific activities for which they have demonstrated competence. Also, as new interventions are added to the armamentarium of medicine, institutions often impose credentialing requirements to guarantee that doctors are adequately trained and have demonstrated their ability to employ the new techniques. All of this attention and development of standards, oversight, and enforcement mechanisms speaks to the profession's acknowledgment of competence as necessary for the trustworthy practice of medicine.

In addition, states ensure that medical education is adequate and that medical professionals are adequately trained by licensing medical professionals. The state's role speaks to the acknowledgment of the potential danger of allowing unqualified individuals to present themselves as doctors and take on the privileges of the profession. It also demonstrates the socially recognized importance of ensuring that doctors have the competence to execute what we count on them to do.

In sum, the profession demonstrates its recognition of competence as a core responsibility by taking a comprehensive approach to ensuring competency in medical practice. Medical schools, accredited by the national Liaison Committee on Medical Education (LCME), make decisions about accepting trainees into their programs. Medical schools then provide the UME education and grant the MD degrees that certify basic competence in medicine. To be accredited, hospitals are required to meet the standards set by the Joint Commission. They then provide GME training in accordance with standards set by the Accreditation Council for Graduate Medical Education (ACGME) and ensure that trainees are competent. Hospitals also ensure the competency of individual physicians by examining and periodically reexamining (e.g., every 2 years) their credentials and performance and granting medical staff admitting privileges as well as privileges for performing a specific set of procedures. Granting privileges also ensures that practicing clinicians are adequately trained and capable of providing training for others. In addition, passing national board examinations that are prepared and administered by specialty boards is required for physician licensing and periodic relicensing (e.g., every 2 years) by states.[6]

As complex as this system appears to be, competence is actually more complicated and subtle than it may at first appear to be. Competence involves a good deal of judgment about clinical details and also about what counts as competent performance. Such discernment cannot be captured in general rules, and the agents of institutions and government are in no position to assess it. Often individual doctors have to make decisions about whether or not they themselves have the required competence and are in a position to treat a particular patient or whether they should instead refer the patient to another physician with greater expertise or resources.

When physicians discuss this sort of choice, they often speak about "feeling comfortable" to undertake the management of a patient's disease or the performance of a medical intervention or surgical procedure. But that should hardly be the measure of a physician's knowledge or skill. Feeling comfortable is a report on physicians' level of confidence, their hubris, or insecurity. Instead, an accurate measure of personal skill and knowledge is required. Because a patient's life and well-being may be on the line, being a doctor is incompatible with grandiosity and inflated self-confidence on the one hand, or insecurity and timidity on the other. Physicians cannot afford to deceive themselves about their competence and wherewithal because someone else

---

[6] I am grateful to Dr. Scott Barnett for reviewing these measures with me.

is relying on their judgment about their own ability and the adequacy of the resources at their disposal.

These factors are critical considerations in making decisions about when a doctor has had enough training and developed sufficient skill to perform a procedure unsupervised, perform a practiced procedure more quickly, try using a new device, perform a new procedure that was described in a journal article, or undertake an intervention that has never been tried before in humans. Similar questions arise about whether a doctor should continue managing a patient with an unusual diagnosis or send the patient to an expert in the field who may be associated with another institution.

The commitment to competence also entails keeping up to date with medical developments. A physician who applies a medical intervention because he or she has not kept up with the literature and learned that the former standard of care has been proven to be ineffective inflicts physical risks and burdens on a patient for no benefit.[7] A doctor who does not inform a patient that a condition that had been thought to involve risks of malignancy has been studied and reclassified as benign subjects patients to needless surveillance, worry, and stress.[8] A doctor who chooses to do an excellent job for a patient using an old technique without explaining that another qualified physician could use a new surgical approach that would involve a briefer period of recuperation and better overall function abuses the patient's trust by withholding relevant information and having failed to develop competence in the new technique. And, doctors who dive into using new products, rather than what has been tried and shown to be effective, or offering new interventions such as transgender surgery or composite tissue transplantation (e.g., face, hand) without adequate practice, preparation, and support also display a failing in competence.

The covenant that empowers medicine is an agreement between society and the profession. Based on the profession's commitments, society reasonably expects medical professionals to competently respond to patients with kindness and mercy, and individual patients rely on physicians to use their medical knowledge and skills to help them with their illness and suffering. In their response, society expects that physicians will not choose their

---

[7] Moseley JB, O'Mallery K, Petersen NJ, et al., "A Controlled Trial of Arthroscopic Surgery for Osteoarthritis of the Knee," *New England Journal of Medicine* 347, 2 (2002): 81–88.

[8] Likhterov I, Osorio M, Moubayed SP, Hernandez-Prera JC, Rhodes R, and Urken ML, "The Ethical Implications of the Reclassification of Non Invasive-Follicular Variant Papillary Thyroid Carcinoma," *Thyroid* 26, 9 (2016): 1167–1172.

treatments by referring to their own personal preferences or aversions, gut feelings, or instincts. We expect doctors to make treatment decisions based on the interests of patients rather than the doctors' own desire for novelty or a marketing advantage. Society and the profession expect individual physicians to look to "the standard of care," that is, the practice guidelines that are supported by evidence and the prevailing procedures within the medical community. Society expects that deviations from the standard of care will only be justified by special considerations, for instance about the patient's values or anatomy that colleagues from the profession would endorse as relevant reasons for a departure from the standard of care given the particular circumstances.

The Duty to Provide Care

The fourth duty of medical ethics is to provide care.
In his article, "Physician's Duty to Treat: Altruism, Self-Interest, and Medical Ethics," Dr. Edmund Pellegrino expressed a view that is very similar to my position.[9] He argued that medicine is not an occupation like any other, and that it is inherently different from work in commerce. Pellegrino offered three arguments for the uniqueness of medicine: (1) He maintained that the vulnerability of the patient requires a protective concern with their well-being. He recognized that medicine is about altruism, the unselfish devotion to patients' welfare; therefore, physicians have a professional responsibility to serve as their patients' trusted guardian. (2) As I explained in the previous chapter, society allows physicians access to special knowledge, powers, privileges, and immunities that it permits to no one else so that they can be used for the good of its members. Pellegrino appreciated that these abilities are not a physicians' private property but social resources granted to them as medical professionals on the condition of their being used to provide benefits to patients and for the social good. (3) Everyone knows these conditions and trusts the medical profession to uphold its part of the bargain.

These three points add up to the central commitment to provide the medical care that people need. It has been well accepted that when a group is granted a monopoly over an activity, the group has the obligation to provide

---

[9] Pellegrino ED, "Physician's Duty to Treat: Altruism, Self-Interest, and Medical Ethics," *JAMA* 258, 14 (1987): 1939–1940.

the service for everyone who wants access to it. That is why the utilities in a region even have to supply their services for those in remote areas. Because society has granted medicine a legal monopoly over the use of its knowledge, powers, privileges, and immunities, the profession and its members are required to provide treatment for everyone who needs it and who wants to avail themselves of the services. Everyone includes the people who are appreciative of the care that they receive, those who are trusting and friendly, and those who are cooperative and adhere to recommended treatment protocols. It also includes those who are not appreciative and those who are neither trusting nor compliant. It includes pleasant and interesting people as well as those who are unpleasant or even frightening, the washed and the unwashed, the generous and the stingy, the insured and rich and those who cannot afford to pay. The spirit of this duty is declared in the Hippocratic oath and more explicitly in the opening statements of the oath of Maimonides, which poetically declares doctors' commitment to all humanity.

> The eternal providence has appointed me to watch over the life and health of Thy creatures.
>
> May the love for my art actuate me all time; may neither avarice nor miserliness, nor thirst for glory or for a great reputation engage my mind; for the enemies of truth and philanthropy could easily deceive me and make me forgetful of my lofty aim of doing good to Thy children.
>
> May I never see in the patient anything but a fellow creature in pain.

To appreciate the implications of this duty, consider some cases from the clinical practice of colleagues at the hospital where I work.

Case 1

Ms. K. is a 32-year-old drug user who eroded the cartilage that separates her nasal cavity from her orbit by snorting cocaine. She has been hospitalized on several occasions for left eye infections caused by her cocaine use, twice in the previous 12 months. Each of these hospitalizations was characterized by her rude, threatening outbursts and struggles with the medical and nursing staff. She now has another serious eye infection. She requires a week of intravenously administered antibiotic treatment to save her sight in that eye.

On this admission, and on each previous admission, Ms. K. has been offered enrollment in a drug treatment program. She consistently refuses it. Ms. K. says that she intends to continue her cocaine use because it makes the pain of life go away. She always comes to the emergency room for treatment when she develops an eye infection. She states that she wants the doctors to cure the infection and save her eyesight, and she accepts all of the recommended inpatient and outpatient antibiotic treatments.

As long as intravenous antibiotic treatment is likely to provide a benefit, and as long as she is willing to accept the treatment, Ms. K. should be provided with it. The fact that her drug use actually caused her repeated infections, that she shows little concern for maintaining her health, or that the drug use was illegal are not relevant considerations in making treatment decisions. The only consideration that is relevant is that without the treatment Ms. K. is likely to lose the sight in her eye. Ms. K. has a medical need, and her physicians have a professional responsibility to address that need by providing excellent medical care, the medical care that would be provided to a pleasant patient with a similar medical need who developed an infection just by bad luck.

Case 2

Mr. H., a 46-year-old Chinese accountant with O blood type, was placed on the liver transplant waiting list. He had hepatitis C with refractory ascites requiring biweekly paracentesis, type 2 hepatorenal syndrome, and hepatic encephalopathy. He had no potential family member or friend who could serve as a living liver donor. He was on the waiting list for a year and his disease progressed, but he received no donor calls despite several recent hospitalizations. Friends suggested that he travel to China, where he could obtain a liver transplant for a fee. He then investigated the option through relatives in China and made the necessary arrangements to stay with them. He received a liver transplant 2 weeks after arriving in China.

Three months after his liver transplant, Mr. H. returned to his previous transplant program, but he was denied care. He then came to our program requesting follow-up care. He explained that he had received a liver transplant in China but, when questioned, stated that he knew nothing about the source of the transplanted organ. He arrived with minimal medical records, and he was about to run out of the immunosuppressive medication that he had received from the transplant center in China.

Before traveling to China for a transplant, Mr. H.'s medical condition was deteriorating. Given the realities of the US liver allocation system, his O blood type, and his New York location, it was likely that he would die from his disease without receiving a transplant organ. It is most likely that Mr. H. received his transplant organ in China from an executed prisoner, but he pursued the only course available to save his life.

Nevertheless, many people, including many medical professionals, find the use of executed prisoners as a source for transplant organs repugnant. Some medical professionals regard providing medical support to a patient who benefited from the execution of a prisoner as collaborating in the practice and therefore refuse medical care to patients who received a transplant from an ethically questionable source. Taking such a stand, however, is not an acceptable option because physicians are obliged to provide needed medical care even though they object to what a patient did to obtain a life-saving liver transplant.

After liver transplantation, patients require ongoing lifelong medical care to manage antirejection medications and to be monitored for other posttransplant medical problems. Although several transplant programs refuse to provide care to patients who have received organ transplants abroad under questionable circumstances, medicine's commitment to provide needed care requires transplant programs to treat these patients as they would treat other patients with similar posttransplantation needs.[10-12]

Case 3

In early May 2009, shortly after New York City officials reported an investigation into a cluster of influenza-like illnesses in a local high school, two classes of children from a nearby elementary school were sent from their school to the hospital for infectious disease (ID) consultations. Many children in this group of 50 were coughing and appeared feverish. The children needed to be evaluated for possible H1N1 swine flu virus, and the school also requested advice on whether or not to close down these classes or the entire school.

[10] Rhodes R and Schiano T, "Transplant Tourism in China: A Tale of Two Transplants" [Target Article], *American Journal of Bioethics* 10, 2 (2010): 3–11.

[11] Schiano T and Rhodes R, "The Dilemma and Reality of Transplant Tourism: An Ethical Perspective for Liver Transplant Programs," *Liver Transplantation* 16, 2 (2010): 113–117.

[12] Rhodes R and Schiano T, "Moral Complexity and the Delusion of Moral Purity," *American Journal of Bioethics* 10, 2 (2010): W1–W3.

Based on reports of widespread influenza-like illness and many severe illnesses and deaths that were different from any other influenza viruses previously seen in either humans or animals, the World Health Organization and the US Centers for Disease Control and Prevention had already issued pandemic warnings about the H1N1 virus.

The children were isolated from contact with other patients and personnel. Six ID attending physicians were sent by their department chair to see the children. One ID attending, suspecting that his spouse was pregnant, refused to see the patients.

Although it is perfectly reasonable to want to avoid contracting swine flu, this case raises the question of whether the preference to avoid personal risk is a good enough reason to justify not providing patients with needed medical services. There are certainly limits to professional responsibility, and risk exposure is a relevant consideration. But, as with other matters of professional ethics, the limit on what counts as an acceptable risk is a matter that must be settled by a determination from the profession rather than each individual physician making a personal judgment. Courageous doctors do not have greater professional responsibilities than timid ones. Every similarly exposed medical professional should have the same duty in a comparable situation.

Some relevant considerations for deciding whether the doctor in this case is justified in exempting himself from his duty include the alternative measures that could prevent his wife from exposure to the disease (e.g., keeping his distance for a period of time), his likelihood of contracting the disease, and the likelihood of serious and enduring consequences from being infected. According to those tracking H1N1, people exposed to H1N1 have about an 8% chance of developing the disease, although young children might have a somewhat greater susceptibility. In the general population, people who contract the disease had approximately a 1% chance of dying from it. Pregnant women who contract H1N1, however, had approximately a 6% chance of dying.

The availability of means to protect people from contracting the disease is also relevant. Personal protective equipment (PPE), including gowns, gloves, shoe coverings, and surgical masks, were available, and the staff involved in the evaluation of the children were practiced in using the equipment. The doctors who were exposed to the children could isolate themselves from others to avoid spreading the disease themselves. Isolation for exposed individuals who do not develop the disease would persist for about 1 day and about 1 week after symptoms develop for those who contract the disease. Also, the use of influenza antiviral medicines for treatment and prevention (chemoprophylaxis) was available for people who were at high risk of flu complications, such as pregnant women.

Taken together, and in light of the department chair and all of the other infectious disease doctors recognizing that the risks involved were consistent with their professional responsibility, participating in the evaluation of the children was required. The doctor who wanted to opt out was shirking his duty.

Another consideration that is often relevant is whether the service of an individual doctor is actually needed. In this case, there were at least five other doctors who were available and competent to perform the evaluations. But every doctor who refuses to perform evaluations leaves the others with more children to evaluate, which translates to greater risk exposure. Although the institution's duty to provide medical services would be satisfied when one doctor refused to participate, each doctor who responded to the call would be at increased risk because of the larger number of evaluations that would be required. Exempting oneself from the professional responsibility would therefore involve imposing an undue burden on a peer.

Just as with those in the military, police, firefighting, law, and teaching professions, some level of exposure to risk is part of the job. By choosing to join the profession, a person accepts a number of risks of different sorts. In full knowledge of information about contagion and infectious disease, doctors accept the risks associated with providing care to patients with communicable conditions.

That is only one sort of hazard that physicians encounter. The behavior of patients with chronic or acute mental illness can introduce other sorts of risks. The medical environment (e.g., sharp instruments, radiation) and the social environment in which medicine is practiced (e.g., war zones, flood zones, disaster sites) can expose doctors to an array of physical risks. Working with people who may become violent when stressed by the circumstances of their lives or the outcomes experienced by their loved ones can put doctors in harm's way. The emotional impact of what doctors witness (e.g., the death of a child) or cause (e.g., a bad drug reaction) by either error or deliberately from a well-justified treatment choice can cause significant psychological trauma. And, providing controversial medical services (e.g., abortion, euthanasia) or treating patients who are despised by society (e.g., a murderer) can expose doctors to risks of social ostracism or even assassination.

In much the same way as physicians refer to the standard of care as the touchstone for their clinical decisions, judgments about the acceptability of risk and other matters of medical ethics are not personal choices but must be based on an understanding of the risks involved, the available remedies, and professional responsibility. The standard for determining when a risk is too great in terms of likelihood or seriousness of harm, and therefore when providing medical care is not a professional obligation, and when a risk is too slight to absolve a physician from the professional duty to provide care, are matters that require the perspective of the profession. In effect, judgments should ideally be rendered by an authorized group of esteemed and experienced medical professionals. In addition, the judgments should be formulated in terms of what any competent, committed medical professional should do under the circumstance, that is, as an ethical standard of care (comparable to medicine's clinical standard of care) or as a medical categorical imperative.[13] In other words, even nonclinical medical decisions should be made by reference to the standard of medical professionalism and duties of medical ethics. The limits of duty are hard to define, particularly when self-interest is likely to affect judgment. Thus, we expect physicians to consult the "ethical standard of care" rather than their personal feelings when making medical decisions.

As Dr. Edmund Pellegrino argued, individual physicians are not entitled to base their decisions on individual, personal judgments about the dangerousness of treating patients who are HIV positive.[14] Instead, each individual physician should be willing to provide treatment for people who are living with HIV because, according to the judgment of the profession, the risk of infection is not significant enough to defeat the professional duty to provide treatment. In the 1980s, many doctors were afraid of contracting HIV. Once enough evidence emerged that universal precautions were effective protections that prevented people from contracting the disease, hospital medical boards, medical societies, and state health authorities required that care be provided for HIV-positive patients who needed the care. The

---

[13] This is a pointed reference to the Kantian criterion for evaluating moral judgments by considering whether a description of the proposed action could be considered a moral law for anyone who was similarly situated. Kant I, *Foundations of the Metaphysics of Morals*, translated by LW Beck (Indianapolis, IN: Library of Liberal Arts, Bobbs-Merrill, 1959).

[14] Pellegrino, "Physician's Duty."

requirement to provide treatment and care extended to all treatments, for elective procedures (e.g., hip replacement surgery) as well as urgent and life-saving treatments. Someone who places personal interests above his patients' interest departs from medicine's standard of altruism and violates a crucial tenet of medical ethics that every physician is duty bound to observe.

Seeing medical ethics from the perspective of a commitment made to society to guide medical practice by profession-wide standards of care has two important consequences. First, it implies that clinician decisions must be informed by professional judgment, not personal judgment. Patients and society rely on physicians to provide treatment according to that standard, and for the most part, they cannot know enough about their doctors' personal values to consider those beliefs in their choice of a physician. The second implication is that becoming a doctor is a moral commitment to give priority to the ethical standard of care over personal interests or values. Becoming a doctor, therefore, is also ceding authority to professional judgment over personal preference. That fact should be recognized and acknowledged so people who are not prepared to accept that condition do not join the profession in bad faith.

Medicine's historical commitments make it clear that physicians accept responsibility to patients and society, and that part of being a doctor is acceptance of the concomitant profession-related risk. For example, the Medical Council of India's Code of Medical Ethics explicitly states, "When an epidemic occurs a physician should not abandon his duty for fear of contracting the disease himself."[15] Although self-preservation limits responsibilities, the ethically crucial issues are whether the danger is great enough to overwhelm the default professional responsibility of responsiveness and who makes the call. Again, the profession does not regard these as matters of personal judgment. Through the ages, one distinguishing feature of medicine has been its reliance on scientific evidence (broadly construed). A gut feeling that something should or should not be done is not enough to justify a medical decision. In medicine, hypotheses have to be supported by theory, judgments have to be supported by observation or data, and positions on whether a risk to physicians is unreasonable should also be determined with scientifically defensible evidence and the endorsement by a consensus of leaders of the

---

[15] Indian Medical Council, *Professional Conduct, Etiquette and Ethics Regulations* (2002), item 5.2. Accessed October 28, 2018, at https://www.mciindia.org/documents/rulesAndRegulations/Ethics%20Regulations-2002.pdf. New Zealand Medical Association, *Code of Ethics for the New Zealand Medical Profession* (May 2014). https://www.nzma.org.nz/publications/code-of-ethics

profession.[16] People who think otherwise miss the significant point that, in the face of risk to physicians, responsiveness should be the default presumption because that is what professionalism requires.

A judgment that responding is too dangerous and should be optional in a particular circumstance has to be left to the consensus of medical experts with the relevant specialized knowledge and experience. In our current age of speedy electronic communication, there is no justification for allowing decisions on recusal or response to turn on the personal fear, lack of courage, or an individual physician's impaired sense of duty. And, if there are particular things that every responsible physician should know in order to effectively respond during disasters, then continuing in ignorance is culpable. Instead of excusing physicians from an important component of their professional responsibility, the profession should take steps to ensure that every physician is prepared. After 9/11 and Hurricane Katrina, no physician and no organization of medical professionals can legitimately turn a blind eye to this crucial aspect of medical responsibility.

By crafting codes and principles of ethics, the profession defines the ethical standard for medical practice. As has been noted, for example, the AMA's Code of Ethics "is intended to put forth a uniform standard of conduct for individuals who belong to a profession."[17] In the critically important matter of response to the victims of a disaster, it is crucial that leaders of the profession accept their responsibility for defining the standard for professional behavior.

Principle VI of the AMA Code of Medical Ethics, which was only added to the code about 50 years ago, stands out in the medical literature by taking a stand in the opposite direction. It states, "A physician shall, in the provision of appropriate care, except in emergencies, be free to choose whom to serve . . . and the environment in which to provide medical care."[18,19] Whereas the rest of the AMA code delineates physician responsibilities, Principle VI anachronistically declares that physicians are free to choose whom to serve and their work condition. This statement means that, except for emergencies, physicians have no responsibility to serve anyone

---

[16] Morin K., Higginson D., and Goldrich M., "Physician Obligation in Disaster Preparedness and Response," position statement from the AMA's Council on Ethical and Judicial Affairs (CEJA Opinion 3-I-04, E-9.067) (2005). This statement presents a laudable account of professional responsibility in the face of a disaster. The CEJA authors explicitly acknowledged "that unique responsibilities beyond planning rest on the shoulders of the medical profession," p. 1.

[17] Morin et al., "Physician Obligation," p. 4.

[18] American Medical Association, *Code of Medical Ethics*.

[19] Similar problematic statements appear in the Canadian Medical Association, *Code of Ethics*, item 17, and the Australian Medical Association, *Code of Ethics*, items 2.1.11–2.1.13.

and no responsibility to provide medical care in a place that they prefer to avoid. Apparently, if I am reading the report correctly, the implications of Principle VI for disasters is that it is up to individual doctors to decide when a situation counts as an "emergency." They have no duty to go to the scene of a disaster, they are free to leave the area, and they do not have to provide care to those who are unable to pay their fees, particularly when the disaster has left people without access to bank accounts, ATMs, or insurance cards. Physicians are free to avoid education about how to respond to a disaster. They are free to avoid means of protecting themselves from hazards. They are free to opt out whenever they feel frightened, repulsed, or disinclined to provide medical care.

Although it is easy to understand why AMA members have repeatedly decided to keep Principle VI in their code as they continue to make revisions and why they feel comforted by the license it allows them, it is legitimate to ask whether that provision is consistent with the ethical responsibilities of being a physician. It is hard to see how Principle VI can be reconciled with the commitments espoused elsewhere in the AMA code (or in the Hippocratic oath, the oath of Maimonides, or the Geneva code) without either eviscerating the concept of physician professional responsibilities or contorting and deflating the meaning of Principle VI. In light of its untoward implications and the fact that Principle VI counters the positions espoused in the ethics statements by the vast majority of other organizations of medical professionals, the AMA statement deserves debunking criticism.

Mindfulness

The fifth duty of medical ethics is mindfulness.
While it is good for people to be mindful of what they say and what they do, most people are free to avert their eyes at least sometimes, put their head in the sand, and ignore things that they ought to do and situations that might be unpleasant. There may be prices to pay for being inattentive, but those burdens are typically personal matters.

Being mindful, however, is a core duty for doctors. In their professional roles, doctors cannot afford the luxury of turning a blind eye. Medical practice requires a remarkable level of awareness and foresight. In a sense, mindfulness can be seen as an element of medical competence or an implication of medicine's fiduciary responsibilities, but specifically identifying mindfulness as a core duty of medicine emphasizes its importance in both decision-making and interactions.

In clinical situations, it is often critical for a doctor to be alert to subtle signals that are easy to overlook. In fact, a mindful doctor may have to search for information that others will prefer to pointedly ignore. For example, geriatrician Dr. Howard Fillit teaches his fellows to have patients remove their shoes and socks in order for the fellows to examine their feet. Doing so is particularly important in geriatrics because a patient's neglect of foot care is often an early sign of dementia or physical impairment. Recognizing such problems at an early stage could be important in providing a patient with appropriate care. Being generally alert to possible disease symptoms or complications of treatment enables doctors to identify them and respond to them in a timely way.

Another element of mindfulness is being observant of problems that trainees or colleagues may be having. If competence is a duty of the profession, each physician has a role to play in the identification of possible difficulties and taking the appropriate steps to address them. Often enough a question can help a colleague rethink a treatment plan. Sometimes a helping hand or discrete word of advice can help to avoid a serious problem. Explanations or demonstrations can be useful measures, and sometimes reporting patterns of problem behavior up the chain of command can be necessary.[20] But without being alert to developing potentially problematic situations, such interventions would not be possible.

Mindfulness is particularly important in the way doctors interact with others and their responses to the situations they encounter. Although being spontaneous and carefree may be desirable qualities in social relationships, doctors have to studiously consider and choose their responses. When most people see blood gushing or physical injuries, they pull back in horror and fear of causing further harm. Doctors have to learn to react in exactly the opposite way: They are required to apply pressure to stop the bleeding and explore the injuries in order to repair them. Nonphysicians may freely display their reactions to the physical characteristics, behavior, and character traits of others; doctors must not.

---

[20] This issue is discussed in some detail in Chapter 8, Physicians' Commitments to Fellow Professionals.

Doctors have to contain their revulsion to the sights, smells, and tactile experiences that others can freely express, and they have to act as if they are not fearful when they are. A doctor also has to be able to convey bad news and compassionately share the grief of one family, then step into the corridor to compose herself before walking into the next room to share the joy of a patient with a good outcome who is cured and leaving the hospital. Being present in the moment and adopting the appropriate demeanor is part of the job. In one sense, these required reactions may seem disingenuous; in another sense, they resemble standard human interactions. Yet, it is the degree to which composure is required and the extent to which unnatural responses have to be cultivated and incorporated into the medical response that makes mindful responses a duty of medical ethics.

Case 4

I entered the elevator on the sixth floor. It was already occupied by a disheveled patient in a wheelchair and a physician in a white coat who was pushing him. The stench emanating from the patient was nauseating and overwhelming. All the while, riding down to the ground floor, the doctor smiled and chatted with the patient in a way that apparently made the patient feel comfortable and relaxed.

When we all emerged from the elevator, they went off in one direction. I stopped holding my breath and exhaled before going off in another direction. There was no way that the doctor had been immune to the reeking odor of the patient in the elevator, but she had overcome her aversion and was able to fulfill her duty to her patient without compromising their relationship in any way.

Someone who boards a subway can easily avoid sitting beside a person who stinks. It is totally acceptable to change your seat or move to another car when you find a fellow passenger obnoxious in any way. But a doctor has to be mindful of the effect that her response is likely to have on a patient and contain her reaction to serve the needs of the patient.

More generally, mindful responses are particularly important in a doctor's communication because doctor-patient interactions tend to occur in a compressed time frame of brief office or hospital visits and because patients anticipate receiving a report during their doctor visit. The combination of the time-pressured conversation and the anticipation of the doctor's report makes every gesture and word that the doctor utters important. Statements are recalled and repeated to friends and family members, and those spoken words often become the patient's grounds for making critical medical choices.

A doctor's fleeting facial expression, a carelessly chosen word, an optimistic overstatement, or a pessimistic understatement can leave a patient with a mistaken impression. Phrasing that is vague invites misunderstanding, whereas language that is blunt can be off-putting or frightening. Some words that are hard to say out loud and face to face (e.g., die) can be especially difficult to voice, so physicians sometimes avoid using them, and their omission leaves patients and family members with false hopes.

Potential problems that can impede mindful communication are often recognized, and medical educators and program leaders actually take measures to address foreseeable difficulties and prevent inappropriate responses. Medical education frequently includes learning what to say and how to say it, and involves practice with standardized patients, actors who play these roles. Senior doctors often include junior doctors in sensitive conversations so that trainees can learn how it should be done. Medical institutions even develop model scripts for directing conversation about unusual issues that are hard to explain accurately and with the right tone, like the discontinuance of ineffective medical interventions.

Also, doctors need to consider how much information should be provided and when. Too much scientific detail in an initial presentation about a new and serious diagnosis (e.g., a rare genetic condition in a newborn) can be overwhelming and actually uninformative. Frequently, a more useful approach involves limiting the initial explanation to the clinical implications and next steps while inviting questions and showing willingness to respond as the questions arise. Going forward, a plan could involve adding layers of the background science to the discussion over a course of several appointments. Overall, mindful doctors will attend to their patients' reactions and try to gauge the level of specifics that their response should include.

4

The Commitment to Science

The sixth duty of medical ethics is the commitment to science.

Medicine's association with empirical methods and science is at the core of the profession's expertise. Doctors are duty bound to base their diagnoses and treatment decisions on their observations and data, and patients seek their advice and care because doctors make decisions based on biomedical science. Although the phrase *evidence-based medicine* is relatively new to the medical literature, patients have long believed that doctors use evidence to guide their practice, and they trust doctor's recommendations on account of that understanding.

This commitment means that when evidence is available, physicians are not free to recommend treatments based merely on a hunch or vague feeling but are obliged to use scientific evidence to guide their practice. They are also required to justify deviations from the standard of care in terms of scientific or patient-specific reasons that their physician peers would find compelling.

Even though patients envision doctors to be making evidence-based medical decisions about their care, there is a great deal that we do not know about the human body, the human genome, the human microbiome, the diseases that afflict us, how those conditions can be cured or ameliorated, and how the human organism and its environment interact. Because medicine needs evidence to guide clinical practice, medicine is ethically committed to pursue knowledge across the vast realm of the great biomedical unknown.

Because doctors have the knowledge and skills that are needed to generate hypotheses based on scientific understanding and clinical experience, to design and conduct studies, and to recruit and monitor study participants, every doctor should be committed to advancing biomedical knowledge. Although this responsibility is not explicitly mentioned in many codes that I have examined, this perspective on research is espoused by medical professionals and medical organizations and enshrined in the mission statement of institutions. It is also articulated in the Australian Medical Association Code of Ethics' direction to "endeavour to participate in properly designed, ethically approved research involving human participants in

The Trusted Doctor. Rosamond Rhodes, Oxford University Press (2020). © Oxford University Press.
DOI: 10.1093/oso/9780190859909.001.0001

order to advance medical progress."[1] Supporting medicine's research agenda can be accomplished in numerous ways depending on a doctor's interests, resources, expertise, and opportunities. Thus, the obligation to advance biomedical knowledge can be fulfilled by initiating studies, collaborating in research, recruiting participants, or encouraging patients to enroll in appropriate studies. The associated virtue related to this duty is the personal commitment to rely on science to guide medical decisions and promote medicine's scientific agenda.

At the same time, two views that oppose the commitment to science are frequently declared in the literature and professional statements. One is the position that physicians should always prioritize the good of their individual patient over research. The other is the belief that the ethics of medicine is radically different from the ethics of research. These positions, which are incompatible with medicine's commitment to advancing biomedical science, need to be recognized, and the conflict needs to be sorted out. In light of the recent movements toward a learning healthcare system, pragmatic trials, and comparative effectiveness research, perhaps an ensconced perspective that regards research and treatment as radically different endeavors should be revised to a view that appreciates research as an activity of the medical profession that is governed by medical ethics and standards of medical professionalism.

Research and the Patient's Best Interest

The popular view that medicine's primary responsibility is to benefit the individual patient derives primarily from the World Medical Association's (WMA's) *Declaration of Geneva*, which was adopted by its General Assembly in September 1948 and revised several times, most recently in October 2017.[2] It would bind physicians with the words, "The health of my patient will be my first consideration." Similarly, the view is expressed in the WMA's *International Code of Medical Ethics*, which was adopted in October 1949 and most recently revised in October

---

[1] Australian Medical Association. *AMA Code of Ethics 2004. Editorially Revised 2006. Revised 2016* (2016), item 2.5.1. Accessed October 28, 2018, at https://ama.com.au/system/tdf/documents/AMA%20Code%20of%20Ethics%202004.%20Editorially%20Revised%202006.%20Revised%202016.pdf?file=1&type=node&id=46014

[2] World Medical Association. *WMA Declaration of Geneva* (revised October 2017). Accessed May 15, 2018, at https://www.wma.net/policies-post/wma-declaration-of-geneva/

2006.[3] It declares that "a physician shall act in the patient's best interest when providing medical care." These views have also been incorporated into the *WMADeclaration of Helsinki—Ethical Principles for Medical Research Involving Human Subjects* section on "Recommendations Guiding Medical Doctors in Biomedical Research Involving Human Subjects, which makes that priority explicit.[4] The original version of this WMA document was produced in 1964 by doctors for doctors. Its Principle III, 4, declares that "in research on man, the interest of science and society should never take precedence over considerations related to the well-being of the subject." The slightly revised 2006 version endorses the same priority in its Principle 8.

> 8. While the primary purpose of medical research is to generate new knowledge, this goal can never take precedence over the rights and interests of individual research subjects. The health of my patient will be my first consideration.

In making these claims for the primacy of the patient, the WMA promulgated a misleading mythological paradigm into the practice of medicine. In effect, the WMA's lofty language advanced the view that doctors should always aim to do what is in the best interest of the individual patient. That position, however, is at odds with exemplary clinical practice, which often considers the benefits of other patients and society, and sometimes legitimately prioritizes such concerns ahead of the interest of an individual patient. For that reason, the claim does not square with good clinical practice, which acknowledges that doctors almost always have duties to multiple individual patients, to groups of patients, and to the population at large.

Consider the patient who has to wait for her appointment because the patient with the earlier appointment has complicated medical needs that require more than the scheduled amount of the doctor's time. While she waits for her office visit, that second patient is not her doctor's "first consideration." And neither is the first patient whose visit time is extended, but curtailed before she would like it to be by the doctor, who rushes on to the next patient. Imagine a patient whose surgery is delayed because another with a more

[3] World Medical Association. *WMA International Code of Medical Ethics* (adopted October 2006). Accessed May 15, 2018, at https://www.wma.net/policies-post/wma-international-code-of-medical-ethics/
[4] World Medical Association. *Declaration of Helsinki: Recommendations Guiding Medical Doctors in Biomedical Research Involving Human Subjects*. Accessed May 15, 2018, at https://www.wma.net/policy/current-policies/?text=Helsinki&type=&year_from=1981&year_to=2018zzz

urgent need is allotted the operating room. The surgeon who accepts the postponement is not acting in the best interest of the patient who was booked for surgery. Reflect on the doctor who refuses to allocate a scarce transplant organ to a patient who has a low chance for long-term survival, even though she is likely to survive longer if she receives the transplant. Envision the physician who quarantines a patient to prevent him from spreading contagious disease. Consider the doctor who chooses which antibiotic to prescribe by considering her patient's needs, costs, and the needs of future patients in light of mounting concern over the evolution of antibiotic-resistant bacteria.

I can go on at length to make the point that these are common features of good medical practice. All of these may be ethically appropriate medical decisions, but they do not put the affected patients' interests first, and they may actually impose unwanted burdens or harms on some patients. Such situations are unavoidable and inescapable for any doctor who has more than a single patient and who is therefore vulnerable to the patients' competing claims to serve their conflicting interests. This shows that the direction to "act in the patient's best interest" is a distorting exaggeration and inconsistent with medical ethics.

By starting with their idealized and unrealistic fantasy view of a physician's clinical duty, that "a physician shall act in the patient's best interest," the WMA compounds its error by extending this inaccurate and misleading model of ethical clinical practice to biomedical research. Ethical medical practice does not always require serving the patient's best interest. The ethical conduct of research, however, always requires investigators to justify the involvement of human participants by balancing the research risks and burdens against the potential benefit. This evaluation is very much like the assessment of burdens and benefits that is always incorporated into clinical treatment decisions. And like good clinical care that does not always serve the patient's best interest, ethically acceptable research will not always serve the patient's best interest.

The Doctor's Role in Research

Being a good doctor is something like being a good parent in that both are complex roles that entail good performance in numerous tasks. A good parent simultaneously has the responsibility for protecting the family, feeding, clothing, and sheltering each of her children, keeping them healthy and safe, promoting their virtue, educating them, disciplining them, nurturing their talents and their civic spirit, providing them with experiences and opportunities, and so on. When a parent has more than one child, duties owed to one can conflict with duties owed to others, and in many circumstances, the different kinds of duties can conflict with each other. In other words, being a good parent is a complex role that involves weighing and balancing a variety of strong obligations. No single obligation has absolute priority, and although some duties are sometimes sacrificed for the sake of fulfilling others, none can be ignored.

The role of a physician is similarly complex. It entails obligations toward numerous patients and a variety of duties to society. It involves treating and educating patients, as well as sustaining medical institutions, training future physicians, contributing to the oversight and advancement of the profession, advocating for health-promoting policies, advancing biomedical science, and so on. Because none of these responsibilities may be neglected, and because attending to some of them can necessitate setting others aside for at least the time being, doctors often have to make decisions to triage one sort of obligation in order to satisfy others. There is no hierarchy that simply resolves the inevitable conflicts always in favor of one role, only factors like harms, benefits, urgency, availability of resources, feasibility, and opportunities that make some choices better than others at a particular time.

Doctors are in the best position to identify gaps in medical knowledge and appreciate the suffering of patients for whom current treatments are inadequate. Given their numerous unanswered questions about the functioning of human bodies, their awareness of both the efficacy and the insufficiency of current treatments, they are prepared to play central roles in advancing biomedical research. The necessity of promoting research is more apparent to them than any other group, and doctors are best situated to appreciate the usefulness of innovations. It is therefore clear that their unique perspective justifies a robust research agenda for medicine and a commitment by physicians to play a role in advancing it.

For some medical conditions, there are currently no effective treatment options. Other diseases are not adequately addressed with current treatments. Sometimes the available treatments are unaffordable, or the treatment itself or its side effects are too burdensome for patients to bear. Sometimes doctors have inadequate understanding of how the body works, how it responds to medical interventions, and the kinds of problems that can ensue from inadequately understood medical interventions. For example, today's medicine has an imperfect understanding of pain and how it should be treated. Too often, this lacuna leads doctors to disregard the abuse potential of opioids and start patients on them. Then, when their prescriptions expire, patients with chronic pain are left to manage their symptoms on their own. The limited alternatives for pain management coupled with inadequate alternative treatment options may have contributed to today's US opioid epidemic, which has produced a startling increase in overdose deaths.[5,6]

Without human subject research, improvements in medical treatment cannot be achieved. This leaves current and future patients vulnerable to death, disease, injury, pain, suffering, and disability. But with research and scientific advances, some of these life burdens may be diminished, and others may be avoidable. For this reason, doctors who are committed to advancing their patients' interests should regard themselves as being committed to the necessary means for achieving that goal, namely, supporting research by doing what they can by collaborating on studies themselves or encouraging patients to contribute to the advancement of biomedical science.

Asking Patients to Participate in Research

Many distinctive features of individuals have neither scientific nor moral significance. Biologically, anatomy and physiological processes in one human are typically very much like those in others. This means that knowledge gained from studying one individual is likely to be applicable to another, and vice versa. Ethically there are no physical differences that are so noteworthy as to mark some of us as fit material for research while exempting others from the moral responsibility of contributing to the communal goal of promoting biomedical science.

Advancing medical science and improving current treatment options can only be achieved by studying human bodies. Whereas other social obligations can be fulfilled in other ways (e.g., by writing a check, by sending a stand-in), at a certain point in biomedical research there is nothing that we can substitute for people, and that includes patients. Study involves some sacrifice of

---

[5] Beauchamp GA, Winstanley EL, Ryan SA, and Lyons MS. "Moving Beyond Misuse and Diversion: The Urgent Need to Consider the Role of Iatrogenic Addiction in the Current Opioid Epidemic," *American Journal of Public Health* 104, 11 (2014): 2023–2029.

[6] Franklin G, Sabel J, Jones CM, et al. "A Comprehensive Approach to Address the Prescription Opioid Epidemic in Washington State: Milestones and Lessons Learned," *American Journal of Public Health* 105, 3 (2015): 463–469.

their flesh, their privacy, their safety, their comfort, and their time. Because these basic goods are precious to everyone, basic moral principles of equality, universalization, and mutual love require people to give of themselves as they would wish to receive from others. The fragility of their bodies, the invasiveness of research, their emotional and genetic interrelatedness, the lack of an adequate alternative, and the commonality of the desire to benefit from the advancement of medical knowledge require us to regard research participation from the perspective of benefitting the human community. Solidarity with our fellow humans tells us that everyone should be willing to do a fair share and be willing to participate in biomedical research.[7]

Almost everyone, including almost all of a doctor's patients, will have a serious medical need at some point in their lives. At the point in time when they have a serious medical problem, they will want optimal treatment to be available, preferably something better than today's treatments, options that are more effective, less burdensome, and more affordable. That goal can only be achieved through biomedical research. Because investigators sometimes need to study people who are ill, people from different genetic groups, and entire populations, the participation of all kinds of people is needed for studying all that needs to be explored. Some studies cannot be conducted without widespread participation, while others would proceed slowly without general participation.

Every patient should be willing to do a fair share in developing effective therapies for conditions that affect them and for medical needs that might befall them or their loved ones in the future. Everyone should also be willing to do a fair share in protecting us all from the promulgation of ineffective treatments or the promotion of inferior treatments. Even though voluntariness is an important criterion for research that involves interfering with people's bodies, we should recognize that those who would refuse to do a fair share of participation in valuable, minimally burdensome, and reasonably safe studies are behaving as free-riders. They are taking advantage of the contributions of others and accepting the benefits of other people's sacrifices without doing their part. This consideration suggests that justice requires all patients to be willing to contribute to the research effort, and that those who refuse to do their part are treating others unjustly. Because we should expect

---

[7] Rhodes R, "Rethinking Research Ethics" [Target article], *American Journal of Bioethics* 5, 1 (2010): 7–28. Reprinted as the "Most Controversial Article" in *American Journal of Bioethics*' 10-year history: *American Journal of Bioethics* 10, 10 (2010): 19–36.

others to behave ethically, and because we are free to ask others to abstain from unethical behavior, asking patients to participate in studies is reasonable, acceptable, and good. Doctors should therefore feel comfortable in inviting patients to participate in studies and regard it as a duty to encourage patients to volunteer when they fit a study's enrollment criteria.[8]

How to Conduct Clinical Research With Human Participants

While unanswered questions persist and call for deeper insight, research on stem cells, gene transfer, immunotherapy, and the human microbiome present new opportunities for advancing biomedical science. The need for improved understanding presses doctors to undertake studies that will enable them to answer open questions and delve into new domains for broadening medical knowledge. In that light, it is useful to consider some of the conditions that studies must meet in order to be ethically acceptable.[9]

The most basic condition is the requirement that investigators employ risk assessment standards in order to identify possible risks to subjects, minimize those risks, and avoid exposing subjects to risks that are not necessary for achieving the study's scientific goals. A related condition involves an assessment of proportionality. Although the risks and benefits involved in studies are rarely commensurable, those contemplating enrolling human subjects in a study must examine all of the risks and burdens involved and compare them to the array of possible anticipated benefits. Overall, investigators must judge whether the risks and burdens to the individual outweigh the anticipated likely benefits and justify their conclusions to reviewers, peers, participants, and perhaps also the public.

It is easier to justify studies that involve only low risks and unlikely potential harms. As the risks increase, the potential benefit to subjects should increase. There may, however, be extreme circumstances in which people have very little to lose by participating. Sometimes people at the brink of

---

[8] A recent study has shown that this may actually be difficult to achieve because people are reluctant to participate in research and do not recognize participation as a moral duty. Weinfurt KP, Lin L, Sugarman J, "Public views regarding the responsibility of patients, clinicians, and institutions to participate in research in the United States," *Clinical Trials* (2019): 1–6.

[9] Emanuel E, Wendler D, and Grady C. "What Makes Clinical Research Ethical?" *JAMA* 283, 20 (2000): 2701–2711.

death may have the possibility of gaining a great deal by participating in a study. When death is imminent, an investigational therapy could offer a slim chance at prolonging life (e.g., a study of a new artificial heart). In other circumstances, there may be no possibility of the patient benefitting directly, but the possibility of contributing significantly to advancing knowledge. In some circumstances, the brief duration of an investigational procedure could justify enrolling subjects in a study that promises them no personal health improvement or life extension.[10]

In addition, research produces knowledge that can benefit any patient. In that sense, taking a long view, anyone who may someday come to rely on what is learned can benefit. When hypotheses are either proved or disproved by a study, we all benefit from advancing the science. From this perspective, we should reject the common view that human subject research must provide direct health benefit to study participants. When we take social benefit seriously and accord it appropriate weight, we can arrive at a reasonable and more balanced overall view of a study's benefits.

Research-Related Risks and Benefits

It is always difficult to compare the risks and benefits of medical interventions because the advantages and disadvantages cannot be measured in the same terms. Pain, disability, inconvenience, and embarrassment are very different from each other, so they cannot be weighed on the same scale. Comparisons are further complicated by having to factor in the likelihood, duration, and severity of each factor. Physicians are, however, regularly engaged in making calculations that involve balancing incommensurable factors. Surgeons must make risk-benefit comparative assessments before every surgery, and oncologists must consider whether the likely risks and benefits of an

---

[10] Like most research ethics policymakers, Emanuel et al. ("What Makes") maintained that the contribution to society is not a sufficient justification for research, but that the individual participants must also receive direct personal benefit from their participation and that only "health-related potential benefits" should count. This position, which reflects the thinking of many authors, has dramatic and counterproductive implications for biomedical science and for society. For example, the requirement that participants receive direct potential health-related benefits eliminates the possibility of recruiting healthy volunteers for studies because, by definition, healthy volunteers have no medical conditions that can be improved by their participation. Yet, the use of healthy volunteers is often critical in developing an understanding of normal human function, for example, in defining a healthy human microbiome. The participation of healthy volunteers is also an essential feature in assessing the safety of products, including probiotics, and sometimes a critical element in establishing study drug dosing and an acceptable limit for risks in clinical trials.

intervention justify the burdens that it imposes. The same type of comparative assessment must be made before undertaking any study that involves human subjects. The balance, however, is somewhat different in research because the risks are borne by individual study participants, whereas the possible benefits will accrue primarily to future patients, a group that may or may not include the current study participants.

Vulnerable Patients

Many authors and policymakers are especially reluctant to allow research involving "vulnerable" populations, presumably to protect them from harms and prevent their exploitation. According to the policies of the Office of Human Research Protection and the institutional review boards (IRBs) that adopt additional policies that constrain research with groups of potential participants, vulnerable groups include the mentally ill, the mentally handicapped, pregnant women, fetuses, products of in vitro fertilization, children, prisoners, the elderly, people who are in the midst of a medical emergency, and the educationally or economically disadvantaged. That's a lot of people.

Sometimes, classifying individuals as part of a vulnerable group and requiring special protections (e.g., for the elderly, the educationally or economically disadvantaged) may be inaccurate. For example, it is disrespectful to presume that an elderly person without a high school diploma cannot make research participation decisions for herself. In any circumstance other than research, we would call the categorization and restrictions disrespectful, ageist, and discriminatory.

Some vulnerable groups include only individuals who lack decisional capacity (e.g., young children, profoundly retarded, demented, or unconscious individuals). Individuals in such groups are vulnerable to being treated thoughtlessly and carelessly. Investigators need to be concerned with their interests and protect them from unreasonable harms. It may be especially important, however, to involve these individuals in research. In some circumstances, it may be important to learn about their underlying debilitating condition, while in other cases, it may be important to learn about how an intervention affects them in particular. And when individuals from vulnerable groups are housed together in group homes or other institutions, it may be especially important to study how communicable diseases are transmitted or prevented or how changes in their microbiomes might make them prone to infection or able to ward off disease.

Certainly, we all accept that children should be protected from avoidable risks and harms, including those associated with research. We all worry that children's small and developing bodies may be especially susceptible to harms. Because children have a longer life span ahead of them than adult subjects, children may have to endure any untoward effects of research longer than other subjects would and experience consequences that would not appear in those with fewer years of life remaining. These are all legitimate concerns.

Regulators have, therefore, restricted studies involving children, particularly studies that involve "more than minimal risk," that is, hazards greater than those encountered in the child's everyday life. Nevertheless, the paternalistic protectionist tenor of today's research environment often leaves researchers reluctant to undertake clinical studies involving children. Yet, children are sometimes injured, and they sometimes become ill. Without study, we cannot improve the healthcare of children.[11] Studies of adults may not be applicable to children because their bodies are smaller, their metabolism is different, they are far more active than adults, their activities are different, and their bodies are still growing and developing. Without data to support the treatment of children, every treatment with an intervention that was not studied in children is an experiment with a single subject. Thus, "treatment" with interventions that have not been studied in children exposes each child to the full spectrum of risks without providing information that might be useful in the treatment of other children in the future. It makes no sense to expose every child to the risks of unstudied treatment when the alternative of enrolling a few in carefully thought out studies with vigilant oversight would expose those few to no greater risks than what would be associated with the unstudied treatment. In effect, the current approach protects no children from risks and harms and prevents every child from receiving the benefits of scientific advance. This approach does not represent a favorable risk-benefit ratio.

[11] Kopelman L, "Health Care Reform and Children's Right to Health Care: A Modest Proposal," in Rhodes R, Battin MP, and Silvers A, editors, *Medicine and Social Justice: Essays on the Distribution of Health Care*, 2nd edition (New York: Oxford University Press, 2012: 335–345.

Research Oversight

Human subject research imposes participants to some risk of harm. Independent review by a panel of experts and community members assures participants and society that the study conforms to the highest ethical standards. In the United States, granting agencies, data and safety monitoring boards, as well as institutional, regional, and private review boards (IRBs) review and oversee the conduct of human subject research. Reviewers have responsibility for approving or withholding approval from proposed studies, amending them, overseeing their activities, and terminating them when appropriate.

Independent review of proposed studies requires scientists to disclose what will be done, to whom, how, when, where, and why. This disclosure allows reviewers to consider all aspects of a proposed study and evaluate its merits in order to reach a decision about whether or not it conforms to regulatory and ethical standards. Although a study may appear very reasonable to a researcher, independent review allows additional eyes to check on researcher bias. By giving reviewers the responsibility to assess the risk-benefit ratio of a study, independent judgment can confirm the reasonableness of the risks and burdens involved in study participation so that unreasonable studies are prevented.

Furthermore, regulatory requirements for institutional review make institutions responsible and accountable for the studies conducted by employees and anyone using their facilities. Severe penalties can be levied for regulatory infractions, and the attendant publicity can have serious ramifications on institutions. This structure of penalizing institutions for the infractions of employees aligns the institution's interests with regulation adherence and helps ensure that investigators will be scrupulous in upholding the ethical standards set out in research regulations.

Independent board review and oversight of studies ensures the trust and trustworthiness of biomedical research. It promotes confidence that nothing about the project is being concealed, that informed reasonable people find the study design to be valid, that the promised results will be valuable, that subjects are fairly selected and treated with respect, and that the risks involved have been minimized and are justified and proportional with the anticipated benefits.

Voluntary Consent

Voluntary participation is a critical ethical requirement for most human interactions. A choice made without knowing the key facts cannot be considered voluntary or autonomous. Because knowing and understanding the relevant facts are critical elements in autonomous choices, people with the capacity to take responsibility for their actions need to have critical information when they make important choices. For that reason, informed consent has become ensconced as the cornerstone principle of research ethics. And, according to bioethicists who see research ethics in terms of common morality, the concept of autonomy explains the centrality of informed consent in the ethical practice of research.[12]

When investigators ask people who are capable of making their own decisions to participate in a study, they must provide the information that participants will need to make participation decisions that reflect their own values and priorities. In effect, when autonomous individuals are well informed about the goals of a study and the burdens and risks involved in participation and consent to enrollment, they take on a responsibility to do what they agree to do and can be considered ethically responsible for their choice. If they had been inadequately informed, whether deliberately or carelessly, or deceived about critical details of the study, their enrollment decision would not be voluntary.

People who enroll in biomedical research typically accept some burdens and some risks. By enrolling, they also express their willingness to promote the social good of contributing to the development of biomedical knowledge. Regardless of the actual scope of participants' motives, participation in research should always be seen as a noble choice that expresses concern and sympathy for the plight of others and solidarity with the community of humanity. People who volunteer to serve as research participants should not be seen merely as subjects being used for the purposes of others. Instead, they should be acknowledged as collaborators in important social projects, as courageous citizens who accept their responsibility to do what they can to further biomedical research. Research participants are entitled to feel proud of doing their part, and that they have earned respect for their sacrifice.

[12] Beauchamp TL and Childress JF, *Principles of Biomedical Ethics*, 7th edition (New York: Oxford University Press, 2012).

Research participants should, obviously, be treated very well. They deserve careful treatment and monitoring during the course of a study to ensure that risks are minimized and that their well-being is maintained. Also, because the burdens of a study may turn out to be more significant than a subject had anticipated, thereby changing the risk-benefit ratio, subjects must be allowed to withdraw from a study at any time and without penalty. Additionally, as meaningful information becomes available during the study period, it should be shared with study participants. Meaningful information regarding the intervention's effectiveness or the subject's condition should be carefully monitored and shared as the study progresses. Beyond that, information that participants disclose to further the research project should be safeguarded according to standards of medical confidentiality.

Once a study is completed and the data analyzed, the findings must be shared to make the contribution of participants worthwhile. Because research participants are collaborators in the research enterprise, they also deserve to be informed of study findings so that they can partake in the pleasure of having helped to produce valuable knowledge. That communication expresses respect for what the participants have done to advance medical knowledge and to benefit others.

Later, if evidence of potential harm associated with the investigational drug, implant device, or other intervention emerges, study participants should be informed of the problem. In addition, if the problems that are consequent to study participation require treatment, this should be made available to the participants. Excellent treatment of research subjects throughout, and sometimes even after the study period, helps to promote and maintain society's trust in the research enterprise.

Contentious Research Issues

Although there is significant agreement among physicians and bioethicists on the need for research and the core ethical requirements for conducting studies with human subjects, a good deal of disagreement remains over some important matters. I sketch two of the issues that I find particularly worthy of attention and especially important as matters of medical ethics.

The Innovation/Research Distinction

Physicians are legally allowed to treat patients with any approved and avail-able medications and prescribe or administer those medications for off-label uses. They are also permitted to provide innovative treatments, that is, untried interventions that a physician hypothesizes may help a patient. No one has to review a doctor's decision to innovate with a novel surgical procedure, an un-studied off-label use of a drug that has been approved for a different purpose, or an entirely original treatment approach. A physician who takes on the respon-sibility of trying to improve clinical practice by undertaking a formal study and systematically evaluating the results is, however, required by the regulations, institutions, and academic journals to first submit the plan for IRB review and secure IRB approval. The time involved and the regulatory burdens associated with IRB review of research sometimes have the effect of inhibiting research.

The requirements imposed on those who choose to conduct "research" do provide the assurance that answering the study question has value, that the study itself is well designed, and that subjects are selected fairly and not subjected to unreasonable risks. In sum, IRB oversight allows society to trust that research is conducted according to the highest ethical standards. At the same time, no similar reassurance or oversight is provided for innovative treatment. While some regulations of research may be overly burdensome and nitpicky, the totally laissez-faire approach to innovation may be too tol-erant and risky.

The radical distinction between the totally unregulated approach to "in-novation" and the highly regulated and reviewed approach to "research" was established in the *Belmont Report*, which was issued on September 30, 1978, and published in the *Federal Register* on April 18, 1979.[13] Its distinction be-tween innovation and research was then maintained in the Department of Health, Education, and Welfare's revised and expanded regulations for the protection of human subjects 45 CFR, part 46, and published in the *Federal Register* in 1979 in what has become known in the United States as the Common Rule.[14] The purported division between innovation and research

[13] National Commission for the Protection of Human Subjects of Biomedical and Behavioral Research. *The Belmont Report, Part A: Boundaries Between Practice and Research* (April 18, 1979). Accessed June 10, 2018, at https://www.hhs.gov/ohrp/regulations-and-policy/belmont-report/read-the-belmont-report/index.html#xbound
[14] In the Common Rule (45 CFR 46 Subpart A), §46.102 Definitions, (d), *Research* means a sys-tematic investigation, including research development, testing and evaluation, designed to develop or contribute to generalizable knowledge. Accessed June 10, 2018, at https://www.hhs.gov/ohrp/regulations-and-policy/regulations/45-cfr-46/index.html#46.102

is both arbitrary and conceptually incoherent. Ideally, both of these physician activities rely on the scientific method and entail formulating and testing a theory-based hypothesis by gathering and analyzing empirical data. Hence there is no scientific distinction between them. It is incoherent because the Common Rule's definition of *research*, which is set to draw a sharp contrast with "innovation," either makes no sense or fails to distinguish the activities. In the regulations, research is defined as "a systematic investigation . . . designed to develop or contribute to generalizable knowledge." Whereas all knowledge is generalizable, this statement falsely suggests that the knowledge gained through innovation is not generalizable. The observed results of a successful innovation are likely to be shared with colleagues and students or even presented in a case report, and the findings are likely to be applied in future situations that would benefit from a similar approach. And while an innovation that is expected to produce marginal benefit might require a meticulous design and an elaborate data-gathering plan to demonstrate its effect, the value of an innovation that is expected to produce a dramatic benefit (e.g., a new way of positioning a patient for maximizing exposure and minimizing the incision size, a novel surgical use for the umbilical vein) may be appreciated immediately.

Placebo Research

Clinical trials involving a placebo arm provide an inert intervention for one group of study participants in order to compare the effect on that group with the effect on others who receive active intervention. Scientifically, this research model is the gold standard for assessing the efficacy of an intervention because it can demonstrate assay sensitivity, that is, whether the intervention actually produces the desired result. Employing an inert intervention as a comparator is important because the administration of any intervention in a medical context, even an inert placebo, has been shown to produce a beneficial result. A clinical trial must be able to demonstrate that the benefit provided by the active intervention is greater than the beneficial result provided by the placebo.

Placebo research is particularly contentious for physicians because many are inclined to regard it as depriving some patients of useful treatment, thereby causing harm. Conceptually, this interpretation of placebo research reflects two misunderstandings. First, the use of a placebo as doing nothing is mistaken because numerous studies have shown that placebos actually confer benefits while imposing no risks of harm. This means that study participants who receive the placebo are likely to benefit while being exposed to less risk than those in the study's active arm. Second, the common placebo aversion that presumes that study participants who are randomized to a placebo arm and endure study burdens with no chance of receiving benefits relies on a shortsighted view of the ultimate study results. Taking a farsighted view of research outcomes, instead of narrowly focusing only on what happens during the study period, means that participants with chronic or recurrent medical problems will benefit from study findings regardless of the study arm that they happen to be randomly assigned.

An example illustrates my criticism of both the innovation-research distinction and the aversion to placebo research. It also reinforces the position on the physician's role in research that I have been urging. Because decisions on these matters often require consideration of complicated clinical and scientific issues, and because discussion of the ethics is often obscured by poorly understood principles from common morality (e.g., justice, vulnerability), explaining my concerns requires a detailed example.

An Ethical Conundrum Over a Placebo Study

In 2014, a controversy arose when a previously approved drug was proposed as a treatment for a rare, debilitating, fatal disease. The US regulators demanded a randomized placebo controlled study to demonstrate the safety and efficacy of the proposed intervention whereas the European regulatory agency considered a randomized placebo controlled study of the new intervention to be ethically unacceptable. Examining the dilemma will explain how such conundrums should be addressed.

The Facts

Consider the ethical acceptability of doctors inviting their patients to enroll in a proposed placebo-controlled trial of a new intervention as a possible relapse prevention treatment for neuromyelitis optica (NMO). NMO is a relatively rare disease. Its prevalence ranges from 1/100,000 to 4/100,000 in

Europe and North America.[15] This means that neurologists' experience with this disease is limited.

In more than 90% of patients, NMO is an incurable relapsing disease involving attacks of optic neuritis or transverse myelitis. It is disabling, with poor remission leading to rapid accrual of irreversible neurological disability. In studies from 1977 to 1997, only 68% of patients survived for 5 years after diagnosis, and 60% of patients exhibited severely impaired ambulation or blindness in at least one eye after 7–8 years.[16]

The natural history of NMO is relatively unpredictable. Disabling damage accrues during acute attacks, and relapses tend to occur in clusters after periods of remission. Periods of remission, however, can last for years even when patients receive no relapse preventing treatment.[17] In a few patients the disease takes a relatively benign course, with only minor disability for up to 10 years.[18]

Patients with NMO have a more severe disease than patients with relapsing-remitting multiple sclerosis (RRMS), including a higher risk of dying from the disease. One study that compared both conditions at the same center found that the age of onset for both diseases was the early 30s, with a mean survival of NMO patients of 7.4 years and 10.3 years for RRMS patients. Disease progression in patients with NMO was higher than in patients with RRMS (0.9 vs. 0.6), and patients with NMO experienced significantly more disability on the Expanded Disability Status Scale (EDSS) than patients with RRMS (39% vs. 17%).[19]

Neuromyelitis optica is and has been commonly misdiagnosed. In 2004 an antibody biomarker for the disease was discovered,[20] and by 2006 it was widely used.[21] Nevertheless, uncertainty regarding the diagnosis persists

---

[15] Jarius S, Wildemann B, and Paul F, "Neuromyelitisoptica: Clinical Features, Immunopathogenesis and Treatment," *Clinical and Experimental Immunology* 176, 2 (2014): 149–164.

[16] Jarius et al., "Neuromyelitisoptica."

[17] Kimbrough DJ, Fujihara K, Jacob A, et al., "Treatment of Neuromyelitis Optica: Review and Recommendations," *Multiple Sclerosis and Related Disorders* 1, 4 (2012): 180–187.

[18] Jarius et al., "Neuromyelitisoptica."

[19] Bichuetti DB, Oliveira EM, Souza NA, Tintoré M, and Gaggai AA, "Patients With Neuromyelitis Optica Have a More Severe Disease Than Patients With Relapsing Remitting Multiple Sclerosis, Including Higher Risk of Dying of a Demyelinating Disease," *Arquivos de Neuro-psiquiatria* 71, 5 (2013): 275–279.

[20] Lennon VA, Wingerchuk DM, Kryzer TJ, et al., "A Serum Autoantibody Marker of Neuromyelitis Optica: Distinction From Multiple Sclerosis," *Lancet* 364, 9451 (2004): 2106–2112.

[21] McKeon A, Fryer JP, Apiwattanakul M, et al., "Diagnosis of Neuromyelitis Spectrum Disorders: Comparative Sensitivities and Specificities of Immunohistochemical and Immunoprecipitation Assays," *Archives of Neurology* 66, 9 (2009): 1134–1138.

because many patients who are diagnosed with NMO do not have the biomarker. Depending on the study, the percentage of patients with NMO without the biomarker can be very low or as high as 80%.[22-25] Furthermore, a multicenter cohort study of 187 patients found that 30% of patients were initially misdiagnosed as having multiple sclerosis (MS). This is problematic because some MS treatments may worsen NMO.[26]

Relapse prevention therapy for NMO has focused on a variety of immunosuppressive medications. None of them has been validated in a rigorous randomized trial.[27,28] Systematic reviews of the literature have produced treatment recommendations, but they are based on studies rated evidence level III or IV because their findings were based on small numbers of subjects or retrospective reviews.[29] In some studies, the number of participants was as few as seven. And the diagnostic uncertainty for NMO undermines the value of older retrospective studies[30-34] because it is not clear whether the diagnosis was correct, particularly for studies that included data obtained prior to 2006. Also, the different retrospective studies used different follow-up periods, criteria for diagnosis, and criteria for defining a relapse. And it is not clear whether the disease state of the participants was comparable, whether the baseline and improvement measures were taken at the same points, and whether disability was measured in the same way. In sum, assay sensitivity, the ability of a study to distinguish between active and inactive (i.e., effective

[22] Jarius et al., "Neuromyelitisoptica."

[23] Thomas T, Branson HM, Verhey LH, et al., "The Demographic, Clinical, and Magnetic Resonance Imaging (MRI) Features of Transversemyelitis in Children," *Journal of Child Neurology* 27, 1 (2012): 11–21.

[24] Mealy MA, Wingerchuk DM, Greenberg BM, and Levy M, "Epidemiology of Neuromyelitis Optica in the United States: A Multicenter Analysis," *Archives of Neurology* 69, 9 (2012): 1176–1180.

[25] Kitley J, Woodhall M, Waters P, et al., "Myelin-Oligodendrocyte Glycoprotein Antibodies in Adults With a Neuromyelitis Optica Phenotype," *Neurology* 79, 12 (2012): 1273–1277.

[26] Mealy et al., "Epidemiology of Neuromyelitis Optica."

[27] Kimbrough DJ, Mealy MA, Simpson A, and Levy M, "Predictors of Recurrence Following an Initial Episode of Transverse Myelitis," *Neurology—Neuroimmunology, Neuroinflammation* 1, 1 (2014): e4.

[28] Trebst C, Jarius S, Berthele A, et al., "Update on the Diagnosis and Treatment of Neuromyelitis Optica: Recommendations of the Neuromyelitis Optica Study Group," *Journal of Neurology* 261, 1 (2014): 1–16.

[29] Sato D, Callegaro D, Lana-Peixoto MA, Fujihara K, and Brazilian Committee for Treatment and Research in Multiple Sclerosis, "Treatment of Neuromyelitis Optica: An Evidence Based Review," *Arquivos de Neuro-psiquiatria* 70, 1 (2012): 59–66.

[30] Lennon et al., "A Serum Autoantibody Marker."

[31] Jarius et al., "Neuromyelitisoptica."

[32] Thomas et al., "The Demographic, Clinical, and Magnetic Resonance Imaging."

[33] Mealy et al., "Epidemiology of Neuromyelitis Optica."

[34] Kitley et al., "Myelin-Oligodendrocyte Glycoprotein Antibodies."

and ineffective) interventions, was not established for the drugs that are used to prevent relapses.

Whereas studies from 1977 to 1997 reported that 60% of patients exhibited severe impairment, with new diagnostic tools and criteria, cases that are less severe can now be identified. This makes it especially difficult to compare recently diagnosed patients to historical controls. It also makes it easy to mistakenly conclude that better outcomes in minor cases provide evidence of treatment efficacy because the previous disease progression is likely to have tracked a very different cohort of patients. Reliance on underpowered or retrospective studies therefore invites investigators to draw deceptive conclusions about the efficacy of the drugs that they employ.

In addition, the six recommended drugs are associated with significant side effects for short-term use, while the side effects of their long-term use have not been studied. Yet, patients with NMO are likely to be treated with these drugs for the rest of their lives, so the drugs' safety for chronic use should be a concern (Table 4.1).

Table 4.1 Drugs Used for NMO Relapse Prevention

Preventive Therapy Drug	Side Effects	Median Follow-up
Azathioprine	Lymphoma, nausea, elevated transaminases, leukopenia, diarrhea, bone marrow suppression, fatigue, hair loss, hepatotoxicity	9–42 months
Mycophenolate mofetil	Headache, constipation, bruising, anxiety, hair loss, leukopenia, diarrhea, fatigue, hair loss, skin malignancies, lymphoproliferative disease, skin malignancies	24–27 months
Rituximab	Recurrent herpes zoster, urinary tract infection, respiratory infection, fatigue, transient leukopenia, transient transaminase elevation, infections, transient hypotension, transient flu-like symptoms, allergic reaction	12–24 months
Methotrexate	Infections	6–62 months
Oral corticosteroids	Hyperglycemia, hypertension, insomnia, mood disturbances, weight gain, osteoporosis, glaucoma	19–45 months
Mitosantrone	Nausea, vomiting, hair loss, amenorrhea, neutropenia, acute myeloid leukemia	12–24 months

Because NMO is a rare, progressively disabling, fatal disease with a relatively unpredictable natural course,[35-37] all of today's patients can be expected to experience additional acute disabling attacks, repeatedly, until death. This means that developing definitive evidence for the efficacy and safety of any relapse prevention therapy is in the long-term interest of every patient with NMO.

The Argument for Conducting a Placebo Study

The inadequate evidence to support the efficacy of available interventions and establish their assay sensitivity, as well as the lack of evidence on safety for long-term use, speak to the need for definitive studies.[38-40] Furthermore, the serious disease burden associated with NMO, its variable natural history, and the rarity of the disease imply that study opportunities should not be squandered. Studies that can provide decisive evidence by enrolling adequate numbers of subjects and running the studies for an adequate duration are needed. Studies should also be efficient; that is, they should enroll the fewest participants necessary for decisively answering the study question and accomplish that goal in the shortest feasible time period to provide patients who need effective treatment and physicians who rely on the scientific evidence with the information that they need in a timely way. Placebo-controlled studies generally meet these criteria.

Nevertheless, relying on their own extremely limited personal patient experiences and the meta-analyses of review panels encourages "experts" to maintain that preventive therapy with the six immune-modulating agents that are in use is effective in reducing the relapse rate and the amount of disability following an acute attack.[41] Yet, because of the variability in the natural course of NMO, all that a physician with a patient on treatment can know is that the patient has not yet had a relapse or that the disability following an attack is not severe. The physician has no scientific reason to believe that the administered drug is playing a role in the patient's disease progression.

---

[35] Jarius et al., "Neuromyelitisoptica."
[36] Kimbrough et al., "Treatment of Neuromyelitis Optica."
[37] Bichuetti et al., "Patients With Neuromyelitis Optica."
[38] Kimbrough et al., "Treatment of Neuromyelitis Optica."
[39] Trebst et al., "Update on the Diagnosis."
[40] Sato et al., "Treatment of Neuromyelitis Optica."
[41] Kimbrough et al., "Treatment of Neuromyelitis Optica."

Without adequate evidence supporting treatment decisions, prescribing any of the six previously tried drugs shouldn't be counted as anything more than innovation. Nevertheless, the inadequately supported claims of efficacy in the literature incline physicians to prescribe the "endorsed" drugs and oppose enrolling patients in placebo-controlled studies of new drugs. This is a significant barrier to research because the rarity of the disease means that there are few potential research participants, and physician reluctance to participate suppresses enrollment.

Determining whether or not to use a placebo-controlled design for studying a new drug as a preventive therapy for NMO requires evaluating the harms and benefits involved and to whom they will accrue. Two populations should be considered: (1) the study participants and (2) the entire population of people living with NMO. Typically, research review focuses exclusively on study participants and only the benefits that accrue to them during the trial. An ethical analysis, however, requires a broader perspective that examines all of the effects on all of those who are likely to be affected by an action. This includes determining whether the risks of harm are reasonable under the circumstances and whether the distribution of burdens and benefits is just, in that people who are similarly situated receive similar consideration.

First, the obvious risk for participants enrolled in a placebo-controlled trial, is the harm of suffering disabling, irreversible damage during acute attacks that might have been avoided by remaining on treatment with one of the six endorsed immune-modulating agents. The key term here is *might*. There is only weak level III and level IV evidence supporting the efficacy of the drugs currently used to prevent attacks, and those drugs are all associated with serious harmful side effects. The uncertainty of the foregone benefits, the drug-associated risks of treatment, and the placebo benefit provided to those in the control arm[42] all have to be balanced in the harms-benefit analysis.

At the same time, all participants who face a lifetime of future disabling attacks benefit from a study that provides a definitive answer to questions about the efficacy of the new study drug. Positive study results will benefit patients by providing information about an effective treatment that could prevent or minimize disabling relapses; negative results will benefit them by eliminating an ineffective potential intervention and thereby save them from

[42] Kolak J, *An Updated Appeal for Placebo Orthodoxy.* Oxford-Mount Sinai Consortium on Bioethics, New York, April 18, 2018.

the costs and burdens associated with its use as well as the possible benefits of being maintained on another drug. This farsighted view of benefits should be the standard in the harm-benefit analysis of any study.

On enrollment and before randomization, all participants in a placebo-controlled study have the same chance of receiving either an inert or an active intervention. Thus, placebo studies instantiate the formal principle of justice by treating similarly situated participants in the same way.[43] And because all participants have an interest in a definitive answer to the study question, participation in a placebo trial furthers their interests and does not oppose them. Furthermore, at the start of a study, no one knows whether the study drug will be ineffective, provide benefits, or be harmful. In that sense, the placebo group, unlike the intervention group, is not exposed to drug-related harmful side effects.

Second, the entire affected population of people living with NMO may be harmed by the absence of adequate evidence for guiding physicians in the treatment of their devastating disease. The entire group would benefit from a placebo-controlled trial by receiving a definitive answer to questions about the study drug's efficacy or lack thereof. That information will benefit all of them over the entire course of their illness. By using a placebo-controlled study, the answer will be obtained sooner and with fewer subjects than what an alternative study design could produce, and thereby it could prevent more relapses and relapse-related disability. Obtaining a definitive negative answer efficiently will prevent patients from investing time and money in an ineffective treatment and needlessly suffering drug-related side effects. In addition, having definite evidence of efficacy could facilitate obtaining insurance coverage for the drug.

Understanding the requirements of justice for the entire affected population involves explaining who should be asked to participate in a placebo trial. Given the significant benefits of a placebo trial to the entire affected population, and to protect patients from the promotion of ineffective or inferior treatments, every physician should be willing to collaborate on a placebo-controlled study and invite their patients to enroll.

---

[43] Issues of justice are discussed in detail in Chapter 9.

Countervailing Arguments

Although what I have said thus far may seem clear and straightforward, others in the research ethics community and the medical community may take issue with my position. Objectors are likely to focus exclusively on the study participants and the period of their study participation. They are also likely to ignore the implications for the participants over their future course and the implication for others in the disease community. Those objections are influenced by two documents. The 2002 version of the *International Ethical Guidelines for Biomedical Research Involving Human Subjects* by the Council for International Organizations of Medical Sciences (CIOMS), guideline 11, was particularly restrictive of placebo-controlled trials. It required that a placebo control may only be used

- when there is **no established effective intervention;**
- when **withholding an established effective intervention would expose subjects to, at most, temporary discomfort or delay in relief of symptoms;**
- when use of an established effective intervention as comparator would not yield scientifically reliable results and **use of placebo would not add any risk of serious or irreversible harm to the subjects.** [emphasis added][44,45]

---

[44] Council for International Organizations of Medical Sciences (CIOMS), *International Ethical Guidelines for Biomedical Research Involving Human Subjects.* Geneva, Switzerland: CIOMS, 2002. Accessed August 26, 2018, at https://cioms.ch/wp-content/uploads/2016/08/International_Ethical_ Guidelines_for_Biomedical_Research_Involving_Human_Subjects.pdf

[45] CIOMS 2002 has exerted its influence for many years. CIOMS 2016 is somewhat more tolerant of placebo research, but its restrictions are still significant. The new guideline 5 states:

"As a general rule, the research ethics committee must ensure that research participants in the control group of a trial of a diagnostic, therapeutic, or preventive intervention receive an established effective intervention.

Placebo may be used as a comparator when there is no established effective intervention for the condition under study, or when placebo is added on to an established effective intervention.

When there is an established effective intervention, placebo may be used as a comparator without providing the established effective intervention to participants only if:

o there are compelling scientific reasons for using placebo; and

o delaying or withholding the established effective intervention will result in no more than a minor increase above minimal risk to the participant and risks are minimized, including through the use of effective mitigation procedures."

Accessed August 26, 2018, at https://cioms.ch/wp-content/uploads/2017/01/WEB-CIOMS-EthicalGuidelines.pdf

Similarly, the WMA's *Declaration of Helsinki—Ethical Principles for Medical Research Involving Human Subjects* (64th WMA General Assembly, October 2013) makes similar pronouncements on placebo-controlled trials.

Use of Placebo

33. The benefits, risks, burdens and effectiveness of a new intervention must be tested against those of the best proven intervention(s), except in the following circumstances:

Where no proven intervention exists, the use of placebo, or no intervention, is acceptable; or Where for compelling and scientifically sound methodological reasons the use of any intervention less effective than the best proven one, the use of placebo, or no intervention is necessary to determine the efficacy or safety of an intervention

and the **patients who receive any intervention less effective than the best proven one, placebo, or no intervention will not be subject to additional risks of serious or irreversible harm as a result of not receiving the best proven intervention.**

Extreme care must be taken to avoid abuse of this option. [emphasis added][46]

Both of these documents take a strong stand on restricting placebo-controlled studies. The crucial issue in an NMO trial would be the risk of disabling irreversible damage during acute attacks. Because of the inadequate evidence for the safety and efficacy of existing therapies, it is hard to say when the risks are features of disease progression or the discontinuation of questionable therapy. Also, because there is no scientifically established effective intervention, it is fair to say that there is still only innovation and no "best proven intervention." People in the research ethics community may, however, take the opposite view because prescription of the "endorsed" drugs is considered the standard of care.

Physicians are likely to raise a variety of concerns. One reflects worry for the suffering of patients who could be in the placebo arm of a study. What these caring physicians seem to overlook is that it's not only study participants, but also patients living with NMO who are destined to suffer

[46] World Medical Association. *WMA Declaration of Helsinki—Ethical Principles for Medical Research Involving Human Subjects.* Accessed August 26, 2018, at https://www.wma.net/policies-post/wma-declaration-of-helsinki-ethical-principles-for-medical-research-involving-human-subjects/

with the consequences of this disease and its treatments throughout the remainder of their lives. Their error is ignoring the bigger picture and failing to appreciate how their reluctance to enroll patients in placebo studies affects their patients beyond the study and has consequences for all patients with NMO over their life span.

In the case of NMO, the most salient consideration is that these patients will continue to suffer attacks and accumulate disability. The possibility of preventing the next attack for a study participant, regardless of how severe the disability resulting from an attack while off medication may be, pales in comparison to the future in store for that patient. The uncertain chance of avoiding the next attack may well be worth the chance of identifying an effective treatment. Misplaced fear of complicity may distort the otherwise-clear thinking of dedicated physicians.

In conversations, I've heard doctors express another concern. They feel unable to tell their patients, "I'm not going to treat you." Again, this concern may be about misplaced guilt over any disability that a patient suffers while enrolled in a placebo study. Again, there is no way to sort out whether an attack suffered by a patient after discontinuing treatment with a drug of questionable efficacy is related to the withdrawal or the natural progression of the disease. The coincidence may feel related and even culpable, but that psychological reaction is just why medicine must rely on science rather than emotions in assessing the value of treatments. Science, not the desire to avoid feelings of guilt, must guide medical practice.

An ancient insight is expressed in the query, "Who benefits?" Posing this question in relation to physicians who are reluctant to enroll patients in a randomized placebo-controlled trial of a new drug for NMO is revealing. As I have argued, no patients with NMO benefit from physician reluctance to undertake these studies. Refusal to participate does, however, benefit physicians who allow themselves to avoid feeling guilty if an off-treatment patient who is in a study's placebo arm suffers an attack. In light of medicine's commitment to advancing the welfare of patients and physicians' duty to put the welfare of patients before their own, adopting a policy that serves the psychic welfare of physicians at the cost of patients' well-being should be troubling.

Physicians who are averse to enrolling patients in a placebo trial can recast how they describe their reluctance. Would they feel comfortable telling their patients this? "I'm not going to try to find an answer to your questions about the efficacy of this drug." It's hard to imagine that a caring physician would dismiss patients' hope for a cure so flippantly. Instead, a physician could describe the invitation to participate in a placebo trial by saying, "I'm going to try my best to find an answer to your questions about whether or not this drug may help you."

Physicians also contend that patient bias makes patients reluctant to participate in studies. For some individuals, that may be true. For many, however, the opposite may be true. Patients with many diseases are the most dedicated and fervent in promoting research on the diseases that affect their lives. Unless their physicians oversell claims for the effectiveness of the existing treatments and understate the risks of long-term use, I see no reason to presume that patients with NMO will be different.[47]

Reflecting on the question of the acceptability of a placebo-controlled study for a new NMO drug as a philosopher reveals that the core issue may be a very old problem that was insightfully addressed by Rene Descartes in 1639 in his famous *Meditations on First Philosophy*.[48] In his Fourth Meditation: The Problem of Error, he explains how we come to make errors. According to Descartes, two intellectual faculties are involved in errors: the intellect, which is the faculty of knowledge, and the will, which is the faculty of choice. As he sees it, human understanding is limited by how we obtain knowledge, but the will is infinite because it can elect to believe anything. So, according to Descartes, we commit error by willing to believe based on insufficient evidence. Over the course of medical history, this appears to be a frequent occurrence, and it appears to be what transpires today when physicians who are eager to help their patients believe in treatments that are not sufficiently supported by evidence.

Philosophers also learn from nonphilosophers. Thomas C. Chalmers, MD, the former dean of my medical school, played a pivotal role in the scientific development of the randomized controlled trial. Chalmers recognized the dangers in physicians' inclination to develop confidence in interventions that were not supported by scientific evidence. He maintained that to avoid the development of attitudes favoring an intervention, patients should be randomized, and the efficacy of interventions should be

---

[47] Based on findings from a placebo controlled trial, Soliris(eculizumab), was approved for the treatment of neuromyelitis optica spectrum disorder (NMOSD) in adult patients who are anti-aquaporin-4 (AQP4) antibody positive by the US Food and Drug Administration on June 27, 2019. https://www.nationalmssociety.org/.../Neuromyelitis-Optica-(NMO)/Treatments. Accessed, 12/9/2019.

[48] Cottingham J, editor, *Descartes: Meditations on First Philosophy: With Selections From the Objections and Replies* (Cambridge: Cambridge University Press, 1996).

studied.[49,50] He argued that in order to provide a sound basis for treatment, studies must be well designed and carefully conducted. He understood that it is better to randomize patients than to administer an intervention as if it were known that it was effective.

In a similar vein, the philosopher Benjamin Freedman published a landmark article, "Equipoise and the Ethics of Clinical Research," in 1987 in *The New England Journal of Medicine*.[51] In it he described a concept that he termed *clinical equipoise* and argued that a study was justified whenever there was genuine uncertainty over whether the treatment would be beneficial. He maintained that even when a clinician or a researcher believes in the efficacy of an intervention, there is clinical equipoise as long as there is no actual proof that the benefit exists. Clinical equipoise existed with respect to the six drugs recommended for NMO, and it certainly existed with respect to new drugs that may be effective. Because a placebo-controlled trial offers the most efficient means to definitively answer the study questions, because there is no scientific reason to believe that enrolling patients exposed them to additional significant harm, and because obtaining clear answers to the study questions in a short period is valuable to both the study participants and others in the affected patient community, placebo studies of promising interventions should be undertaken. Because NMO is a rare disease and because a great deal about the disease and potential treatments is yet to be learned, to the extent possible, every patient should be treated in the context of a study so that physicians may learn about the disease and its treatments as they also provide care for their patients.

Conclusions

The practice of medicine is advanced by research, and those who choose to initiate studies need to guide their investigations by the rules that must be upheld for the ethical conduct of human subject research. All patients rely on the medical community to support the scientific research that informs evidence-based practice. Their reliance creates a moral imperative to use the

---

[49] Chalmers TC, "Randomize the First Patient," *New England Journal of Medicine* 296 (1977): 107.

[50] Chalmers TC, Celano P, Sacks HS, and Smith H, "Bias in Treatment Assignment in Controlled Clinical Trials," *New England Journal of Medicine* 309, 22 (1983):1358–1361.

[51] Freedman B, "Equipoise and the Ethics of Clinical Research," *New England Journal of Medicine* 317, 3 (1987): 141–145.

scarce resources that are available as effectively as possible. When physicians acknowledge and accept that treatment in the context of research offers our best hope for advancing the field, we have our best chance at improving medical knowledge. This means that physicians should be supportive of studies and willing to collaborate in research as a frequent and common companion of medical practice.

5

Duties of Behavior Toward Patients

Commitment to medicine involves a person developing the necessary knowledge and skills and honing character to become an exemplary physician.
The core duties of medical ethics revolve around physicians' commitments
to patients. This chapter elaborates on three of the duties that physicians have
to their patients: nonjudgmental regard, nonsexual regard, and confidentiality. These basic duties were pointedly identified as essential to medical
practice as far back as we can identify records describing the responsibilities
of physicians. The Hippocratic oath, for example, alludes to all three of these
requirements.[1] The Hippocratic oath commits physicians to provide care to
everyone without distinguishing the most from the least worthy—even slaves
were to be accorded good medical care. It mentions the necessity of doctors
refraining from exploiting their intimacy with patients for sexual advantage
and notes the critical requirement to maintain the confidentiality of information imparted during a medical encounter. It is somewhat surprising that
of all of the codes of ethics included in this book's Appendix, only the World
Medical Association International Code of Medical Ethics[2] acknowledges
all three of these duties. The insights that justify all of these requirements of
medical ethics therefore need to be made explicit as both duties of action and
personal character commitments for physicians.

Nonjudgmental Regard

The seventh duty of medical ethics is nonjudgmental regard.
Medicine is committed to providing treatment based on patients' medical
needs. This suggests that patients with similar medical needs should be
treated in much the same way when their medical circumstances are similar.

---

[1] Miles SH, *The Hippocratic Oath and the Ethics of Medicine* (New York: Oxford University
Press, 2004).
[2] World Medical Association. *WMA International Code of Medical Ethics* (2006). Accessed December
13, 2018, at https://www.wma.net/policies-post/wma-international-code-of-medical-ethics/

The Trusted Doctor. Rosamond Rhodes, Oxford University Press (2020). © Oxford University Press.
DOI: 10.1093/oso/9780190859909.001.0001

Unfortunately, that is not always the case, at least in part because nonjudgmental regard has not been clearly identified and articulated as a medical
duty. Its importance plays out in at least two problematic contexts: the acceptance of patients' reports as truthful and doctors making judgments
about patients' worthiness.

Nonjudgmental Regard of Patient Truthfulness

Physicians elicit information from patients about their medical history, the
history of their current illness, and their symptoms. Some of these reports
are easily verified by examination or with medical instruments such as
thermometers, x-rays, and blood tests. Other reports are unverifiable and
based entirely on patients' subjective experience. No instruments can confirm that a patient's report of pain or fatigue is accurate. Yet, pain and fatigue
are frequently symptoms of illness.

Usually, doctors accept their patients' descriptions of their subjective
symptoms, but the reports of some groups of patients tend to be disbelieved.
Doubted patients are most typically women, especially single women; people
of color; the elderly; the homeless; people living with sickle cell disease;
people with a psychiatric diagnosis; and people with enigmatic chronic
conditions. Even though their testimony is challenged for different reasons,
because we can readily identify the groups whose reports are rejected, it is
reasonable to conclude that some prejudiced judgmental attitudes are in
play. We also see the judgmental attitudes toward different groups reflected
in documented medical care and health disparities.[3-5]

To appreciate this problem, consider the experience of a patient living with
sickle cell disease. The first crisis of a person with this heritable disease typically occurs in the first year of life, and for the rest of their lives, these individuals suffer one to six crises per year. The disease has a variable course,
but it is associated with intermittent lifelong need for medical care, disability,
and early death. People living with sickle cell disease experience numerous

[3] Ubri P and Artiga S, *Disparities in Health and Health Care: Five Key Questions and Answers*, Henry J. Kaiser Family Foundation (2016, August 12). Accessed July 25, 2018, at https://www.kff.org/disparities-policy/issue-brief/disparities-in-health-and-health-care-five-key-questions-and-answers/

[4] American Medical Association. *Reducing Disparities in Health Care*. Accessed July 25, 2018, at https://www.ama-assn.org/delivering-care/reducing-disparities-health-care

[5] Centers for Disease Control and Prevention. *CDC Health Disparities & Inequalities Report* (CHDIR) (2013). Accessed July 25, 2018, at https://www.cdc.gov/minorityhealth/chdireport.html

medical problems, including strokes, eye problems, heart disease, kidney problems, and pulmonary hypertension.

Patients with sickle cell disease are typically people of color, and they are often raised in a community that is somewhat distrustful of medicine.[6,7] The distrust of medicine has its roots in the mistreatment of blacks in southern medical institutions for more than a century, the revelations of the Tuskegee Study of Untreated Syphilis in the Negro Male, and the early history of aggressive promotion of genetic testing for sickle cell disease in their communities. This history has melded together to produce persistent beliefs that people of color will be abused by doctors.

There is also the personal experience of patients who live with the disease. Acute episodes of intense, stabbing, or throbbing pain are the principal symptom of sickle cell disease, and many adolescents and adults with the disease also experience chronic pain.[8] Crises occur when the sickle-shaped blood vessels clump together and block blood flow and oxygen delivery. Patients then seek treatment in hospitals for their pain, and there the problems begin.

Distrust goes both ways. Doctors are cautioned to avoid causing or enabling drug addiction. They have also been made aware of drug abuse within the African American community. And, by temperament, doctors typically like to be incontrol and tell patients what they need and what to do. So, when a knowledgeable patient with sickle cell disease arrives at a hospital emergency room requesting a specific dose of a specific opioid to treat his pain and encounters a new doctor, suspicions are likely to flare.

Often the patient's pain is not accompanied by signs that the doctor can independently detect. A stoical patient may bear his pain in silence, giving the doctor reason to doubt that he is actually experiencing pain. A patient who groans, screams, and thrashes about may give the doctor reason to suspect that the patient is putting on a show. The physician has qualms about complying with the patient's demands and contributing to addiction, and the doctor may also be resistant to accepting orders from a patient. An adult patient who has had numerous similar experiences of being doubted in the

---

[6] Gamble VN, "A Legacy of Distrust: African Americans and Medical Research," *American Journal of Preventive Medicine* 9, 6 (1993, November–December): Supplement, 35–38.

[7] Schroeder MO, "Racial Bias in Medicine Leads to Worse Care for Minorities," *US News and World Report*, February 11, 2016. Accessed July 25, 2018, at https://health.usnews.com/health-news/patient-advice/articles/2016-02-11/racial-bias-in-medicine-leads-to-worse-care-for-minorities

[8] National Heart, Lung, and Blood Institute. *Sickle Cell Disease.* Accessed July 25, 2018, at https://www.nhlbi.nih.gov/health-topics/sickle-cell-disease

past anticipates the skepticism of the doctor. Rage (in the doctor) is a predictable and normal reaction to being manipulated and made vulnerable to institutional and legal penalties. Rage (in the patient) is a predictable and normal reaction to having your veracity questioned, particularly when you are in agony.

Thoughtful doctors and hospital administrations prevent this sort of problem by maintaining records of their patients' medical history, contact information for their primary care doctor, and the effective treatment for meeting their urgent needs. They also train staff to consult those records when a patient arrives in crisis. In the case of a patient who is new to the institution, however, the only way to avoid a predictable interpersonal crisis is to be nonjudgmental and believe the patient.

As a patient, it is infuriating to have your honesty doubted, particularly when the suspicious party is your doctor and you need the doctor's medical attention. Awareness of the doctor's distrust undermines the trust that is necessary for establishing a well-functioning doctor-patient relationship. It makes for difficulty in the doctor establishing an effective treatment plan, and it interferes with the patient's willingness to comply with recommended treatment.

Writing in *The New Yorker*, Lydija Haas described books by several women with illnesses that are hard to diagnose, such as Lyme disease, who recounted their experiences with incredulous doctors.[9] But the phenomenon of doubting the truthfulness of a patient's reported symptoms extends further to well-studied conditions that doctors would be able to diagnose if they believed their patients' reports, such as heart attack, severely herniated disks, and multiple sclerosis. Instead, based on prejudiced presumptions about women, people of color, people with a psychiatric diagnosis, the elderly, and homeless people, some doctors assume that these patients are experiencing anxiety, depression, or hysteria; hypothesize that the patient craves attention; or posit that the patient is malingering or manipulating the system to get a warm bed with room service for a few winter nights.

Physicians need to be committed to maintaining nonjudgmental regard and accept their patients' reports of symptoms because women, people of color, people with a psychiatric diagnosis, the elderly, and homeless people can all have serious medical problems that require medical attention. Standard medical thinking requires doctors to consider and take measures

---

[9] Haas L, "The Disbelieved," *The New Yorker* June 4, 2018, pp. 93–97.

to avoid the worst outcomes. Failing to diagnose and treat a medical problem that requires attention is far worse than allowing oneself to be manipulated for a short time. So, nonjudgmental acceptance of a patient's reported symptoms is required by medical ethics.

With time and sincere effort on their behalf, most patients will come to trust their doctors. There will be times when the medical problem cannot be identified and times when identified problems have no known effective treatment. Still, patients will appreciate their doctor's taking their symptoms seriously and the doctor's genuine effort to identify the cause and find a solution. There will also be times when it turns out that a patient has been malingering or fabricating, and evidence will come to light that supports such a conclusion. The default presumption, however, should be nonjudgmental belief in the reports of patients, coupled with a high threshold for doubting a patient's veracity.

Nonjudgmental Regard of Worthiness

Our parents have taught us to be careful of the friends we make, and parents today teach the same lesson to their children. The advice amounts to an instruction to be judgmental. In everyday life, this caution is important because the wrong friends can lead you astray. It is often prudent to quickly assess unsavory characters and distance oneself from them.

In criminal law, when punishment is being contemplated, we require a great deal of evidence before making a judgment about the guilt of an accused party. Our standard for judgment is evidence that gives us confidence in our conclusion beyond any reasonable doubt. In ordinary circumstances, however, we make judgments very quickly and with little evidence. We make snap judgments about who looks nice and who we should try to befriend. Based on appearance or slight behavioral clues, we size up people who might be dangerous and take aversive actions, from avoiding eye contact, crossing the street, or reaching for a cell phone in readiness for dialing 911. And patients make quick judgments about which doctor to trust, often based on dress, age, gender, race, or accent. In some contexts, these judgments can be extremely valuable, but sometimes they are inaccurate and misleading. In any event, it's what people do.

Great wits are often especially adept at identifying flaws in others and making them the butt of jokes and objects of derision. We also feel free to keep our distance from immoral people, like the murdering, lying, cheating, and bullying character, Tony Soprano, and see no need to extend social invitations to anyone like them. In times of war, people feel free to hate the enemy. And, sometimes, we think that others should be held accountable for their own misfortune.

Yet, when it comes to medical care, we want doctors to attend to us and our loved ones' needs regardless of whether or not we or they were somehow at fault for a current medical condition and regardless of one's worth in the eyes of others. In fact, we expect physicians to provide excellent medical care for prisoners with medical needs, for wounded enemy soldiers, for terrorist bombers, and even for Tony Soprano.

In medicine, in contrast to everyday life, doctors are committed to the nonjudgmental regard of their patients. This means that physicians should entirely avoid making judgments about patient worthiness. By allowing a distinctive set of powers, privileges, and immunities exclusively to medicine, society, in effect, grants the profession a monopoly over medical services. Therefore, medicine is required to provide medical services for everyone with a medical need, and medical professionals are not free to refuse services for anyone based on a personal aversion or self-serving reason.

Because we never know how unworthy we or our loved ones may appear in the eyes of others or where or how disheveled one of us is likely to be when we happen to need medical attention, we expect doctors to promote the medical interests of those in need of medical attention without first judging their worth or worthiness. Physicians have to be nonjudgmental in their allocation of caring concern and medical attention, and they have to try hard to avoid feeling frustrated by a patient's noncompliance or angered by a patient's deception, disrespect, or demandingness.

When patients receive behavioral clues that their worthiness is being assessed and that the judgment regarding their worthiness could result in care being withheld, they are likely to be less than forthcoming in providing their medical history. Without an accurate history and forthright sharing of symptoms, a doctor may not be able to make an accurate diagnosis or develop an effective treatment plan. Patients who have the sense that they are being judged, and possibly disqualified from treatment, are not likely to disclose information about their habits, behavior, past adherence to recommended treatment, or symptoms.

One emergency medicine doctor with a good grasp of this issue explained that he tries to treat every patient as he would treat the president of the

United States. Such physician behavior is likely to indicate to patients that in their doctor's eyes they are deserving of high-quality medical care. That attitude in turn inclines patients to be forthcoming and cooperative. Thus, the commitment to nonjudgmental regard is required in medicine because without it, physicians' ability to fulfill their core responsibility, the duty to provide medical care, will be impeded.

Another colleague explained that he obtains a relatively accurate picture of a patient's alcohol use by framing questions with exaggerated expectations. "So, how much do you drink a day, about a case of beer and a quart of booze?" he asks with a chuckle.[10] Putting the question that way shows the patient that an honest response will be accepted. It allows a patient to shrug and reply, "No, not so much, only a six pack and sometimes a pint." In other words, doctors have to convey their openness to the truth about their patient's behavior and their willingness to provide needed medical care regardless of what that truth may be.

Being judgmental is not only anathema to medicine but also dangerous. Judgments of deservingness are complicated and layered, and doctors lack the skills and wherewithal to make accurate assessments. A situation encountered in our liver transplant program illustrates the hazard in making judgments about patient worthiness.

Case 1

On a Wednesday evening, I was working late in my office when I received a call from the chief liver transplant surgeon and a hepatologist, the medical director of liver transplantation. They had received a call from a city hospital about a patient with acute hepatic failure who was in urgent need of liver transplantation. They were told that the patient was a murderer who had become ill while in jail. The question for me was whether we should accept the transfer of this patient to our transplant program and list him for liver transplantation. The corrections department officials had guaranteed that they would cover the transplantation-related expenses and provide the patient with any needed antirejection medications posttransplant, but a more proximal transplant program had already refused to accept the patient.

---

[10] This example was provided by Dr. Avi Barbasch.

The hepatologist and I argued that unless the patient had a death sentence, he should be treated as we would treat any other patient in need of transplantation. As long as the patient met our transplant criteria, we should accept him. The surgeon was not convinced.

The next afternoon, the patient's case was presented at the weekly Thursday afternoon meeting of the Liver Transplant Recipient Review Committee. By that time, the information on the patient's legal status had changed somewhat. It was reported that he had only been charged with murder, but he had not yet been tried for the crime. The multidisciplinary committee of about 40 members was sharply divided on what to do. They were ultimately swayed by the chief surgeon, who argued that we should not take the part of judge and jury, and that at this point, before a verdict had been reached, it was our job to regard him nonjudgmentally, as any other patient would be. If his medical condition was stable enough, he should be transferred to our program for transplantation.

By the next day, Friday morning, the team had additional information. They had learned that the patient was not accused of murder, he was merely accused of attempted murder of someone who he had caught assaulting his sister.

This case shows how difficult it can be to determine who is worthy and who is not. As the details of the case came into view, judgments changed. One issue is that an accurate assessment of worthiness should reflect all of the elements of a person's life. Physicians are not in a good position to gather all of the relevant information, and partial views are likely to yield inaccurate conclusions. In our case, we did not know if the accused attempted murderer was also an excellent student, a musician, a valuable friend, an important support for his younger siblings, and a devoted son. Similarly, we are in no position to know if some apparently worthy transplant candidate is also a tax cheat, a wife beater, an exploitative boss, and a repeat sex offender. The point is that doctors should not venture down the foxhole of trying to sort out who is worthy of care and who is not. Medicine does not have the authority, the resources, or the perspective to make those calls.

Contrary to the American Medical Association's Principle VI of its code of medical ethics, physicians should not be free to choose their patients.[11] Factors such as poverty, minimal insurance, or any characteristic that may incline a physician against accepting a patient do not justify withholding care. The same holds for a physician's personal discomfort, disagreement, aesthetic qualms, concern over sleepless nights, or a guilty conscience. Only patient-centered medical reasons (e.g., unfavorable risk-benefit ratio) or physician competence reasons (e.g., lack of relevant expertise), and sometimes legal prohibitions, justify turning away a patient with a medical need. Even then, when it is acceptable for a doctor to refuse to provide a requested service, the doctor may still have a professional obligation to make an appropriate referral. Whereas ordinary morality allows people to distance themselves from the unpalatable choices of others, that luxury is incompatible with the practice of medicine. Medicine's fiduciary responsibility requires physicians to use their knowledge and skills to promote their patients' good.

Nonsexual Regard

The eighth duty of medical ethics is nonsexual regard.
Everyone knows that sexual abuse is a horror. When a doctor engages in sexual abuse, however, the offense is more shocking, and it seems much worse than the same behavior by a nonphysician. In ordinary morality, the wrongness of sexual abuse comes from the violation of autonomy. In medicine, the wrongness of physician sexual involvement with patients comes from the breech of the fiduciary relationship and trust.

Doctors are allowed special license, powers, privileges, and immunities that are denied to others. They are trusted to use that special set of rights only in the promotion of their patients' interests. So, for a doctor to take advantage of opportunities to acquire knowledge of intimate details about a patient's

[11] Similar problematic statements appear in other codes of medical ethics. Australian Medical Association. *AMA Code of Ethics 2004. Editorially Revised 2006. Revised 2016* (2016), items 2.1.11–13. Accessed October 28, 2018, at https://ama.com.au/system/tdf/documents/AMA%20Code%20of%20Ethics%202004.%20Editorially%20Revised%202006.%20Revised%202016.pdf?file=1&type=node&id=46014; Canadian Medical Association. *CMA Code of Ethics (Update 2004)* (2004), responsibility 17. Accessed October 28, 2018, at http://www.cpsa.ca/wp-content/uploads/2019/01/CMA_Policy_Code_of_ethics_of_the_Canadian_Medical_Association_Update_2004_PD04-06-e.pdf; New Zealand Medical Association. *Code of Ethics* (2014), responsibility 17. Accessed October 28, 2018, at https://www.nzma.org.nz/publications/code-of-ethics

life, capitalize on occasions for observing nudity or sexual touching, or exploit the effect of drugs on a patient is an abuse of both trust and the fiduciary relationship. Doctors need their patients to trust that the intimacy of the doctor-patient relationship has no sexual overtones in spite of the revelation, the nudity, and the touching.

Anxiety or suspicion about a doctor's sexual or romantic intentions would seriously undermine the doctor's ability to provide patient care. The well-established practice of carefully draping a patient during examinations and procedures expresses the importance of nonsexual regard. Medicine has even developed its own terms to distinguish sexual behavior from nonsexual behavior. In common parlance, people speak of ogling, fondling, and caressing. In medicine, behavior that looks very similar is described in nonsexual terms as inspection, palpation, and examination.

Beyond the obvious prohibited sexual behaviors, the rule that requires nonsexual regard extends its prohibition across the entire spectrum of romantic entanglements. An instructive story was shared by a psychiatrist in a teaching a session for residents on this topic.

Case 2

Years before, the psychiatrist had treated a patient for situational depression. The therapy was successful, and they were bidding each other farewell after their final session. She then asked, now that her treatment was concluded, would he like to have dinner with her?

The psychiatrist refused her request, even though it was clear that he had been more than fond of her, and the depth of his feelings was still obvious years after that conversation. He explained to the group that his patient's feelings for him were the product of projections. Psychiatrists carefully safeguard their personal information because it is likely to interfere with the doctor-patient therapeutic relationship. Therefore, he was confident that she knew very little about him, so her interest and attraction were, in a sense, an illusion. He added that their doctor-patient relationship had not been terminated because the future is long, and his patient had to feel free to return to him as a patient if and when she should need psychiatric treatment in the future.

This poignant vignette illustrates important points about nonsexual regard. It shows the subtle ways in which the obligation of nonsexual regard can
be relevant in clinical practice. It also illustrates how important upholding
that duty is. Patients have to feel free to interact with their doctors without
any thought that either sex or romance is part of the agenda.

Confidentiality

The ninth duty of medical ethics is confidentiality.
The ninth duty of medical ethics is confidentiality.[12] Because doctors need
their patients to divulge intimate personal details about their behavior and
their history in order to make an accurate diagnosis and develop an effective
treatment plan, patients must be able to trust their doctors to keep the information that they share confidential.[13] The justification of physicians' obligation
to uphold confidentiality is related to the trust that is necessary for patients to
share secrets of their history and bodies in the course of their treatment. The
duty of confidentiality requires safeguarding the information that patients may
consider secret and share with their doctors. The profession's commitment to
confidentiality means the information can only be shared with other medical
professionals within the medical context and on a need-to-know basis.

Confidentiality is different from the ordinary morality concept of *privacy.*[14] Privacy marks an individual's protected domain of activity that is
shielded from the intrusion of others.[15] The boundaries of privacy are, typically, physical spaces, like what is inside my thoughts, inside my body, behind my bedroom door, behind the locked door of my home, preserved in
my diary, or saved on my personal computer.

---

[12] Gillon R, "Confidentiality," in Kuhse H and Singer P, editors, *A Companion to Bioethics* (Malden, MA: Blackwell, 1998: 425–431).

[13] Beauchamp and Childress, *Principles*, 2013, 320–321. Beauchamp and Childress and others who followed their lead explained confidentiality in terms of respect for autonomy. In contrast, I justify the medical ethics duty of confidentiality in terms of trust. This difference should be noted.

[14] Gert, Culver, and Clouser discussed what physicians typically consider to be confidentiality in terms of privacy. They justified privacy in terms of the rules of common morality, such as not causing harm. Gert B, Culver CM, and Clouser KD, *Bioethics: A Systematic Approach* (New York: Oxford University Press, 2006).

[15] Public Law 104-191. The Privacy Rule protects all "individually identifiable health informa-tion" held or transmitted by a covered entity or its business associate, in any form or media, whether electronic, paper, or oral. The Privacy Rule calls this information "protected health information (PHI)." 45 C.F.R. §§ 160.102, 160.103. https://www.hhs.gov/hipaa/for-professionals/privacy/laws-regulations/index.html

The concept of *confidentiality* delineates a socially defined protected space for sharing specific information among a cohort of medical professionals who are committed to using that information in the service of that individual patient. We find similar protected spaces in other professions, namely, law and the ministry. The boundaries of confidentiality are not physical spaces. Without violating confidentiality, information can be transferred between the doctor's office, a hospital emergency room, the medicine and surgery services, and the pharmacy. And the medical professionals who care for a patient 24 hours a day and 7 days a week need access to confidential patient information in caring for a patient. They are therefore free to communicate the information to one another, and none of that information sharing counts as a violation of confidentiality. Information is legitimately shared among medical professionals on a need-to-know basis. Those who may need access to the information in the service of a patient include doctors, medical trainees, nurses, social workers, physical therapists, pharmacists, laboratory technicians, and so on. In today's world of electronic communication, a good deal of the shared information is accessed through electronic medical records. In addition, it should also be noted that information shared with the permission of the patient does not violate confidentiality. Those who are given access by a patient to otherwise-confidential information may include family members, insurers, employers, schools, sports team officials, and so on.[16]

At least since the time of Hippocrates, the need for doctors to be trusted with personal information has been recognized, and confidentiality has been identified as an essential duty of medical ethics. Without assuring patients of confidentiality, doctors' ability to serve their patients would be impaired. This perspective explains why violations of confidentiality put the public's trust of medicine in jeopardy and show that confidentiality is a significant medical duty that needs to be accorded moral weight within clinical practice. Patients and society expect physicians to preserve patient confidentiality, and they rely on physicians to uphold it as a core responsibility of the profession.

For the most part, the responsibility to uphold the promise of confidentiality is unproblematic, but difficulties do arise. Even though doctors are aware of confidentiality as a medical duty, and even though the Health Insurance Portability

---

[16] Mark Siegler took the opposite view and regarded all of the information that is shared among medical professionals to be a violation of confidentiality. Siegler M, "Confidentiality in Medicine—A Decrepit Concept," *New England Journal of Medicine* 307, 24 (1982): 1518–1521.

and Accountability Act of 1996 (HIPAA) and research ethics regulations make a big deal over privacy, they tend to be more willing to compromise confidentiality than other professional duties. Perhaps confidentiality is regarded as less critical than other medical obligations because in everyday ethics, people are free to share whatever they know unless they have made a specific promise not to or signed a nondisclosure agreement. Perhaps the obligation appears less binding because life and death are rarely on the line. Perhaps the obligation to uphold confidentiality has been rendered optional by bioethicists who emphasize the ruling in the *Tarasoff* case, in which a state court ruled that a psychologist whose patient had threatened to kill a young woman had a "duty to warn" her or protect her from harm.[17] Even though there have been court rulings in other states that upheld medicine's duty to safeguard patient confidentiality, and even though the California rule was specifically limited to disclosures made to mental health professionals, it has become common to read the ruling as having far-reaching applicability. The resulting relatively casual attitude toward confidentiality justifies an effort to make its stringency vivid.

One kind of problem arises when the breach of confidentiality is not obvious. For example, the label on a ward (e.g., Oncology Service), a posted list of patients together with their doctors' names displayed on a board behind the nurse's station, or the nurse who calls a patient's name in a waiting room— all of these standard practices disclose information to visitors and others that a patient may have preferred not to be made known. Information that a patient regards as sensitive may be communicated to an unwelcomed audience through an overheard conversation on a speakerphone or even through the return address on an envelope. And electronic medical records that are rightly available to all treating physicians allow for the sharing of information that a treating doctor may not actually need to have. For example, a patient's ophthalmologist may not need to know about a patient's abortion history.

Doctors and medical institutions need to be vigilant and aware of the ways in which confidentiality may be breached inadvertently. The message is to be attentive to the ways in which confidential information may be disclosed and evaluate measures that are likely to protect confidentiality without imposing a more serious burden on patient care.

Another problem arises when something about a situation invites presumptions about what information a patient is willing to share or some

---

[17] Tarasoff v. Regents of the University of California, 17 Cal. 3d 425, 551 P.2d 334, 131 Cal. Rptr. 14 (Cal. 1976), was a case before the Supreme Court of California. The Court held that mental health professionals have a duty to protect individuals who are being threatened with bodily harm by a patient.

feature of an interaction makes it awkward to uphold confidentiality. It is easy for a doctor to assume that a patient who appears for an appointment accompanied by a relative or friend is willing to have her information shared with that person. Although that is usually the case, sometimes it is not. It is, therefore critical to make sure that an occasion is created, such as during a physical examination, for a private conversation in which a pointed question about information sharing can be asked. In a typical example, an 18-year-old female is brought to the emergency room by her mother. She has been experiencing nausea and vomiting, and the examining physician is concerned that she may be pregnant. The presence of the mother may suggest that the patient is willing to share her medical information with her mother. At the same time, the patient may actually want her confidentiality to be upheld. Also, asking the mother to step outside the room for the physical examination may feel awkward, and it may even be met with some resistance. This is the occasion for the doctor to summon his authority and ask the mother to wait outside during the examination. The presence of a female assistant for the examination would help to overcome the mother's protective reluctance. Once the mother is no longer within earshot, the issues of sexual activity and sharing future medical information can be raised with the patient so that confidentiality may be upheld.

The duty to preserve confidentiality may also conflict with other important physician responsibilities. In such cases, any breach of confidentiality must be justified. It is important to consider all of the foreseeable implications of a breach of confidentiality, the long-range implications as well as the immediate ones, the harms to those immediately involved in the situation, as well as the implications for society or a group that may be affected. The standard should be that the decision to violate confidentiality would be consistent with upholding the trustworthiness of the profession and that experienced and esteemed medical professionals would agree that the particular violation of confidentiality was justified. Another way of approaching a confidentiality decision would be to consider whether a consensus of respected and experienced colleagues would endorse incorporating such exceptions into the institution's confidentiality policy. And even when disclosing confidential information can be justified, the justification does not provide a broad license to share it.

Some situations in which the duty to uphold confidentiality is especially important are relatively unusual. Often enough, the answers to questions that arise related to upholding confidentiality or disclosing information are not obvious, and these situations can challenge the doctors who confront them with difficult ethical dilemmas. Because confidentiality issues have not been given as much attention as other more dramatic issues in medical ethics, I provide several examples to illustrate the kinds of situations in which questions about violating confidentiality arise.[18]

Case 3

A 38-year-old woman with advanced AIDS was dying from AIDS-related disease. She was admitted to the hospital after she had collapsed in the subway. She had been traveling from her home in Brooklyn to a doctor visit in the Bronx, a subway trip that usually takes 2 hours. Shortly after her admission, and just before lapsing into a coma, the patient provided the team with the critical points of her medical history, including her underlying disease, the name of her doctor, and the institution where she had been receiving care. She emphatically insisted that she did not want anyone in her family to know her diagnosis. Based on her medical condition and her physical appearance, the doctors at the admitting hospital, which is located in Manhattan at approximately the halfway point in her travel, believed that this would be her final hospital admission.

The patient's boyfriend of many years, her adult children, and her sisters all lived in Brooklyn. They were contacted and informed of the patient's admission. When they arrived at the hospital, they were attentive and concerned. They also claimed to have no knowledge of the patient having any underlying medical problems even though they had noticed that she had been getting very thin.

That said, the team had the sense that the boyfriend was more informed than he let on. Records from the Bronx hospital, where the patient had been receiving treatment for the previous 10 years, did mention that the boyfriend was aware of the diagnosis. Those records also clearly stated that the patient did not want her diagnosis disclosed to her family.

The team appreciated that the family needed to be informed about her condition in order to make decisions about the patient's end-of-life care. The unconscious patient was not able to participate in the decisions, and there was no advance directive to provide information about the patient's preferences.

---

[18] These cases are also useful examples of clinical moral reasoning, the approach to resolving ethical dilemmas that is presented in Chapter 11.

Which medical information should be shared with this patient's family? Confidentiality was obviously important to this patient. Even though there are hospitals and clinics in Brooklyn where she could have received HIV treatment, she chose to repeatedly travel a great distance in order to avoid being recognized and having her secret revealed. The assurance of confidentiality allowed her to accept treatment and enabled her to survive with the disease as long as she had.

Two factors are important to consider in this situation. First, it is not obvious that anyone else's life would be either put at risk or benefited from the disclosure of the information. The patient's sisters and daughters were not at risk of contracting the disease. We also have good reason to believe that the boyfriend was already informed about the patient's disease status. It is therefore likely that either he had been taking disease protection measures throughout his relationship with the patient or was HIV positive himself and possibly also receiving treatment.

Second, the team needed to assess what information the family was entitled to receive and what they needed to know in order to make appropriate decisions on behalf of their loved one. They were not entitled to the information that the patient wanted to have safeguarded by confidentiality, that is, the name of her underlying disease. They did need to know that the patient was dying, and that there was no further treatment that was likely to change her course. Although some interventions might prolong the dying process and extend her life somewhat, they should be informed that there was no expectation that she would regain consciousness. In other words, the name of the underlying disease was not needed for making end-of-life decisions on behalf of this patient. In this case, there was no moral justification for disclosing the information.

Case 4

A 43-year-old woman, employed as a home health aide for an elderly man, was admitted to the hospital with a cocaine-associated myocardial infarction. She had been admitted 3 months earlier with the same diagnosis. There was no grossly evident heart damage from the infarctions.

The inpatient medical team was concerned that the patient's cocaine use exposed her elderly client to harm. They were also concerned that notifying her employer would violate her confidentiality.

Medical professionals are committed to upholding society's trust in the profession. Thus, when the behavior or impaired skills or cognitive function of another medical professional is found to endanger patients, those who discover the problem are obliged to report it to their institution or their local medical board. In such circumstances, confidentiality would have to be violated even though confidentiality would have to be safeguarded in similar circumstances involving a patient who was not a medical professional.

In this case, however, no one was sure about what kind of situation this was. More information was needed in order to know how to proceed. Questions had to be asked and answered because the answer to the disclosure issue lay in the details.

Was this patient a medical professional? No, she was a woman from the neighborhood, a relative of a granddaughter's friend. She had previously worked as a nanny, and as her previous clients' children had grown, she had been looking for a new job when this employment opportunity became available. Once the team was assured that the situation did not involve professional reporting responsibilities, they were able to focus on determining the risks of harm to others.

What was their patient's pattern of drug use? Prior to the two cocaine episodes, the patient had never used cocaine. She now knew better and was too frightened of what could happen to ever try it again. She had smoked marijuana a few times at parties on weekends. She had never purchased it herself, and she had never smoked while taking care of a client. This information gave the team some assurance that their patient was not impaired when she was working.

What was the environment like for the patient's client, and what were her responsibilities with him? The client lived in a house together with several members of his extended family, including adult children and several grandchildren. He needed assistance with activities of daily living, such as feeding, bathing, dressing, taking his medications, and walking in the neighborhood. These added details allowed the team to appreciate that their patient's client was not isolated, but surrounded by loved ones who were able to monitor the care that he was receiving. The team was then in a position to conclude that they had no justification for violating their patient's confidentiality, and they had to protect her medical information.

Case 5

A 23-year-old man with a spinal cord injury was treated for several months after a gunshot injury. Although he would be confined to a wheelchair, his doctors believed that with further rehabilitation he would have greater function and be capable of more independent activity. Recently, he has been refusing to participate in rehabilitation therapy, and he says that he just wants to be left alone. The rehabilitation medicine physician believes that the patient's mother would be able to persuade him to continue with therapy. The patient has refused to allow his doctor to inform his mother that he has been refusing to participate or apply himself in rehabilitation.

In this case, the doctor has both a duty to promote the patient's medical interests and a duty to preserve his confidentiality. The decision about whether to sacrifice confidentiality turns in part on the impact that violating confidentiality will have on this patient's future interactions with medical professionals. His medical condition makes it certain that he will have a lifelong need for medical care. Therefore, it is critical that the patient's trust in medicine not be jeopardized. Two other important considerations are the likelihood of the mother's intervention making a difference and how significant a difference additional therapy would make toward enabling this patient to live independently. It is also important to recognize that this situation does not require an urgent response. Over time and with encouragement, people often do change their minds. Also, a psychiatrist could explore whether the patient is depressed, demoralized, living with mistaken beliefs about what rehabilitation is possible for him, or how his mother will interpret his need for her involvement. Perhaps treatment for depression would make him more amenable to rehabilitation or having his mother more involved in discussions about his treatment. In sum, the certainty of the importance of maintaining this patient's trust in his doctors by preserving his confidentiality coupled with the uncertainty of the need for violating his confidentiality to perhaps create a medical benefit for him add up to the conclusion that his confidentiality must be maintained.

Case 6

After moving to the city with her family, a 24-year-old woman made an appointment to visit her new primary care doctor. When she was asked about her family history, she revealed that she was the eldest of four children, and their father had died of some kind of cancer at age 44. The doctor explained that genetic diseases, including susceptibility to cancer, can run in families. He then recommended genetic testing and genetic counseling.

After completing the testing, the genetics counselor informed the patient that she had tested positive for familial adenomatous polyposis (FAP), an inherited disorder that is characterized by cancer of the large intestine (colon) and rectum. People with the classic type of FAP begin developing multiple polyps, noncancerous growths in their colon, as early as their teenage years. Their condition has to be monitored because the polyps tend to develop cancer.

The genetics counselor further explained that members of her immediate family were also at risk for FAP. They needed to be informed so that they could be tested for the gene. In her follow-up visit with her doctor, he emphatically repeated the urging of the genetics counselor. The patient insisted that she did not want her confidentiality to be violated. She declared that she didn't want her siblings to be told because she didn't want them to know her business, and she didn't want to ruin their lives with the knowledge.

The doctor was inclined to inform the patient's three siblings, who were also his patients. They were all over 18 and at risk for the disease. He saw withholding the information as harming them, so he regarded it as his duty to share the information with them. Two points need to be considered. Will withholding the information actually be harming them? Is there a way to provide the needed testing and monitoring without violating confidentiality?

Harm involves making someone worse off. In this case, no relatives would be made worse off by not revealing the patient's diagnosis; the situation of the other siblings will be exactly what it had been before their eldest sister received her test results. If she were to share her personal genetic information, the communicated information should be regarded as providing her relatives with a benefit. It might be kind for her to share the information, but because no one is at risk of harm from her silence, the doctor has no duty to warn.

The siblings are not aware of their disease risk, and they have either inherited the disease gene or not. As the primary care doctor for the other siblings, the doctor will have the opportunity to ask each of them questions about their family history and offer advice for genetic testing. None of that will violate the eldest sister's confidentiality.

This doctor's initial patient has an ongoing medical need. He will need to periodically monitor her condition, and to do so, he will need her continued trust. Also, as time passes and the shock of the genetic diagnosis wears off, the doctor will have further opportunities to discuss the benefits of sharing her diagnosis with her family, help her to rethink her decisions, and support her in finding a way to communicate what she has learned with at-risk relatives.

A further consideration is the implication of his betrayal of confidentiality. Sharing the eldest sister's information without her permission will inform all of the siblings that doctors violate confidentiality. That revelation would undermine the trust of each of them in doctors upholding their duties. After testing, it may turn out that none of the other siblings has the FAP gene. In that respect, none of them would benefit from the doctor's violation of confidentiality. They would all, however, be harmed by having their trust in confidentiality eroded by the doctor's revelation.

In order for doctors to be able to promote the welfare of their patients, patients have to disclose private information about their history, their behavior, their health, and their habits. Because patients would be reluctant to disclose some of that information (e.g., about drug use, sexual habits, diet) without the assurance of confidentiality, the promise of confidentiality must be upheld as a central tenet of medical ethics. That commitment means that when a patient wants information about a medical condition to be kept private, the physician must accept that position even when the physician considers the choice to be wrong. Although there are some circumstances that justify violating confidentiality (e.g., situations involving impaired physicians or other medical professionals), the bar has to be set very high.

6

Duties to Respect Patients' Autonomy and Assess Capacity

The duties that I have discussed thus far are all rather straightforward and relatively clear. The next two interrelated duties, to respect autonomy and assess decisional capacity, are conceptually more difficult to sort out and explain. The first is acknowledged in most codes of medical ethics, while the second is not mentioned in any. Explaining them and how they are linked to each other will require making conceptual distinctions, sticking to precise use of language, and getting into the weeds of some ongoing philosophical debates.

Respect for Autonomy

The tenth duty of medical ethics is respect for autonomy.
The concept of "autonomy" is a useful theoretical tool of moral philosophy, but it is difficult to comprehend because the concept is used in a variety of applications with significantly different meanings. It is also important to be aware that people often use the term in ways that show little understanding, and even misunderstanding, such as when they speak of "giving someone autonomy" or "taking away" their autonomy. Because autonomy is a capacity that someone either has or does not have, it can neither be given nor taken away. Someone's autonomy can be constrained, for example, if the person is imprisoned or tied up, but even then the person retains the capacity for autonomous action. When physically restrained, liberty or freedom is restricted, but not the capacity for autonomous decision-making and action.

To navigate this subtle but important conceptual domain, it is crucial to recognize and distinguish three related but distinct ways in which the concept of autonomy is employed: (1) the ideal of autonomy, (2) respect for autonomy, and (3) nurturing autonomy. Each of these senses of autonomy has a distinct role in medical ethics that clinicians need to comprehend in order

The Trusted Doctor. Rosamond Rhodes, Oxford University Press (2020). © Oxford University Press.
DOI: 10.1093/oso/9780190859909.001.0001

to understand their moral duties as physicians and identify their professional responsibilities in encounters with their patients.

Autonomy as an Ideal: The First-Person Concept

Autonomy is employed as a first-person concept to describe what Ruth Faden and Tom Beauchamp call a lofty "ideal."[1] In this first-person sense, the concept of autonomy expresses the core content of a person's own moral obligation to the oneself. As an ideal, it shows **me** (first person) just how I should act; that is, it directs me to determine my own actions by the moral laws or the personal commitments that I create for myself. In other words, to be autonomous is to be a good ruler over oneself. To act autonomously is to act from the rules, principles, or reasons that one creates for governing one's own actions. It requires **me** to conform my actions to **my** decision about what to do, to **my** own ideas of what anyone in a situation like mine should do. In that respect, I regard my own actions as instantiating **my** values, **my** commitments, and **my** goals. I see **my** choices in terms of obedience to the rules that I believe should determine the actions of anyone else who is in a similar situation.

Autonomy, in this core Kantian sense, is a lofty standard that I should aim to meet in all of my actions and the criterion for my self-evaluation of what I do.[2] Autonomy in this first-person sense involves my reflecting on the issues involved in my situation, considering my options in terms of my values and moral commitments, making a decision that reflects the ethical standards I embrace, and abiding by the conclusion of my own reasoning.

In this sense, autonomy is a threshold concept. It amounts to the ability to be held responsible for my actions and to be eligible for moral praise or blame for what I do. In the bioethics literature, a number of authors have provided detailed accounts of the several abilities that comprise autonomy.[3-5] Drawing on their accounts, I take it that to be autonomous an individual must have the specific abilities to:

[1] Faden R and Beauchamp TL, *A History and Theory of Informed Consent* (New York: Oxford University Press, 1986).

[2] Kant I, *Foundations of the Metaphysics of Morals* (Indianapolis, IN: Bobbs Merrill, 1959).

[3] Buchanan AE and Brock DW, *Deciding for Others: The Ethics of Surrogate Decision Making* (Cambridge: Cambridge University Press, 1989).

[4] Gert B, Culver CM, and Clouser KD, *Bioethics: A Systematic Approach* (New York: Oxford University Press, 2006).

[5] Appelbaum PS and Grisso T, "Assessing Patients' Capacities to Consent to Treatment," *New England Journal of Medicine* 319, 25 (1988): 1635–1638.

- adopt values, principles, and goals, and continually reconstruct and re-order them in light of changing circumstances and developing moral insights;
- understand the relevant facts of the situation, appreciate their likelihood and significance, and appreciate that they are relevant to the individual and her situation;
- combine those facts with the individual's values, principles, and goals and reach conclusions that make sense;
- communicate a choice and explain the decision with relevant reason;
- constrain one's behavior in accordance with the conclusions about what should be done.

In addition, an individual must also be

- free of a serious volitional disability (i.e., a mental malady or mood disorder).[6]

Respect for Autonomy: A Second-Person Concept

The other two senses of autonomy are involved in explaining how we ought to regard and act toward **others**. Respect for autonomy reflects the appropriate moral attitude toward others who are capable of autono-mous action. As Richard Arneson explained, "The root idea in autonomy is that in making a voluntary choice a person takes on responsibility for all the foreseeable consequences to himself that flow from this voluntary choice."[7] In other words, it is the ability to act autonomously that makes someone a moral agent. That is what distinguishes moral agents from other creatures both human and nonhuman, and that ability requires the actions of moral agents to be treated with respect. When we show respect for the action of a moral agent, we hold them responsible for what they do and the consequences that result from their choices. In sum, we show respect for their choices by leaving them alone and avoiding interference with what they choose to do.

---

[6] Gert et al., 2006, 226–230. It should be noted that these authors use the term "competence" which most bioethicists reserve for legal decisions. As they define it, "competence is the ability to make a rational decision" 226.

[7] Arneson R, "Mill Versus Paternalism," *Ethics* 90, 4 (1980): 475.

In this sense, respect for autonomy is very different from the sense of respect as a social concept that conveys veneration, esteem, or reverence.[8] Respect for the autonomy of moral agents denotes the legal sense of recognizing an individual to be sufficiently "competent" to stand trial and the medical sense of having decisional "capacity" to make medical decisions. We show respect to moral agents and their choices when we hold them accountable for what they do.

Conversely, we recognize that regardless of the harm that their behavior may cause, chickens, wolves, young children, demented adults, and people with profound depression are incapable of taking on responsibility for what they do. It is because they lack autonomy that we don't regard them as moral agents and we don't punish them for their behavior. And, it is because they are incapable of taking on responsibility for what they do that we may interfere with their behavior. In the legal sense of recognizing that a fellow human is not sufficiently competent to stand trial, the court declares the individual to be "incompetent." In medical interactions, doctors identify those who lack decisional capacity and rely on others to make medical decisions on their behalf. In other words, it is a mistake to show respect for the behavior of the incompetent or accept the medical decisions of an individual who lacks decisional capacity.

The idea of respect for the autonomy of others is related to the first-person sense of autonomy as self-rule, but it is a distinct concept that requires us to **presume** that others are acting from the values and principles that they embrace and to leave them alone. In other words, as long as it is reasonable to consider another person to be capable of acting autonomously, we should treat him *as if* he is autonomous by allowing him to make choices for himself and allowing him to live by his own lights.

Moral theorists Immanuel Kant[9] and John Stuart Mill[10] instructed us on how we are to act toward others: We are to respect their choices and the actions that flow from their autonomous decisions and voluntary choices. For Kant, the capacity for autonomous action marks persons as moral agents and distinguishes them from other beings. In this Kantian sense, *person* is a moral term that signifies special moral status and implies that what persons do belongs to the realm of morality. Their actions deserve respect in that they

---

[8] Failing to appreciate the significant difference in these two meanings of *respect* leads to serious confusion on a number of issues in medical ethics.

[9] Kant, *Foundations*.

[10] Mill JS, *On Liberty*, edited by Elizabeth Rapaport (Indianapolis, IN: Hackett, 1978).

may be praised as laudatory or condemned. Beings who are not capable of autonomous action are not persons, so what they do is not judged in moral terms. Because they are not moral persons, bees, vipers, tigers, 4-year-old humans, and demented elderly humans are not blamed for their inappropriate behavior, not even when there are terrible consequences.

According to my reading of Kant, for the most part, we are required to presume that other adult humans are moral persons and acting autonomously unless we have compelling evidence to the contrary. We therefore have to allow them to make their own choices. In other words, respect for autonomy is the ethical default position that we are morally bound to take toward other people and their choices. Typically, we cannot know whether some particular other adult human is in fact reflecting on the issues involved, considering his options in terms of his own values and moral commitments, making a choice that reflects the ethical standards that he embraces as moral laws for himself. Nevertheless, Kant told us that we should adopt the hypothetical attitude of assuming that the other is acting autonomously and treat the individual as if that were the case. He explained that we have

> a duty to respect man even in the logical use of his reason: not to censure someone's errors under the name absurdity, inept judgment, and the like, but rather to suppose that in such an inept judgment there must be something true, and to seek it out.[11]

He instructed us to "cast a veil of philanthropy over the faults of others, not only by softening but also by silencing our judgments,"[12] and to try to find a way of seeing their actions as informed and autonomous. Respect demands that we try to think of what another does as something we also could find reasonable if only we knew the facts of the situation as we try to imagine the other does.

Mill's discussion of respect for autonomy occurs in his famous essay, *On Liberty*.[13] There, he argued to defend individual liberty against government intrusions. According to Mill's "harm principle," limitations on liberty are justified only by harm to others. Respect for autonomy in this Millian

[11] Kant I, *Immanuel Kant: Ethical Philosophy (The Metaphysical Principles of Virtue*; Part II of *The Metaphysics of Morals* [hereafter, *MPV*]), translated by JW Ellington in *Ethical Philosophy* (Indianapolis, IN: Hackett, 1983 [§39, 463] 129).

[12] Kant, *MPV*, [§43, 466] 132.

[13] Mill, *On Liberty*.

sense marks a boundary for law and public policy rather than a standard for judging or interfering with the actions or choices of other individuals. Nonetheless, Mill's concept of respect for autonomy is compatible with Kant's use of the phrase and prescribes the attitude that we should have toward the actions of others.

Physician's Duty to Respect the Autonomy of Patients

The concept of respect for the autonomy of others translates into the physician's duty to respect the autonomy of patients. In terms of common morality and the ethics of Kant and Mill, the duty to respect the choices of patients is explained by the patients being adults who appear to be capable of making autonomous decisions and taking responsibility for their actions. The justification for doctors' distinctive duty to respect their patients' autonomy is somewhat different, and the content of the doctor's duty is also somewhat different from the responsibility that other people have in their everyday lives.

Most people, most of the time, want to do things their own way, and they want to decide what to do for themselves based on what they regard as best under the circumstances. People tend to become angry or at least annoyed when others try to impose their will and make them do things that they choose not to do, and people tend to avoid others who are likely to force things on them. Because patients need to trust their doctors to take seriously their views on what is best and not impose a different view on them, doctors must respect their patients' values, priorities, and choices.

Because doctors want to help their patients, they must avoid actions that would give them a reputation for imposing unwanted treatment on their patients. Without assuring patients that their refusal of offered interventions will be respected, patients would be less likely to seek or accept their care. Thus, respect for a patient's autonomy can mean that a surgeon will have to accept a patient's refusal of a surgical intervention that would leave the patient with an ileostomy and the refusal of a blood transfusion by a patient who is an observant Jehovah's Witness. Without the trust that the doctor will yield to the patient's choice, the patient who refuses the ileostomy would not be able to rely on the surgeon to perform the alternative surgery (e.g., a J-pouch), which in this patient's case would be more likely to involve complications than the ileostomy. And without trust, the patient who refuses the transfusion would not be able to rely on the doctor to employ other life-preserving interventions that might enable the patient to survive without receiving blood.

Nurturing Autonomy: Another Second-Person Concept

The third sense of autonomy is nurturing autonomy. This concept is also other-regarding, but it provides direction for how we should treat those who, in some way, lack autonomy. When autonomy is absent, individuals' choices and what they do should not be blamed or praised because they are not morally responsible. They are incapable of autonomous action primarily because of insufficient cognitive development, a natural or induced cognitive impairment, or a volitional impairment. Children; the demented; individuals who are intoxicated, in the grips of psychosis, a phobia, or a mood disorder, or even a cognitive bias may be exempt from moral disapprobation precisely because their acts are not autonomous. The fact that someone lacks autonomy does not give anyone license to treat that individual rudely or callously. It does show that we recognize their behavior as ineligible for moral censure and, more importantly, that their expression of preferences does not merit the respect that autonomous choices must be accorded. Even while we are morally obliged to treat those who lack autonomy politely and with caring concern, we should not unquestioningly yield to their preferences. Instead, we must regard their likes and dislikes with some hesitation and be prepared to intervene to protect them from harming themselves or others.

The duty to nurture autonomy is addressed to those others who presently lack autonomy globally, for some specific decision, or about some particular matter but who, presumably, might be autonomous in the future. This concept of nurturing autonomy is less recognizable than the concepts of self-regulating autonomy and respect for autonomy. It even lacks a standard label and slips into discussions under the mantle of other concepts. Nurturing autonomy frequently is subsumed into discussions of paternalism, and because the term *paternalism* connotes immoral authoritarian overreaching and is a contentious feature of the liberal agenda, champions of liberalism only mention it sotto voce.

In the tradition of liberal political philosophy, however, the need to create citizens who are capable of reason-guided, self-controlled action justifies measures that are aimed at nurturing the capacities that are essential for autonomous action.[14] Even Kant discussed the obligation to inculcate the habits that will make human beings into autonomous persons. Indeed, for Kant, a person needs moral instruction to the extent that he is ignorant of duty and incapable of taking duty as his end.[15] And John Rawls, the twentieth-century's leading philosophic champion of liberalism, also argued for cultivating the abilities and habits (i.e., virtues) that would allow citizens to be autonomous.[16]

Nurturing autonomy is a distinct other-regarding, future-oriented concept that directs us to create, restore, or preserve autonomy, in the first-person sense, for others who we cannot presently presume to be fully autonomous or who we cannot presume to be autonomously confronting a particular decision. Because this concept rests on the judgment that the other is not presently autonomous but has the potential for future autonomy, it presents a justification for intervention, what has been called "soft paternalism."[17]

Physicians' Duty to Assess Decisional Capacity

Although nurturing autonomy is a duty for everyone in their interaction with children, it rarely comes into play in interactions with other adults. In fact, the general duty to regard other adults as if they are acting autonomously and to respect their choices means that we seldom interfere with what others do. If we try to intercede, we open ourselves to criticism of being condescending or patronizing.

The determination of capacity, however, becomes an especially critical issue in medical ethics because of physicians' commitment to acting for the patient's good and their fiduciary relationship to their patient. An autonomous person defines her values for herself in her own terms. She creates her own rankings of her priorities among those things that she considers to be "good," and she makes her choices in ways that reflect the things that she prizes, cherishes, and esteems. Physicians should respect those values and comply with the choices of patients who have decisional capacity.

[14] Berkowitz P, *Virtue and the Making of Modern Liberalism* (Princeton, NJ: Princeton University Press, 1999).

[15] Kant, *MPV*, [§49, 477] 145.

[16] Rawls J, *Political Liberalism* (New York: Columbia University Press, 1993).

[17] This is a more general, and therefore more useful, concept than the reigning models for justified paternalism offered by Gerald Dworkin, in terms of future-oriented consent, and Harry Frankfurt, in terms of higher order desires.

When a patient's decisions threaten the patient's life or function, however, it becomes the physician's responsibility to assess the patient's decisional capacity. Instead of going as far as possible to presume that a patient is acting autonomously and respecting the patient's choices as if they were autonomous and leaving them alone. Physicians have the opposite responsibility. It is the physician's duty not to presume, but to actually assess the patient's decisional capacity. And when a patient's autonomy is found to be impaired, and to the extent justified, the doctor is ethically required to intervene and act to promote the patient's interests.

While in ordinary life people are obliged to presume, as far as possible, that others are autonomous, features of medical decisions and patients make medical decisions a different matter. Often, medical decisions are very serious; life or function may be on the line. Often the consequences of a medical decision are enduring. Furthermore, impairment of decisional capacity is far more likely in medical situations than in everyday life. A patient may be under a cloud of depression, in a state of euphoria, or in the grips of fear or be experiencing hallucinations. Mood disorders and psychosis impair judgment. A patient may be in denial, repressed, or simply operating with judgment distorted by a variety of psychological biases. A patient's reasoning may be impaired by a disease state, drugs, pain, or fear. At the very time when clear judgment is needed, decisional capacity is vulnerable, and patients may be decisionally incapacitated. All of this amounts to the fact that medical decisions can be significantly different from other decisions. Thus, when a patient refuses a clinically important medical intervention, distinctive features of the medical situation make it appropriate, and actually a professional responsibility, for clinicians to assess the patients' decisional capacity.

Assessing Patients' Decisional Capacity

The eleventh duty of medical ethics is to assess patients' decisional capacity. Judgments about decisional capacity in the clinical practice of medicine tend to make doctors uncomfortable precisely because making such judgments is at odds with common morality, and doctors often miss making the diagnosis that a patient lacks decisional capacity. This may be due to their lifelong habituation to presuming that other adults are acting autonomously. It may also be related to medical school training in the four principles approach to bioethics, which often leaves trainees with an oversimplified and distorted understanding of respect for autonomy.[18] Yet, the evaluation of patients' inability to make a particular medical decision is so clearly a medical responsibility that it is given its own term. In philosophy and ordinary parlance, we speak of autonomy, but doctors determine a patient's lack of decisional capacity, and when the matter has to go to the courts, the judge can declare a patient to be incompetent.

A patient's capacity to accept recommended treatment is rarely challenged. That is as it should be because ethical regard requires others to presume that an adult can make decisions that reflect her own values. In contrast, a patient's capacity to refuse recommended treatment should be questioned and assessed, particularly when there are significant consequences to the refusal of treatment and when most reasonable people would accept the treatment. Although these contrasting responses of accepting the decisions of patients who agree with medical recommendations and challenging the decisions of those who refuse recommended care may seem confusing or even appear ethically inconsistent, the distinction is well justified. When patients' choices are consistent with their welfare, the duty to respect their autonomy requires a charitable attitude that presumes the patient to be making an autonomous decision. When patients' preferences are likely to subvert their welfare, physicians' duty to promote the benefit of patients requires an assessment of capacity and willingness to intervene to the extent justified.

Buchanan and Brock discussed a "decision-relative variable standard" of decisional capacity.[19] I take their remarks to express the two points that I have been trying to make. The more detrimental it would be to a patient to refuse treatment, the more robust his demonstration of autonomy must be. Refusals of treatment that involve few and insignificant negative consequences for patients should not require them to demonstrate autonomy. This variable standard should *not* be taken to mean that there are degrees of autonomy. Someone either has the ability to take responsibility for a particular decision or lacks it.

Inherently, a determination that an individual patient lacks the capacity to make some particular decision or any medical decision at all is accompanied by consideration of whether it might be appropriate to impose an intervention on the patient, including one that the patient clearly prefers

---

[18] The failure to identify impaired decisional capacity has been reported. Sessums LL, Zembrzuska H, and Jackson JL, "Does This Patient Have Medical Decision-Making Capacity?" *Journal of the American Medical Association* 306, 4 (2011): 420–427.

[19] Buchanan and Brock, 60–61.

not to have. In ordinary life, outside of medical situations, except for the most extreme circumstances, such as coming across someone standing on a high-floor window ledge apparently on the verge of jumping off, questioning another's autonomy or imposing something on another over her objection would violate the standard moral rule of respect for autonomy. Yet, the assessment of a patient's decisional capacity is an important medical responsibility.

Even though it is fair to assume that every adult knows to take prescribed medications, exercise, and avoid smoking cigarettes, when a patient's behavior shows inadequate appreciation of those facts, a doctor may assume that the patient's thinking with respect to that issue is impaired. Denial or repression may be involved. In such cases, an appropriate physician response may involve imposing something that the patient would prefer not to have, such as reminding the patient to take medications, to exercise, or to stop smoking. Coming from an acquaintance or an employer, that prodding would be paternalistic and probably rude. When spoken authoritatively by a doctor, it is accepted as professionally required, and it is often effective in helping to modify the patient's behavior. Studies have shown that admonitions, even mild recommendations, or just handing a patient a pamphlet can lead a patient to change behavior. Because such paternalistic interventions can achieve significant benefits for the patient, and because the interventions do not impede liberty, they are well justified.[20]

Although doctors typically prefer to characterize their admonitions as "education," their reminders and repetitions are paternalistic. In that the physician's words, scowls, or encouraging smiles are used to promote the good of patients, and in that they are often imposed when the physician has reason to believe that they may be unwelcome, they are properly termed acts of paternalism. Paternalistic interventions span the entire range from verbal reminders, to nudges, to bringing in the patient for extra office visits, to encouraging a patient to bring a family member along to an appointment, to urging a patient to stay an extra day in the hospital, or to imposing a medical intervention in opposition to the patient's stated preferences. The more serious and enduring the imposed paternalistic intervention, the more justification it requires. In other words, reminders and encouragement are

[20] Center for the Advancement of Health, "When Doctors Tell Patients to Quit Smoking, They Listen," *Science Daily* May 1, 2008. Accessed August 27, 2018, at https://www.sciencedaily.com/releases/2008/04/080430205039.htm

often justified because they are fleeting and do not physically interfere with a patient's liberty.

The importance of physicians' assessment of capacity, coupled with doctors' discomfort and common morality engendered tendency to avoid paternalistic interventions, make the development of a clear understanding of the concepts of autonomy and respect for autonomy crucial elements of medical decision-making. Furthermore, physicians need a clear understanding of these concepts to give them confidence in sorting out how to respond when they suspect that a patient may lack the capacity to make a decision that needs to be made. A two-step procedure is involved. First the patient's decisional capacity should be assessed. The more serious and enduring the consequences of refusing a medical intervention are, and the more urgent the need for the intervention, the more important it is for the doctor to ensure that the patient's refusal is autonomous. When the medical decision has to be made quickly and when the patient's refusal of the recommended intervention is likely to have terrible consequences while acceptance of the treatment is likely to produce a beneficial outcome, physicians should require the patient to demonstrate robust decisional capacity and explain why they find the proposed treatment unacceptable. Without providing reasons that make sense of the choice, the patient should not be judged capable of making the decision. A doctor will have to determine whether the patient lacks decisional capacity globally or whether the problem is more situational and related to the decision at hand. Although all licensed physicians have the authority to make the determination that a patient lacks decisional capacity, when there is significant doubt, a consultation with a psychiatrist may be in order. If the patient is found to have capacity, then, out of respect for autonomy, the patient's choices to forgo a treatment should be accepted, but that finding does not rule out revisiting the issue and continuing the discussion. When the patient is found to lack the capacity to make some specific critical decision, it is the physician's duty to ask an available surrogate to decide on behalf of the patient, and when no surrogate decision maker is available, to treat the patient in opposition to an expressed preference.

If the patient is found to lack capacity globally or for the specific decision that has to be made, the second step involves a determination of the paternalistic measures that may be imposed in the face of the patient's refusal. In dire and urgent circumstances, when the patient is incapable of making the necessary treatment decision, the doctor must determine the course that serves the patient's interests and act accordingly. This is medical paternalism, but it is justified by the absence of decisional capacity and the degree and likelihood of the harm that will be suffered. The more drastic the proposed intervention, the stronger the justification must be. It is relatively easy to justify verbally urging or encouraging a patient to stop smoking because that sort of paternalistic intervention (i.e., words, encouraging smiles) is not particularly drastic or enduring. And when a patient refuses the standard of care and the difference between the best and nothing is not very significant, there is little justification for imposing a test or a treatment even when the patient clearly lacks decisional capacity. The decision to take a patient to surgery without consent is harder to support. It may, however, be justified by meeting two conditions: (1) the patient's inability to demonstrate the capacity to refuse the intervention with clear and coherent reasons and (2) a life-threatening emergency and the substantial likelihood of providing a significant benefit with treatment.

For patients whose decisional capacity is impaired only with respect to some particular object (e.g., cigarettes, needles, surgery), the doctor's unwanted intervention is only justified with respect to that particular object. For patients with impairment of a limited scope or duration, the doctor's overall goal should be to nurture or restore the patient's capacity. In such cases, to the extent that treatment can be delayed, it should be postponed until the patient's decisional capacity has been restored.

Assessing Decisional Capacity: Cases to Consider

Some cases will help to clarify the implications of the duty to assess decisional capacity and the types of nuanced differences that require different responses. Doctors' duty to respect patients' autonomy means that they have to accept the choices of their patients who have decisional capacity. At the same time, doctors' fiduciary responsibility commits them to safeguarding their patients' well-being and overriding expressed preferences that expose patients to significant danger when the preference does not arise from an autonomous choice. Inherently, the determination that a patient is making an autonomous choice or lacks decisional capacity will be the critical issue in answering questions concerning whether it is appropriate to impose unwanted interventions and treat a patient in opposition to expressed preferences.

Case 1

J. F. was brought to the emergency department by the police after collapsing in pain in a nearby subway station. A scan revealed a large aortic aneurysm, and bypass surgery was strongly recommended. If the aneurysm should burst, he was expected to bleed out and die. If he should have the surgery, a period of rehabilitation and lifelong blood-thinning medication would be necessary.

J. F. had been a boxer, and his face and ears showed signs of that career. He had significant hearing impairment, which made it difficult to communicate with him. His condition was explained to him several times, and he seemed to understand. Nevertheless, J. F. refused to have the surgery. When he was questioned about his refusal, he offered no reasons for refusing, saying that he never really wanted surgery, and that he doesn't like taking medicine. He repeatedly declared that he wanted the doctors to just let him be. He wanted to leave the hospital because he was feeling better.

J. F. reported that he received the same diagnosis of his condition some time ago at the Manhattan Veterans Affairs (VA) hospital. When contacted, the VA records confirmed his story. The aneurysm now does not seem much larger than it was 6 months ago. The VA had no record of any next of kin, and J. F. said that he has no relatives or close friends.

J. F. provided several different addresses for his residence, but none of them actually exist. He said that he had to go home and feed his dogs. He gave inconsistent answers about how many dogs he had and what their names are.

Should the doctors involved provide bypass surgery over J. F.'s objections?

The lack of insight into his condition and his inconsistent responses that do not square with reality indicate that J. F. lacks decisional capacity. Nevertheless, surgery should not be imposed over his objections because it is highly unlikely that he would comply with the postsurgical rehabilitation or the required blood-thinning medication. Under these circumstances, it is unreasonable to expect that bypass surgery would provide a significant enough benefit to justify forcing the treatment on him. Furthermore, when there is no emergent need for treatment, as in this case, the court must be petitioned to determine whether or not the patient is *competent*—a legal determination—and decide whether the treatment may be imposed over the patient's objection. Without the legal determination, and lacking the emergency justification for proceeding without a court decision, imposing unwanted treatment on J. F. would be unlawful and amount to battery.

Whereas many details of this case are unique, the pattern of a cognitively impaired patient refusing beneficial medical interventions arises in many different settings. Often the promised benefits of treatment are neither significant nor likely enough to justify imposing them on an unwilling patient.

- There is the emotionally compromised patient who steadfastly refuses to continue hemodialysis. Because liberty is an important value, indefinitely constraining his freedom in order to provide renal dialysis treatment cannot be justified.
- There is the disagreeable and difficult patient with chronic obstructive pulmonary disease who refuses to take care of himself and continues heavy smoking and drinking while taking prescribed medication only intermittently. He may not be denied his liberty so that a safer routine can be imposed on his life.
- There is the previously discussed patient who has been inhaling cocaine for years, causing the destruction of the cartilage separating the nasal passage from the orbit and causing repeated eye infections. When she comes into the hospital for intravenous antibiotics, she complies with treatment and she keeps her post hospitalization scheduled appointments, but she refuses to enter a drug treatment program. She should not be forced to enter a program because she appears to have decisional capacity, because there is no urgent need for treatment, and because enrollment in a treatment program does not promise a likely and significant benefit for a reluctant patient.

Case 2

N. K. is a 26-year-old female patient who presents to the operating room for scoliosis repair. She is otherwise healthy, and her preoperative hematocrit is 39%. She is a Jehovah's Witness, and she refuses to have any blood or blood products during or after the surgery. She has been fully informed of the likely outcomes, and she is willing to cooperate with any treatment that does not involve receiving blood.

Although N. K.'s religious commitments are not mainstream, many people rely on faith and religion to guide their lives. Because the inclination to accept religious beliefs is so common, we extend the presumption of autonomy to people who make decisions based on long-held religious values. In this case, it is important to explore N. K.'s religious beliefs more fully. Do they form an important part of her identity? Have these commitments been long standing? People sometimes take a position to impress their audience, so it is important to ask these questions in a private interview and ascertain whether she is prepared to accept death rather than violate this belief. When her doctors conclude that N. K. has decisional capacity and that refusal of blood is an element of N. K.'s core values, her refusal of the blood transfusion should be honored.

Even though this is not a life-preserving intervention, N. K. and her doctors regard the scoliosis repair to be in her interest. As long as the decision to accept the increased risk of death that transfusion refusal entails, the decision to undergo the repair expresses N. K.'s priorities. The choice of a patient who has decisional capacity must be respected when it involves a request for an intervention that falls within the range of reasonable risks. Similarly, the refusal of treatment by a patient who has decisional capacity even life-preserving treatment) or a decision to discontinue a treatment that is already being administered (even when death is likely to result) must be respected.

Furthermore, N. K.'s trust that her physicians will respect her choice allows her to accept all of the recommended interventions that do not entail blood products. That assurance provides her with significant benefits. The confidence that unwanted treatment will not be imposed on patients also extends across society, and it allows people of faith and people with strong personal priorities to accept medical treatment with the confidence that it will be provided on their terms. Trust in physicians' commitment to respect patients' autonomous decisions allows patients, for example, to accept medical treatment (e.g., for appendicitis or gangrene) with the assurance that the rejected surgery will not be performed.

That said, whenever a physician decides to question a patient's choice and assess the patient's capacity to refuse treatment, paternalistic intervention is contemplated. Consider this more nuanced case:

Case 3

C. J. is a 76-year-old woman who arrives in the emergency room complaining of pain in her lower abdomen. She is diagnosed as having a strangulated hernia and told that surgery is urgently necessary. Without it, she will die within hours. Because her overall medical condition is quite good for a person her age, the doctors assure her that the surgery is likely to be successful, and that they expect her to have a full recovery after a brief hospital stay.

C. J. responds that she was not prepared for having surgery today, and that she will be going home. When she is questioned about why she is choosing not to have surgery when it is expected that she will die very soon without it, she replies, "It's not your business." When she is asked about why she wants to go home and whether there is something there that she has to do, she responds defensively, "It's not your business." When the doctors press her with the question, "Do you want to live?" she again answers, "It's not your business." She refuses to provide any more of an explanation but remains adamant in her refusal of surgery.

Even though C. J. can speak, the little that she says does not suggest that she fully understands her situation or that she is acting from coherent reasons. She is alone, and the need for surgery was not expected. In this circumstance, she may be overwhelmed by fear of surgery. She may be in denial. Her medical condition may be impairing her cognitive function. In any case, her decision is highly unreasonable because she has a great deal to lose by refusing surgery. Also, she has not explained her refusal by offering personal values or facts about her situation that could suggest that her choice was reasonable.

Because surgery is likely to provide this patient with a great benefit and withholding surgery is likely to result in her imminent death, she would have to demonstrate her capacity to refuse the intervention by showing her doctors robust evidence of her decisional capacity. She would have to provide an explanation that was coherent and persuasive in showing that refusing surgery was consistent with her values. Because of the urgency of the situation and the significant doubts about her decisional capacity, it is reasonable to err on the side of life and conclude that C. J. lacks decisional capacity. If there is time, psychiatry should be consulted, and if not, C. J. should be anesthetized and taken to surgery.

Determining that a patient lacks decisional capacity is sometimes clear and obvious. Patients who are obtunded, hallucinating, or delirious clearly lack decisional capacity. Decisions for them should be made in accordance with their advance directives or previous wishes, if known, or by their court-appointed guardian or the person with the highest standing on the state surrogacy list. In an emergency situation when no surrogates are available, the doctors involved should proceed with treatment.

Sometimes, however, determining whether a patient is capable of making an autonomous choice is a challenge.

Case 4

S. K. is a 32-year-old woman. Seven months ago, she was diagnosed with ulcerative colitis and treated medically. A month ago the condition returned with a vengeance. This time, the medical treatment was not effective. As the only alternative to colostomy, her physician referred her to a gastroenterologist who was pioneering a new treatment with cyclosporine and steroids. After a week on the new treatment, it was clear that it was not effective in S. K.'s case. Surgery was now urgently necessary to avoid a ruptured bowel. S. K. had lost a lot of weight and was down to 80 pounds. Several times and at great length over several days, her medical doctors and surgeon carefully explained the morbidity and mortality of a ruptured bowel and the surgery that was required. After each discussion, S. K. responded, "I can't decide."

What should her physicians conclude about S. K.'s capacity to make a medical decision in this urgent situation? It may be tempting to presume her statement means that she is refusing the recommended surgery. As I see it, S. K. is actually reporting insight into her lack of capacity for making the needed decision, and someone else will have to be the decider because, as she recognizes, she is unable to decide.

Many of us have been in situations where we cannot decide. Being unable to decide is real, and it can be a distressing predicament. But being unable to decide which item to choose on a menu, what to wear to a party, or even which of two attractive job offers to accept are very different from the decision that S. K. faces. Her doctors need the courage to conclude that she lacks the capacity to make the decision that is before her. If time allows, psychiatry could be involved to help S. K. overcome her decisional paralysis. If not, either a surrogate or her physicians will have to make the decision on her behalf.

Another situation where decisional capacity ambiguity arises involves patients who reverse their previous treatment decision. In those cases, it may be hard to determine which choice should be respected. Patients are certainly free to change their minds, but it is important for the doctor to assess the soundness and consistency of the reasons behind the new decision. Is the patient now overcome by fear or denial, or has the patient come to a better understanding of the implications of the prior choice? To assess the patient's capacity, the physician will need to ask the patient to explain why what previously appeared to be the better option now seems to be the worse option.

There are many occasions in which a patient's treatment decisions should not be overridden and when paternalism is not justified. Even if the patient's choice is not one you would want your patient to make, and even if the choice may lead to an earlier death than the recommended treatment would, an autonomous decision should be respected.

Case 5

M. R. is a 28-year-old pharmacist and mother of an 8-month-old baby boy. Her husband is also a pharmacist. Five years ago she had been treated for carcinoma of the breast. Six months ago she was diagnosed with metastatic disease that has been unresponsive to treatment. She has spent most of these last 6 months in the hospital, where she has been supervising her own medication. The disease has spread to her lungs and her bones. Yet, despite her extreme pain, she and her husband have been refusing pain medication in fear that it might suppress her respiration and cause her to die.

For the past three nights, M. R. has been unable to sleep because of constant coughing. She has just telephoned her husband and told him that she cannot continue any longer, and that she will ask for a morphine drip. He accepts her decision.

Although there are many circumstances in which a patient who chooses to die seems to show a lack of decisional capacity, there are also many circumstances in which such a decision is an autonomous choice and a reasonable response to the patient's situation. This is clearly such a case. It is, therefore, a medical responsibility to support M. R.'s decision. Even though it is clear to M. R. and her husband, as well as the medical team, that the morphine drip will hasten M. R.'s death, her doctors should provide the requested morphine to ease her pain and allow her suffering to end.

In other end-of-life situations where a patient still has a good chance of surviving with a good quality of life for months or years, the autonomy of a sudden decision to discontinue treatment may be more uncertain. In such a case, it may be appropriate to consider whether the patient's decision reflects some transient mental state, depression, demoralization, or settled values. These questions should be raised, and the patient's decisional capacity should be assessed. When the patient's remaining life expectancy with or without treatment is brief because continuing treatment (e.g., on a ventilator) is not likely to provide a significant benefit, it is hard to justify refusing to comply with the request to discontinue treatment even when there are lingering questions about the patient's decisional capacity.

The Concept of Autonomy and Creating Physician Duties

At this point, there is a tangential issue that I want to raise. The ideal of autonomy plays another critical role in medical ethics. It explains the moral force that creates the duties that physicians assume. No one has to become a doctor. Applying to medical school is a voluntary choice, so are entering medical school, participating in all of the stages of training, as well as the decision ultimately to take an oath or accept a license to practice as a physician. The choices to don a white coat and sign one's name followed with the letters MD are all voluntary.

When a person chooses to become a doctor, in that decision she commits herself to acting in accordance with the ethics of medicine and resisting the inclinations to behave in ways that would violate those professional standards. The commitment to abide by the rules of medical ethics comes from the voluntary choice to be a doctor. In that decision, and the acts that publicly proclaim it, a person autonomously accepts the responsibilities of being a doctor and binds herself to abide by the duties of a medical professional in her future actions and from then on to direct her character in ways that support the fulfillment of her profession obligations.

Because she autonomously accepts the responsibilities of being a physician by making a promise to fulfill them, she then has all of the duties that are incorporated into that role. Ethically, her choices, actions, and character are to be governed by her commitment, and henceforth, until she sets aside the professional role she has freely undertaken, she is morally bound to abide by the ethics of medicine by her free choice to join the profession.

Conclusions About Autonomy and Medical Ethics

As I have tried to explain, the concept of autonomy is a central moral concept in medical practice. The autonomous commitment of physicians to join the profession constrains their future actions by requiring doctors to abide by the ethics of medicine. The voluntary choice that doctors make to guide their actions by the rules of medical ethics allows patients and society to trust doctors to wield their special powers and privileges in their service.

The duty to respect patients' autonomy is a central moral obligation of the profession because it allows patients to trust that their personal values will be honored when they accept a treatment that a doctor offers. At the same time, assessing decisional capacity is also a critically important medical responsibility. Because of the profound consequences of some medical decisions, and because fear, misconceptions, pain, physical and somatic disease, medication, drugs, mental disorders, and mental illness can all effect judgment, physicians must assess patients' decisional capacity and sometimes oppose patients' stated preferences, sometimes in order to restore a patient's autonomy and sometimes to provide a significant benefit or prevent a serious harm.

Further Thoughts on the Concept of Autonomy

In the contemporary philosophical literature, numerous authors have tried to refine the concept of autonomy and clarify what it means to be a moral agent. They have put forward an array of different accounts, some very similar to others and some that present a more distinctive view of what autonomy entails.

Harry Frankfurt famously maintained that an autonomous action conforms to a higher order volition. He asked us to consider whether we would will ourselves to be guided by the desire that we are acting on. In Frankfurt's view, autonomy is about being the master of one's desires. Someone who is dragged about by desires is a slave to passions and not free.[21] Gerald Dworkin offered a similar account of autonomy that uses the concept of future-oriented consent. In determining whether you or another is acting autonomously, Dworkin asked you to imagine whether the agent would be happy with her decision tomorrow.[22]

Christine Korsgaard relied on a Kantian notion of autonomy. She explained autonomous action as the acts that are considered and reflectively endorsed.[23] For her, an impulsive or thoughtless choice is not autonomous. Only an action that has been duly considered, evaluated, and found to be something that a person would not consider wrong when done by another in similar circumstances would count as autonomous and worthy of respect.

Several authors have explained autonomous action in terms that suggest being true to oneself or consistent with one's values, goals, and commitments. Bernard Berofsky used the terms *self-authorization, self-realization,* and *self-expression* to explain that someone acts autonomously when his action coheres with his view of who he is.[24] Similarly, J. David Velleman explained autonomous action as an expression of identity.[25] For him, an action is autonomous when I can identify myself with the action and when it fits with how I describe myself as self-narrator of my life. In Marina Oshana's account, an action is autonomous when there is an absence of alienation.[26]

Each of these views has something to it that rings true, but also has some shortcomings. For example, Frankfurt's higher order desire model and Dworkin's future-oriented consent model work well with the Jehovah's Witness whose priorities are clear and fixed or the parents who volunteer to be living organ donors for their child because doing what is best for their

---

[21] Frankfurt HG, "Freedom of the Will and the Concept of a Person," in Christman J, editor, *The Inner Citadel: Essays on Individual Autonomy* (New York: Oxford University Press, 1989: 63–76).

[22] Dworkin G, *The Theory and Practice of Autonomy* (New York: Cambridge University Press, 1988).

[23] Korsgaard CM, "Reflective Endorsement," in Korsgaard CK, editor, *The Sources of Normativity* (New York: Cambridge University Press, 1996: 49–89).

[24] Berofsky B, "Identification, the Self, and Autonomy," in Paul EF, Miller FD, Paul J, editors, *Autonomy*, (New York: Cambridge University Press, 2003: 199–220).

[25] Velleman JD, "The Self as Narrator," in Christman J and Anderson J, editors, *Autonomy and the Challenges of Liberalism: New Essays* (New York: Cambridge University Press, 2005: 56–76).

[26] Oshana MAL, "Autonomy and Self-Identity," in Christman J and Anderson J, editors, *Autonomy and the Challenges of Liberalism: New Essays* (New York: Cambridge University Press, 2005: 77–97).

child is always most important to them. When an agent is more ambivalent and then makes a choice, it's not at all clear that the higher order volition or future-oriented consent models are useful. Thus, many of our actions and choices do not fit neatly into the Frankfurt and Dworkin schemes. If pressed, they might conclude that choices reflecting ambivalence are not autonomous. That stand would go too far in the direction of excluding adult actions from responsibility.

Korsgaard's view also seems too demanding. Although we may carefully deliberate about what to do when we face difficult dilemmas, most of what we do throughout the day is far more spontaneous. Most of the actions we perform are not carefully considered in terms of moral rules that we might reflectively endorse. Ultimately, this neo-Kantian view appears to set too high a standard and to exclude most of what we do from counting as autonomous.

Berofsky, Velleman, and Oshana's views seem to have the opposite problem. Instead of limiting the actions that merit respect, they would excuse actions from responsibility whenever the agent subsequently denied identity with them. According to their positions, whatever I do when I'm not feeling myself couldn't be counted as autonomous, and I could not be blamed for those actions. That response seems far too cavalier.

Perhaps the concept of "autonomy" does not fit one narrow definition and trying to describe what is essential to agency or what an autonomous decision is does not account for the full range of human experience. Rather, autonomy appears to be a nest of concepts with a family resemblance, and the broad array of voluntary choices that people make may reflect different senses of autonomy. People who are in control of their choices, actions, and wills are autonomous, they can be held responsible for what they do, and their decisions are worthy of respect.

7

Medicine's Commitment to Truth

Truth-telling is the twelfth duty of medical ethics.
The tenth duty of medical ethics obliges doctors to respect their patients'
autonomy by being truthful with them. That obligation is derived from the
fact that patients are not likely to trust their doctors and accept their care unless doctors commit themselves to allowing patients to make decisions about
the medical care that they will accept or refuse in light of their own values,
commitments, and goals. Truth-telling is a corollary of the duty to respect
patient autonomy.

Physicians are obliged to be truthful and provide their patients with the information that they will need in order to conduct their lives according to their
own values. In other words, to allow patients to make autonomous decisions,
patients need to know their diagnosis and prognosis even when there are no
medical decisions that turn on the information. A patient's choices about
spending or saving money, where to live, what job to take, which personal
commitments to take on, and so forth may turn on information about their
medical condition. Patients need to know because the information may be
relevant to their own responsibilities and goals, and the physician has no
way of knowing what those are or how they might be related to the patient's
diagnosis, prognosis, or other medical information. Patients who have information about their medical condition may change the ranking of their
priorities, and without the information patients may opt for different options
than what they would have selected if they had been informed.

Again, the chief medical justification for the duty to respect a patients' autonomy is trust, and the same reasoning supports the duty of truth-telling.
Patients need to trust that their physician is providing honest and ample information for making the decisions that they need to make. Without being
able to rely on the report of one's physician, patients are left in a quandary
of not knowing what to believe or not knowing if the doctor's statements

The Trusted Doctor. Rosamond Rhodes, Oxford University Press (2020). © Oxford University Press.
DOI: 10.1093/oso/9780190859909.001.0001

exaggerate or minimize the facts. For example, when a patient is unable to trust a doctor's optimistic report that a lumpectomy for breast cancer is likely to be curative, she may leap to the conclusion that her actual prognosis is death and therefore refuse curative surgery and its burdens for what she mistakenly imagines to be no benefit. And when a patient doubts the veracity of a physician who cautions her to take a medication daily or not to remove bandages for a several days, she may rashly ignore the advice and do things that cause her harm.

The trust in physician veracity is fragile, and secrets or lies have a way of coming out.[1] When physicians withhold information from patients, over time, the facts are often revealed. This frequently occurs because many different medical professionals are engaged in a patient's care, and, particularly as staff changes, some of those involved may not be fully cognizant of which information is supposed to be shared and what is intended to be kept secret and from whom. Furthermore, the nature of disease often makes efforts to withhold a diagnosis or prognosis futile. As disease progresses, patients increasingly feel ill. Then they reasonably conclude that the doctor who left them with a false understanding of their condition either was not very bright or was lying. Both of those insights can be expected to undermine trust in their physician.

In addition, trust in physician veracity is jeopardized by what patients learn from one another. British physician Roger Higgs has explained that patients tend to share their medical experiences with friends and acquaintances.[2] In today's world of social media, those reports can be transmitted widely and rapidly. To the extent that an experience of being deceived by a physician is shared with others and, in turn, their entire network of acquaintances, other patients' trust in the truthfulness of physicians is compromised. Eroded trust undermines the effectiveness of medicine because without trust patients are less likely to seek help from doctors and less likely to follow their recommendations. As philosopher Sissela Bok explained, "Trust and integrity are precious resources, easily squandered, hard to regain. They can thrive only on a foundation of respect for veracity."[3]

By now, many US doctors have come to the conclusion that truth-telling is required in communication with patients, and that is the official message

---

[1] Bok S, *Lying: Moral Choice in Public and Private Life* (New York: Pantheon, 1978).
[2] Roger Higgs, "On Telling Patients the Truth," in Lockwood M, editor, *Moral Dilemmas in Modern Medicine* (Oxford: Oxford University Press, 1985: 621–627).
[3] Bok, *Lying*, 63.

presented in US medical training.[4-8] It has not always been the case. Prior to the mid-nineteenth century, withholding serious information from patients was standard practice. In fact, Connecticut physician Worthington Hooker, writing in 1849, was one of the first to advocate for the radical idea of avoiding lies and sharing serious news with patients who asked pointed questions.[9] Until not too long ago, many doctors believed that it was their duty to protect their patients from the painful truth. From the mid-nineteenth century until late in the twentieth century, the question of whether doctors should be committed to truth-telling was open for debate. For instance, in the 1985 Hollywood film, *Cat on a Hot Tin Roof*, the admirable family physician, Doc Baugh, withheld the information from his patient, Big Daddy, that his medical workup revealed inoperable metastatic cancer, and that Big Daddy did not have long to live. In fact, Doc Baugh had told Big Daddy that he had a spastic colon, and he was otherwise fine. When questioned about the deception by Big Daddy's son, Brick, Doc Baugh explained that he was obliged to do so by "medical ethics."

Why Some Doctors Avoid Truthful Disclosure: Three Physician Reasons

According to Sissela Bok,[10] physicians offer three arguments to support withholding bad news from patients. They maintain "that truthfulness is impossible; that patients do not want bad news; and that truthful information harms them."[11] Although patients cannot understand all of the physiological and medical details the way doctors who have received intensive clinical

[4] Sisk B, Frankel R, Kodish E, and Isaacson JH, "The Truth About Truth-Telling in American Medicine: A Brief History," *The Permanente Journal* 20, 3 (2016): 74–77.

[5] Rich BA, "Prognosis Terminal: Truth-telling in the Context of End-of-Life Care," *Cambridge Quarterly of Healthcare Ethics* 23, 2 (2014): 209–219.

[6] Sarafis P, Tsounis A, Malliarou M, and Lahana E, "Disclosing the Truth: A Dilemma Between Instilling Hope and Respecting Patient Autonomy in Everyday Clinical Practice," *Global Journal of Health Science* 6, 2 (2014): 128–137.

[7] Bruera E, Neumann CM, Mazzocato C, Stiefel F, and Sala R, "Attitudes and Beliefs of Palliative Care Physicians Regarding Communication With Terminally Ill Cancer Patients," *Palliative Medicine* 14, 4 (2000): 287–298.

[8] Sisk BA, Bluebond-Langner M, Wiener L, Mack J, and Wolfe J, "Prognostic Disclosures to Children: A Historical Perspective," *Pediatrics* 138, 3 (2016): e20161278.

[9] Hooker W, *Physician and Patient; or, A Practical View of the Mutual Duties, Relations and Interests of the Medical Professions and the Community* (New York: Baker and Scribner, 1849).

[10] Bok, *Lying*.

[11] Bok, *Lying*, 293

training and decades of clinical experience can, physicians with the requisite communications skills for clinical practice, who have genuine sympathy and the imagination to appreciate the experience that lies ahead for their patients, who devote enough time and make a sincere effort to honestly share the relevant information, should be able to convey all that their patients need to know in order to make their treatment and life decisions. Furthermore, a 2014 study by Nancy L. Solowski and colleagues found that cancer patients are even able to understand concepts and statistics about their patient-specific survival that are presented in an online program by Prognostigram, and 39 of the 40 patients who were interviewed found the information to be useful.[12] So, while it may be impossible to share everything that the physician knows about a patient's medical condition and treatment options, truthful and honest communication is feasible.

The other standard objections, that patients do not want bad news and that truthful information harms them, have been debunked by empirical findings. For example, a 2001 study of 337 patients by Robert J. Sullivan, Lawrence W. Menapace, and Royce M. White found that the vast majority of patients stated that they want to know about their condition (99%). They also thought that physicians had an obligation to inform patients of their condition (99%), and they would want to be told if they had a life-threatening illness (97%).[13] Another 2001 multicenter study by Val Jenkins, Lesley Fallowfield, and Jacqueline Saul with a heterogeneous sample of 2,331 patients showed that 87% (2,027) wanted **all** possible information, both good and bad news, and 98% (2,203) preferred to know whether or not their illness was cancer.[14]

A 2015 study by Jonathan Pugh, Guy Kahane, Hannah Maslen, and Julian Savulescu with 200 lay participants found that "respondents supported fully informing patients about distressing medical information in different contexts, especially when the patient is suffering from a chronic condition."[15] Similarly, a 2018 study by Nicola Oswald et al. showed that patients want to know about not only their diagnosis, but also how to recover and cope with

[12] Solowski NL, Okuyemi OT, Kallogjeri D, Nicklaus J, and Piccirillo JF, "Patient and Physician Views on Providing Cancer Patient-Specific Survival Information," *Laryngoscope* 124, 2 (2014): 429–435.

[13] Sullivan RJ, Menapace LW, and White RM, "Truth-telling and Patient Diagnoses," *Journal of Medical Ethics* 27, 3 (2001): 192–197.

[14] Jenkins V, Fallowfield L, and Saul J, "Information Needs of Patients With Cancer: Results From a Large Study in UK Cancer Centres," *British Journal of Cancer* 84, 1 (2001): 48–51.

[15] Pugh J, Kahane G, Maslen H, and Savulescu J, "Lay Attitudes Toward Deception in Medicine: Theoretical Considerations and Empirical Evidence," *AJOB Empirical Bioethics* 7, 1 (2016): 31–38.

issues once they have gone home after surgery.[16] Furthermore, a systematic literature review of 22 studies of cancer patients' preferred decision-making role found that they wanted a more shared or an active role versus a less passive role.[17]

These findings, that people actually want to be informed about their medical condition, are consistent around the world. Even in Japan, a country that is widely presumed to favor a paternalistic model of medical practice, a 2004 survey of 243 Japanese respondents by H. Miyata et al. found that 69.6% "wanted full disclosure about the diagnosis without delay" while only 26.5% "preferred to have the diagnosis and prognosis withheld."[18] And even among Hispanic patients in the United States, who are also reputed to prefer a paternalistic approach, a 2018 study by Jhosselini Cardenas et al. found that "the majority of patients agreed or strongly agreed that they wanted to hear all of the information regarding their diagnosis (94%), treatment options (94%), treatment expectations (92%), and treatment risks and benefits (96%).[19] And a study of 30 consecutive patients with dementia by Marek Marzanski found that a majority of participants who still had adequate insight "declared that they would like to know more about their predicament." That said, Marzanski remained equivocal on telling the truth to patients.[20]

While a small percentage of patients say that they do not want to know serious medical information, this sampling of the literature provides robust evidence that most patients do want to know. Because doctors are required to guide their practice by scientific data, the findings of these studies suggest that physicians should accept the recommendations that these studies provide: The numbers indicate that truth-telling should be regarded as a duty in medical practice.[21]

[16] Oswald N, Hardman J, Kerr A, et al., "Patients Want More Information After Surgery: A Prospective Audit of Satisfaction With Perioperative Information in Lung Cancer Surgery," *Journal of Cardiothoracic Surgery* 13, 1 (2018): 18.

[17] Tariman JD, Berry DL, Cochrane B, Doorenbos A, and Schepp K, "Preferred and Actual Participation Roles During Health Care Decision Making in Persons With Cancer: A Systematic Review," *Annals of Oncology* 21, 6 (2010): 1145–1451.

[18] Miyata H, Tachimori H, Takahashi M, Saito T, and Kai I, "Disclosure of Cancer Diagnosis and Prognosis: A Survey of the General Public's Attitudes Toward Doctors and Family Holding Discretionary Powers," *BMC Medical Ethics* 1, 5 (2004): E7.

[19] Cardenas J, Infante P, Infante A, Chuang E, and Selwyn P. "Decisional Control Preferences in the Hispanic Population in the Bronx," *Journal of Cancer Education* 9 (2018 February): 1–6. Emphasis added.

[20] Marzanski M, "Would You Like to Know What Is Wrong With You? On Telling the Truth to Patients With Dementia," *Journal of Medical Ethics* 26, 2 (2000): 108–113.

[21] American Medical Association, *Informed Consent: Code of Medical Ethics Opinion 2.1.1.* Accessed August 28, 2018, at https://www.ama-assn.org/delivering-care/informed-consent

It is clear that, despite the evidence, some physicians remain reluctant to provide patients with the truth about their diagnosis or prognosis,[22] and they are sometimes hesitant about sharing the risks of recommended medical interventions.[23] They worry that the information will upset the patient and therein do more harm than good, even though, as far as my search of the literature has shown, no evidence of a pattern of harms related to truth-telling exists. Yet, as Lesley Fallowfield, Val Jenkins, and H. A. Beveridge argued, well intentioned "ambiguous or deliberately misleading information may afford short-term benefits while things continue to go well, but denies individuals and their families opportunities to reorganize and adapt their lives towards the attainment of more achievable goals, realistic hopes and aspirations."[24]

In a similar vein, American sociologist and palliative care physician Nicholas A. Christakis reported that when serious information is withheld, patients may make medical choices that they would not have made in light of the information and communicate mistaken information to loved ones that leaves them no time to say their goodbyes.[25] Nevertheless, psychotherapist Averil Stedford found that most of the patients who she treated for disease-related anxiety management and adjustment disorders had not receive honest information about their disease.[26] An article from 1960 by Bo Gerle, Gerd Lundén, and Philip Sandblom found that of 101 patients with inoperable tumors, those who had not been told the truth about their condition had the highest drug use, anxiety, and depression.[27] Also, psychologists have shown that most people adapt rather quickly to serious news, whereas enduring uncertainty is harmful.[28,29]

[22] Annas GJ, "Informed Consent, Cancer, and Truth in Prognosis," *New England Journal of Medicine* 330 (1994): 223–225.

[23] "Truth Telling in Clinical Practice" [Editorial], *The Lancet*, 378, 9798 (2011): 1197.

[24] Fallowfield LJ, Jenkins VA, and Beveridge HA, "Truth May Hurt But Deceit Hurts More: Communication in Palliative Care," *Palliative Medicine* 16, 4 (2002): 297–303, 2297.

[25] Christakis NA, *Death Foretold* (Chicago: University of Chicago Press, 1999).

[26] Stedford A, *Facing Death* (London: Heinemann, 1984).

[27] Gerle B, Lundén G, and Sandblom P, "The Patient With Inoperable Cancer From the Psychiatric and Social Standpoints. A Study of 101 Cases," *Cancer* 13 (106- November/December): 1206–1217.

[28] Hamilton JG, Lobel M, and Moyer A, "Emotional Distress Following Genetic Testing for Hereditary Breast and Ovarian Cancer: A Meta-Analytic Review," *Health Psychology* 28, 4 (2009): 510–518.

[29] Oberguggenberger A, et al. "Psychosocial Outcomes and Counselee Satisfaction Following Genetic Counseling for Hereditary Breast and Ovarian Cancer: A Patient-Reported Outcome Study," *Journal of Psychosomatic Research* 89 (2016 October): 39–45.

In addition to the harms that patients may experience in their personal lives, withholding information is likely to have destructive effects on the physician-patient relationship and augment the burdens on patients:

- When people are engaged in a deception, they try to avoid disclosure of the truth. Distancing helps protect the deceit, but distancing also deprives the patient of the comfort of the doctor-patient relationship.
- Information that is withheld, as well as outright lies, tends to leak out. When the information is revealed, the patient will have to deal with two problems: the information and a deceitful physician. The deceit-related problem is iatrogenic, that is, it is caused by physician behavior and entirely avoidable. It is a betrayal of trust and a gratuitous harm inflicted on a patient by the physician.
- When patients learn that they were deceived by their doctor, they are rightly angry at having been treated like a child and manipulated. Most people experience anger as a burden, and they would prefer to avoid it as they deal with all of the other difficult emotions associated with a serious illness.
- When a physician withholds information and leaves the patient to figure out the bad news on his own, the patient also gets the message that the physician is unwilling to discuss the matter. That leaves the patient to struggle through without the benefit of the physician's knowledge, support, and guidance.

Why Some Doctors Avoid Truthful Disclosure: A Psychological Explanation

The powerful evidence that patients actually want to know their medical diagnosis and prognosis and findings that withholding information can be harmful, coupled with doctors' persistent fears about disclosing the information, calls for another kind of explanation to explain physicians reluctance about forthcoming communication. The 1970s work by Daniel Kahneman and Amos Tversky established that human errors in judgment often arise from heuristics and biases.[30] Building on their work, psychologists Timothy

---

[30] Tversky A and Kahneman D, "Judgment under Uncertainty: Heuristics and Biases," *Science* 185, 4157 (1974): 1124–1131.

D. Wilson and Daniel T. Gilbert[31-37] and others[38-43] have demonstrated that our judgments about what our future mental states will be are contaminated by a variety of different psychological distortions that they termed *affective forecasting*. Their studies with normal volunteers provided robust evidence that we are all vulnerable to the distortions of affective forecasting.

In these studies, the researchers asked subjects to predict their own future emotional responses to a particular event. The vignettes that they used were taken from the common experiences of university students and faculty. For example, subjects were asked to predict how they would feel if their favorite sports team won or lost a game, if their preferred candidate won or lost an election, if they were offered or turned down for a job, or if they were granted or denied tenure. When the event actually occurred, the same subjects were asked to report their reactions and the predicted responses were compared with the actual responses. The comparisons showed that people were frequently off target in estimating their future reactions.

Gilbert and Wilson discussed a number of elements related to affective forecasting. When people imagine their future reactions, they tend to focus on some specific feature of the future outcome. That singular focus allows them to overlook concomitant aspects of their life in the future and thereby exaggerate the importance of that singular element. Gilbert and

[31] Wilson TD and Schooler JW, "Thinking Too Much: Introspection Can Reduce the Quality of Preferences and Decisions," *Journal of Personality and Social Psychology* 60, 2 (1991): 181–192.

[32] Wilson TD and Brekke N, "Mental Contamination and Mental Correction: Unwanted Influences on Judgments and Evaluations," *Psychological Bulletin* 116, 1 (1994): 117–142.

[33] Wilson TD, Wheatley T, Meyers JM, Gilbert DT, and Axsom D, "Focalism: A Source of Durability Bias in Affective Forecasting," *Journal of Personality and Social Psychology* 78, 5 (2000): 821–836.

[34] Gilbert DT, Brown RP, Pinel EC, and Wilson TD, "The Illusion of External Agency," *Journal of Personality and Social Psychology* 79, 5 (2000): 690–700.

[35] Gilbert DT and Ebert JEJ, "Decisions and Revisions: The Affective Forecasting of Changeable Outcomes," *Journal of Personality and Social Psychology* 82, 4 (2002): 503–514.

[36] Gilbert DT and Ebert JEJ, "Decisions and Revisions: The Affective Forecasting of Changeable Outcomes," *Journal of Personality and Social Psychology* 82, 4 (2002): 503–514.

[37] Dunn EW, Wilson TD, and Gilbert DT, "Location, Location, Location: The Misprediction of Satisfaction in Housing Lotteries," *Personality and Social Psychology Bulletin* 29, 11 (2003): 1421–1432.

[38] Arntz A, "Do People Tend to Overpredict Pain? On the Asymmetries Between Underpredictions and Over-predictions of Pain," *Behaviour Research and Therapy* 34, 7 (1996): 545–554.

[39] Taylor S and Rachman S, "Stimulus Estimation and the Overprediction of Fear," *British Journal of Clinical Psychology* 33, Pt. 2 (1994): 173–181.

[40] Buehler R and McFarland C, "Intensity Bias in Affective Forecasting: The Role of Temporal Focus," *Personality and Social Psychology Bulletin* 27, 11 (2001): 1480–1493.

[41] Taylor S and Rachman S, "Role of Selective Recall in the Overprediction of Fear," *Behaviour Research and Therapy* 32, 7 (1994): 741–746.

[42] Mitchell TR, Thompson L, Peterson E, and Cronk R, "Temporal Adjustments in the Evaluation of Events: The 'Rosy View,'" *Journal of Experimental Social Psychology* 33, 4 (1997): 421–448.

[43] Sieff EM, Dawes RM, and Loewenstein G, "Anticipated Versus Actual Reaction to HIV Test Results," *American Journal of Psychology* 112, 2 (1999): 297–311.

Wilson labeled this sort of distortion *focalism*. A related problem arises in people's estimation of how intense a future feeling will be and how long it will last. People systematically overpredict the intensity and duration of their emotions and exaggerate their negative emotional reactions most markedly.[44] This distortion is called *durability bias*. People also fail to take into account how much their own psychological "immune system" will ameliorate their response to negative events. People are remarkably able to adjust their thinking to accept reality. Also, denial and repression are powerful mechanisms of mental life that help us cope with whatever befalls us. Yet, even in the face of personal experience to the contrary, we tend to ignore our ability to cope and thus fail to take it into account in predicting our future affect. This distortion is termed *immune neglect*. Taken together, these findings show that people have a remarkable ability to adjust to whatever happens, but they often fail to recognize just how resilient they are.

While these studies all focus on people making exaggerated predictions about their own future feelings, two articles, one by Monique M. H. Pollmann and Catrin Finkenauer and another by Jeffrey D. Green and colleagues, dealt with people making predictions about how others will feel.[45,46] They called this bias *empathic forecasting*. In the Pollman and Finkenauer studies, friends were asked to forecast their own and their friend's affective experience for four positive and four negative emotion-eliciting events (e.g., win $10,000 in the lottery, fail an exam). People overestimated their own and their friend's positive and negative affective experience. In sum, they found that people committed the impact bias for themselves and others, and they did so to the same extent for themselves as for others. In fact, they noted that "empathic forecasts more strongly resemble the pattern of affective forecasts than the patterns of affective experiences, even if the affective experience is readily available in people's memory when making the empathic forecasts."

---

[44] Gilbert and Wilson have also found that people have exaggerated expectations about the intensity and duration of their response to positive events. They have found that the affective forecasting bias is, however, more extreme in the reaction to negative outcomes than positive outcomes. Because of its relevance to truth-telling, in this discussion, I focus only on the reaction to negative outcomes. Although some doctors are occasionally reluctant to share good news with patients out of a desire to encourage healthy habits, doctors do not typically withhold good news.

[45] Pollmann M and Finkenauer C, "Empathic Forecasting: How Do We Predict Other People's Feelings?" *Cognition and Emotion* 23, 5 (2009): 978–1001.

[46] Green JD, Davis JL, Luchies LB, et al., "Victims Versus Perpetrators: Affective and Empathic Forecasting Regarding Transgressions in Romantic Relationships," *Journal of Experimental Social Psychology* 49, 3 (2013): 329–333.

Medical situations can be strikingly different from situations in which people on college campuses find themselves and from nonmedical interpersonal relationships. Although these psychological studies on affective and empathic forecasting did not include medical examples and made no claims about their application to medicine, they do offer an explanation of the phenomenon of physicians' reluctance to disclose serious information to patients. Once we recognize that affective forecasting is part of normal human psychology, we are alerted to consider just who in the medical environment is susceptible to its effects. Appreciating that affective forecasting and empathic forecasting are normal human distortions should alert us to how these biases play out in the judgments of patients, clinicians, family members of patients, and even policymakers.

We can recognize the effect of affective forecasting in patients' reluctance to hear a serious diagnosis and prognosis. A patient who is in denial or one who focuses on some untoward consequence or unlikely risk is likely to refuse treatment or fail to comply with a treatment regimen. While a denier may fail to appreciate the need for the intervention, a patient who is in the grip of focalism is likely to have a distorted overestimation of the costs and risk involved in treatment (e.g., the scar, the disability, the hair loss) because the burdens are magnified and the benefits to be had are overlooked or minimized. Focalism contributes to patients' exaggeration of the negative impact on their emotional well-being, and durability bias inclines them to exaggerate how long their bad feelings will persist. Immune neglect inclines them to fail to appreciate how well they are able to adjust to new and even dreaded circumstances. Some patients may avoid seeing a doctor out of a distorted fear of not being able to bear hearing bad news, while others may avoid disclosing problems or symptoms to their physician out of augmented anxiety over being rejected for complaining. Such biased reactions show the effects of affective forecasting, and the combined impact of these distortions can lead patients to make unreasonable judgments about their own capacity to accept the facts.

Without explicitly identifying the affective forecasting phenomenon, doctors actually display awareness of the tendency by encouraging their fearful patients to take some time to reconsider, return for another office visit along with a family member, discuss the matter with friends, or speak with other patients who have had to deal with a similar medical condition. Again, without explicitly noting that affective forecasting can be overcome with cognitive behavioral therapy (CBT), these interventions play the role of CBT and help patients overcome their exaggerated anticipation of overwhelming despair and arrive at reasonable decisions.

Appreciating that empathic forecasting is as pervasive a phenomenon as affective forecasting should also alert us to how this bias can have an impact on others in ways that are particularly relevant to this discussion of physicians' attitudes toward truth-telling. Because of their vulnerability to the empathic forecasting bias, doctors are likely to fear that their patients will be overcome by serious news and unable to handle it. They tend to exaggerate the duration of their patients' bad feelings (how devastated they will feel living without a breast) and ignore the full context of their lives, which are likely to go on without any dramatic transformations. They also tend to overlook their patients' ability to cope with whatever happens (e.g., receiving a diagnosis of cancer). When a physician considers that a particular patient may be unable to cope with bad news, it is therefore important to consider just why that seems to be the case and whether affective forecasting may be distorting the judgment.[47]

Extrapolating from studies of empathic forecasting, we can predict that the feared fallout from giving bad news is likely to be less dramatic and more short-lived than doctors expect because doctors' prediction of patients' reactions are exaggerated and patients' powerful coping mechanisms are overlooked. Yet, because of these common distortions in estimating patients' future responses, doctors reach unjustified and negative conclusions about their patients' emotional responses to future events in the same way that other mortals are likely to distort their predictions of other people's affective reactions.

The ubiquitous phenomenon of biased estimates of anticipated emotional reactions tends to make doctors' decisions about sharing medical information with patients irrational. Empathic forecasting distortions lead doctors to regard sharing serious news as destroying hope and courting disaster and incline them to lie, speak in ways that obscure understanding, or withhold information to avoid harming patients.

In sum, empathic forecasting seems to account for the fact that even though truth-telling is a critical duty of medical ethics, withholding the truth from patients remains all too common.[48] Numerous studies showed that doctors still

---

[47] Empathic forecasting can also incline some physicians to become overly concerned that speaking frankly will lead a patient to reject them in favor of another physician who will be more guarded and dissembling.

[48] Surbone A, "Persisting Differences in Truth Telling Throughout the World," *Support Care Cancer* 12, 3 (2004): 143–146.

are not as forthright as patients want them to be.[49] This is true around the world and even in the United States. For example, a 2012 US study by Jane C. Weeks et al. showed that 69% of 710 patients with incurable lung cancer and 81% of 483 patients with colorectal cancer who received palliative chemotherapy were unaware that their treatment was not intended to be curative.[50] A 2015 Dutch qualitative study by Janine de Snoo-Trimp et al. revealed that some physicians are still reluctant to share information for the same old reasons.[51]

What Should a Patient Be Told?

Most of today's US physicians say that they endorse shared decision-making with their patients, and in response to the question, "What has the patient been told?" will respond, "Everything." By everything, they typically mean all that a patient needs to know has been shared. That answer sounds straightforward and simple, but it is surprisingly vague. Physicians have vastly different views on what everything includes. Does everything mean telling as much as the physician considers sufficient, or does it require sharing all of the immediate and long-term consequences? Does the duty to inform patients dictate how and when the truth should be told? Does it imply sharing only as much as the patient asks to know now and leaving the rest for later? Does telling everything mean that doctors must provide the diagnosis and prognosis even when there is no treatment? Does it mean that numbers have to be used (e.g., number of years, percentages), or are descriptive adjectives sufficient? Does it require revealing incidental findings? Does it mean that small details should be shared when surgery is recommended, such as the number of days following a procedure that the patient will need to forgo showering?

Ethically, patients need to be informed about anything that the physician (or her agents) will be doing to the patient. This is important so that the patient may be prepared for what is to come and so that the patient can make a decision about whether or not to accept the intervention (e.g.,

---

[49] Anderlik MR, Pentz RD, and Hess KR, "Revisiting the Truth-Telling Debate: A Study of Disclosure Practices at a Major Cancer Center," *Journal of Clinical Ethics* 11, 3 (2000): 251–259.

[50] Weeks JC, Catalano PJ, Cronin A, et al., "Patients' Expectations About Effects of Chemotherapy for Advanced Cancer," *New England Journal of Medicine* 367 (2012): 1616–1625.

[51] De Snoo-Trimp JC, Brom L, Roeline H, Pasman W, Onwuteaka-Philipsen BD, and Widdershoven GAM, "Perspectives of Medical Specialists on Sharing Decisions in Cancer Care: A Qualitative Study Concerning Chemotherapy Decisions With Patients With Recurrent Glioblastoma," *Oncologist* 20, 10 (2015): 1182–1188.

examination, diagnostic study, treatment, surgery). The 1990 Federal Patient Self-Determination Act as well as state laws also require patients' informed consent for any treatment or test. Anything that is done to a patient who has decisional capacity without the patient being fully informed can therefore be illegal as well as immoral.

To make an informed decision, it is most important for the patient to understand the rationale for accepting it. So, the physician has to explain *what* it is being offered, *why, when, where,* and *by whom.* Then the patient has to understand the risks of the procedure and the alternatives, including the alternative of what will happen if the condition is not treated. While it may not be feasible to go through all of the risks in detail, it is important to explain those that are most likely (and their likelihood), most serious (and their likelihood), and those that the patient is likely to find most significant (and their likelihood). Truth-telling and eliciting informed consent are ethically necessary for every procedure, not just those that require a signature.

To appreciate the scope of what is not specified by telling everything, consider an example. When pediatricians and a pediatric surgeon recommend, based on a few case reports and their combined experience with two patients, thymectomy for an adolescent with a diagnosis of myasthenia gravis, does telling everything include sharing the uncertainty about the biologic function of the thymus and its role in adolescent development? The thymus gland seems to have a role in controlling immune function, but neither its operation nor its connection to myasthenia gravis is fully understood. The gland is large during childhood and grows gradually until puberty and then becomes smaller. A recent study in adults suggested that thymectomy may be effective in treating myasthenia gravis.[52] But thymectomy could be more or less effective in adolescents, and it is not known if thymectomy before puberty involves additional consequences. Does telling everything include the explanation that there have been no studies of the effectiveness or side effects of the procedure in adolescents?

It is understandable that the physicians involved are likely to feel uncomfortable about sharing these details with their patient and the patient's parents. Doctors are likely to be concerned that the family will react with dismay and then refuse the procedure that they believe is the best course.

---

[52] National Institute of Neurological Disorders and Stroke, National Institutes of Health, *Myasthenia Gravis Fact Sheet* (NIH Publication No. 17-768). (Bethesda, MD: National Institutes of Health, May 2017).

Those worries can make them hesitant about revealing all of the uncertainties. Appreciating the effect of empathic forecasting could help to allay some of the physicians' fears. Appreciating the importance of developing the communication skills that are needed for sharing serious news and accurately conveying the uncertainty that medical care involves should inform physicians' training and help ensure that doctors are adequately prepared for engaging in the needed conversations.

In more standard situations where physicians know a good deal about what can be expected from a medical condition and its treatment, there is still huge variation in how much detail is and should be shared. It is most important to share those risks that are most likely and their likelihood and those that the patient is likely to consider most significant and their likelihood and to explain that other complications are possible but unlikely. (I keep repeating *likelihood* because, in my experience, that critical element is frequently omitted.) It is also important to inform patients of the untreated natural course of the disease as well as alternative recommended treatments. But should that information include disclosure of the level of evidence behind the recommendations? Should it include information about disagreement in the field over the acceptability of different treatment alternatives? Should it include information about whether a treatment approach that would be an option for a more skilled physician is not offered by the physician who is providing the information and expects to be performing the procedure? I'm suggesting that all of this should be explained because a high degree of transparency is needed to promote trust in physicians' reports and enable patients to rely on and accept recommended treatments.

There is also the question of timing. When does information have to be disclosed? Some information should be communicated as soon as the physician receives it, for example, when timely action may be medically necessary. Sometimes a brief delay, of a day or so, in conveying information can be justified, such as waiting for a more definitive laboratory report, postponing a conversation until the doctor will have time for a thorough discussion, or holding off the talk until the patient can be accompanied by a supportive family member. Because any delay in communication is withholding information, the delay has to be justified. Brief delays of hours or days are easier to justify than longer delays, and withholding serious information for more than the length of a weekend should be a rare exception.

To more fully grasp the implications of truth-telling in the physician-patient relationship, consider the issue as it arises in some typical but challenging situations.

Case 1

M. B., a 52-year-old man, arrives at the Emergency Room with crushing chest pain and shortness of breath. The doctor determines that he is having an acute myocardial infarction (MI), and M. B. is admitted to the hospital's coronary care unit (CCU). Despite intravenous medication, his chest pain persists. The cardiologists believe that he is continuing to infarct myocardium and requires cardiac catheterization and possible coronary stenting or angioplasty.

The patient is awake, alert, and aware of his predicament, but he is quite anxious about being in the CCU and the possibility of needing catheterization. His father had a cardiac catheterization 1 year ago and suffered a stroke during the procedure.

Potential complications of cardiac catheterization include the very small risk of stroke, distal embolism, kidney failure, coronary artery rupture or dissection, MI resulting from the procedure, and a few others. The doctor understands the risks of coronary angioplasty to be as follows: death 0.3%; MI 0.3%; stroke 0.1%; need for emergency bypass surgery 1.2%; life-threatening arrhythmia 0.6%; coronary rupture 1.5%; allergic reactions (e.g., to dye) 0.6%. Should M. R.'s cardiologist share all of these risk profile details with him?

In this case, the cardiologist should explore the details of M. B.'s and his father's medical histories. The doctor may need to investigate whether a heritable condition might be involved that could make stroke more likely than usual or make cardiac catheterization an inappropriate intervention for M. B. The doctor will have to consider the risks and benefits of the alternative interventions to determine which treatment is most appropriate for him. If the cardiologist concludes that cardiac catheterization is the recommended intervention, an explanation of the rationale and disclosure of the specific risks of cardiac catheterization should be provided to M. B. because that is what concerns him most.

It is understandable that his cardiologist may be reluctant to disclose the information and anxious that the information might lead M. B. to refuse the needed intervention. Sharing the information, including the actual percentage chance of stroke as well as further heart damage without the procedure, is important for enabling M. B. to make a reasonable decision. It will also help to preserve M. B.'s trust in the truthfulness and competence of his cardiologist.

In light of the high risk of significant heart damage or death without the procedure, the small risk of stroke, and the ability to minimize stroke damage in the hospital setting, refusing the procedure would be an unreasonable decision. Under the circumstances, it is hard to imagine that a person with decisional capacity and a well-functioning psychological "immune system" would refuse. So, even though the doctor is fearful of M. B's reaction to the information, it all needs to be explained. Understanding how the empathic forecasting bias may be inflating the doctor's worry can help to reassure the doctor in making the decision to be forthright in disclosing the medical information.

As in making the decision about which treatment to recommend, the truth-telling decision should reflect the anticipated immediate and long-term consequences and their probability. It is highly likely that M. B. will need future medical care, including follow-up care from a cardiologist. Trust in his doctors will be necessary if he is to avail himself of the care that he will need, and deceiving him about the risk of his pending procedure could be expected to undermine his trust. It is also unlikely that MB will refuse the recommended procedure once the risks and benefits of the alternatives are explained and his specific concerns are addressed. Therefore, it is clear that he needs to be informed, the numerical details should be provided, his questions should be answered as fully as time permits, and no information that is relevant to his decision-making should be deliberately withheld or minimized.

People sometimes need time to take things in and overcome their fears and aversions. If time permits, the treatment could be delayed so that M. B. could be allowed to come to grips with his situation. Compassionate support from his family and physicians or psychiatric intervention with CBT could help to move the process along.

If his need for intervention turns out to be a medical emergency, and if M. B. should refuse treatment without providing a reason that would make sense of his refusal, it is likely that he would be found to lack the capacity to make the decision. Under the circumstances, it is hard to imagine a sound reason that M. B. could offer to justify a refusal of treatment. He might, however, be overcome by fear or denial and therefore unable to appreciate the risks to his life and health. In such a circumstance, the patient's legal agent or surrogate or, if none was reachable, the treating physician would make a surrogate decision[53] that would authorize the necessary treatment.

---

[53] Almost all states have some sort of surrogacy law that stipulates who may make decisions on behalf of a patient who lacks decisional capacity when medical intervention is needed. In New York State, the relevant laws are the Proxy Law and the Family Health Care Decision Act, which provides a ranked list of authorized surrogate decision makers and also allows two physicians to make treatment decisions in medical emergencies when no listed surrogates are available.

Case 2

B. T., a 20-year-old woman, was involved in a car accident and hit her head. Although she did not suffer obvious injuries beyond a bump, her family physician recommended that she see a neurologist.

The neurologist ordered magnetic resonance imaging (MRI) to rule out any brain injury. The MRI revealed that B. T. has lesions on her brain that are consistent with a diagnosis of multiple sclerosis (MS). B. T. does not have any symptoms of MS, so her condition would be classified as radiographic isolated syndrome (RIS). Patients with RIS are not usually offered medication, but they are routinely followed by a neurologist and by interval MRIs and clinical examinations.

There is only limited treatment for this illness, and the prognosis is indeterminate. Multiple sclerosis is a disease characterized by exacerbations and remissions, and the clinical course is quite variable. The patient may suffer severe disability over the next 5 years or may experience only occasional transient symptoms and no functional deficit over the next 30 years. B. T. does not ask for her diagnosis.[54]

Why might a patient not ask? The patient might presume that if there was anything to know, the physician will tell it. Perhaps no questions occurred to the patient. The patient may not consider it appropriate for a patient to question a physician. The physician might have conveyed the impression that questions would not be welcome; with a more creative imagination, I could go on. Nevertheless, whether or not B. T. asks for her diagnosis and prognosis, the information should be shared. B. T.'s silence does not constitute a request for the information to be withheld.

When the neurologist set up the appointment for sharing the MRI results, it would have been a good idea to suggest that B. T. bring along a family member or friend to the office visit because someone close might raise relevant questions and could later help to remind B. T. of conversation details that she might not recall. In any event, respect and caring should be the guiding considerations for the neurologist during the conversation. As he explains the likely course of the disease and advantages and disadvantages

---

[54] This case was described by Dr. Daniel A. Moros.

of alternative treatments, he will also need to consider how to convey the information.[55] His tone, words, eye contact, body language, and timing will all be important elements in fulfilling his truth-telling obligations. Sometimes, even after a sincere effort to communicate what needs to be heard, a doctor is left with the sense that a patient did not adequately understand what was said. Often enough, the psychological immune system prevents serious news from sinking in immediately. As the Marvin Hamlisch song from the film *The Way We Were* goes, "What's too painful to remember, we simply choose to forget." The failure to remember is far less voluntary than the song suggests, but the doctor may need to formulate a plan for trying again to communicate.

Because B. T. is only 20 years old, this case also raises the question of whether a serious diagnosis should be shared with a young adult, an adolescent, or even a child. In almost every case, truth-telling is the best approach even though the language and the level of detail may be tailored to the child's age and ability to understand. It should be noted that the Ethics Committee of the American Academy of Pediatrics acknowledges that deception or withholding information from children can be harmful, and they recommend truth-telling even about matters such as adoption.[56] Similarly, other pediatric organizations recommend informing children of their HIV-positive status, and they report finding no evidence of psychological or emotional harm for disclosure of HIV status to HIV-positive children.[57] Young patients with a serious diagnosis will need ongoing relationships with medical professionals. They will also have to cooperate with medical interventions along the way. The success of all of those interactions will require that the young patients believe and trust their doctors.

Often parents are reluctant to inform their child of a serious diagnosis and prognosis. Understandably, parents want to do whatever they can to protect their child from any avoidable harms. Understandably, they fear that the information will destroy the child's possibility for finding joy in life and thereby inflict great harm. So, under the effects of the empathic forecasting bias, they

[55] Bailea WF, Buckman R, Lenzia R, Globera G, Bealea EA, and Kudelkab AP, "SPIKES—A Six-Step Protocol for Delivering Bad News: Application to the Patient With Cancer," *The Oncologist* 5, 4 (2000): 302–311.

[56] American Academy of Pediatrics, *When to Tell Your Child About Adoption* (last updated November 21, 2015). Accessed August 28, 2018, at https://www.healthychildren.org/English/family-life/family-dynamics/adoption-and-foster-care/Pages/When-to-Tell-Your-Child-About-Adoption.aspx

[57] Krauss B, Letteney S, De Baets A, Baggaley R, and Okero A, "Disclosure of HIV Status to HIV-Positive Children 12 and Under: A Systematic Cross-National Review of Implications for Health and Well-Being," *Vulnerable Children and Youth Studies* 8, 2 (2013): 99–119.

may prefer to shoulder the burden of keeping the secret without appreciating the untoward consequences associated with that choice.

The next case discussion elaborates on family reluctance to have a loved one informed of a poor prognosis and further explores the untoward consequences of what such a well-intentioned preference might involve.

Case 3

N. V., a 56-year-old woman, was admitted to the hospital with metastatic colon cancer, fever, bleeding, ascites, and nodular densities in her lungs. It is expected that this might be her final hospital admission. N. V. is a recent émigré from Russia. A year earlier, when she was still in Europe, she had undergone surgery to resect the cancer. At that time liver involvement was diagnosed, but the complete extent of her diagnosis was not revealed. She was only told only that her liver was big.

N. V. speaks reasonably good English, and she has the capacity to make decisions. In fact, when her father died 2 weeks before this admission, she was the one who signed his do not resuscitate order.

Her husband and her adult children do not want N. V. to be told that she is dying. They report that "in their culture patients are not told a fatal diagnosis."

Should N. V. be told the complete extent of her diagnosis? Should she be informed of her prognosis? Family members often tell the treating physician that they know the patient far better than the physician does, and that their loved one will lose the will to live if confronted with the truth of the diagnosis or prognosis. Doctors are inclined to regard patients as being unable to bear bad news and are therefore disposed to being convinced, without evidence, of claims by loving family members that their relative should be kept in the dark. Yet, as psychologists have shown, people are inclined to make exaggerated predictions about how others will feel. Those findings should make doctors aware that relatives who are reluctant to have information shared with a patient may be in the grips of the empathic affective forecasting bias. Focalism and the durability bias can lead them to the conclusion that their loved one will not be able to bear any bad news.

This common response from families is frequently bolstered by a politically correct (and frequently trumping) appeal to culture. Family members report that in their culture it is disrespectful to speak with a patient about a serious diagnosis or prognosis. The claim is made by the Spanish, Russians, Greeks, Italians, Croatians, and French, and in fact, by families from almost everywhere in Europe. This claim is commonly made by the Japanese, Chinese, Filipinos, Indians, and in fact, by families from anywhere in Asia. The claim is made by families from all over Africa, the Caribbean, and Latin America. And the claim is made by Orthodox Jewish families from around the world. And because almost everyone in the United States and Australia comes from one of these other continents or groups, family members typically invoke the claim that in their culture patients should not be told bad news. Despite the claims by anxious family members, when this common phenomenon is seen through the lens of empathic forecasting, it looks more like a broadly shared feature of human psychology than an exotic feature of a unique culture.

We are all aware of how vastly different people can be in their preferences. The differences may arise from someone's culture or personal beliefs, reasons, or values, and those differences influence people's choices and priorities. There are also likely to be differences between the preferences of a doctor and a patient. Discrepancies can certainly include differences in how people want their medical information to be communicated. This point suggests that even though studies have shown that the vast majority of people want to know their diagnosis and prognosis, one shouldn't presume how any particular patient will want the communication of their medical information to be done.

Although I have been arguing that most patients want full disclosure of their medical information and that patients should be given the truth, the data tell us that there are a few outlier patients who will not want to hear the truth. Even though truth-telling should be the default position in medicine, when there are reasons to doubt that the truth-telling is in order with a particular patient, doctors can avoid a blunder by asking patients to state their preference. For example, as part of taking a patient's medical history, a doctor can explain that in the course of providing her medical care, information about the patient's condition and how it is likely to progress will be received. The doctor can mention the general fact that different people have different attitudes about the management of their medical information and ask the patient how she would like her medical information to be communicated: Would she want to privately receive the information, have it shared in the company of some family members, or prefer that the doctor just speak with one or some of them?

Even though N. V. lived in a society where bad news was frequently withheld from patients, her doctors have no way of knowing her views of the practice or her opinion on how she wants to be treated. Asking N. V. will provide her answer, and her view should govern how her doctor should proceed. If N. V's preference to be kept informed is elicited before the family makes its request for concealment, they should be informed of her desire and explained that federal[58] and state laws require full disclosure.

If N. V's relatives issue their demand before anyone on the team has the opportunity to ascertain her position, and unless they provide significant evidence to suggest that N. V. is likely to suffer significant and likely imminent harm from the revelation, the team will have to address their psychological reluctance and explain the rationale for truth-telling as well as the legal requirements for obtaining the patient's informed consent to any treatment.

People (including doctors and patients' relatives) are often hesitant about disclosing bad news because they do not know whether sharing the information is the right thing to do. The doctor's role is to reassure them that his experience through years of practice has shown that sharing information is the best course. People should be reminded that secrets have a way of coming out, and as N. V's medical situation inevitably continues to deteriorate, the deception will become obvious. Typically, the deceived party is angered by the deception, and anger is alienating. So just when she needs the support of her family most, there will be distance between them that makes it hard to offer one another comfort.

Furthermore, people (including doctors and patients' relatives) are concerned about not knowing what to say or how to answer patients' questions. They also fear the patients' anger or grief in response to news and are uncertain about how they should react to the anticipated intense emotions. The doctor's role is to relieve the family of these burdens by offering to lead the conversation. He can explain that having communicated serious information innumerable times, he knows how to do it. He can propose that they all sit together with the patient as he explains the situation, describes the remaining options, and answers all of their questions.

---

[58] H.R. 4449—Patient Self Determination Act of 1990, 101st Congress (1989–1990). Accessed December 18, 2018, at https://www.congress.gov/bill/101st-congress/house-bill/4449

At this point, it should also be noted that, in addition to doctors and relatives, patients and policymakers are vulnerable to empathic forecasting distortions. This insight illuminates and explains why patients, young and old, can be reluctant to share their diagnosis, their thoughts, and their concerns with loved ones. They worry about the distress that the revelation will cause and therefore choose to keep secrets. It's likely that such fears are exaggerated by the empathic forecasting bias.

Of more general concern, some policy positions from well-meaning medical associations, advisory committees, and particularly the genetics community might be the result of empathic forecasting bias. . Paternalistic policy statements limit the kinds of genetic testing, or impose elaborate time-consuming procedures before testing, or restrict disclosure of incidental genetic findings for diseases that cannot be prevented or ameliorated (i.e., conditions that are not "actionable") and genetic testing of children for adult-onset conditions,[59] are explained by fears of imposing "the unbearable certainty of knowing."[60] These stands oppose the usual view of geneticists that favor genetic testing and sharing genetic information. The inconsistency exhibits telltale marks of empathic forecasting biases.

Case 4

C. M. is a 74-year-old woman who was diagnosed with schizophrenia 10 years ago. She is paranoid and particularly distrustful of doctors and drugs. With medication she has been able to be maintained at home, where she lives with her daughter. C. M. is brought to the Psychiatry Clinic every 6 months for an examination and to renew her medication prescriptions.

Dr. Williams, a new doctor in the clinic, is taking over C. M.'s care. He reviewed C. M.'s chart in preparation for her visit and noticed that C. M.'s daughter has been administering the antipsychotic medications surreptitiously in her mother's morning juice. Dr. Williams is reluctant to give C. M. any drugs without her being informed of what she is taking and

[59] Rhodes R, "Why Test Children for Adult-Onset Genetic Diseases?" *The Mount Sinai Journal of Medicine* 73, 3 (2006): 609–616.

[60] Burson CM and Markey KF, "Genetic Counseling Issues in Predictive Genetic Testing for Familial Adult-Onset Neurologic Diseases," *Seminars in Pediatric Neurology* 8, 3 (2001): 177–186.

*why the drugs are prescribed. He is particularly concerned because pro-
longed use of the antipsychotic drug causes ataxia. The chart notes report
that C. M. displays some movement disorder, but that she does not seem
to notice, and she has not mentioned it as a problem. Dr. Williams is also
aware that if C. M. discontinues the medication she is very likely to severely decompensate. In that case, Dr. Williams expects that C. M. would
be unable to return to her functional baseline even if the medication was
later resumed.*

Should CM be informed about the medication that is prescribed? Should
C. M. be informed that her previous doctors have been ordering it for the
past 10 years and that her daughter has been administering it surreptitiously?
Dr. Williams wants to do what is right, and in his training he learned that
patients should be told the truth. He recalls a conversation with his peers
about informing a 24-year-old patient that his sigmoidoscopy exam and
recent history suggested a diagnosis of Crohn disease that informed his
thinking about truth-telling. That patient had come to see a doctor because
of abdominal pain, diarrhea, fatigue, and recent weight loss, and while the
discussion had begun with some people voicing concern about causing the
patient undue harm, after someone asked others in the group if they would
want to know, they all concluded that the truth should be told.

Dr. Williams is confident that the duty equally applies to psychiatric
patients even though a diagnosis of mental illness or loss of cognitive function can be received as being worse than other chronic or fatal illnesses. He
rightly recognizes that a 73 year-old widower who lost weight, appeared depressed, wore several sweaters on a warm day, responded to questions repeatedly saying that he couldn't recall, and arrived hours late for his appointment
should be told that he needs to be evaluated for dementia and depression.
Dr. Williams also appreciates that a 19-year-old college student who was
hospitalized following a fraternity hazing ritual when he started shouting
insults to other pledges, yelling at them to stop talking behind his back, and
declaring that he was going to the roof to show everyone that he could fly
should be told that he has schizophrenia.

Truth-telling is an important duty of medical ethics, but it is just one
of many duties. Determining whether the truth should be disclosed to
C. M. requires the consideration of all of the relevant duties in the context of
the specific features of the situation. In this case, it is likely that C. M. would

face imminent and enduring serious harm if the information were disclosed because her paranoia would be exacerbated, and she could be expected to refuse her antipsychotic medications. The anticipated degree of deterioration would make it difficult to keep her at home with her daughter and thus inflict a social harm as well.

C. M.'s situation meets the "therapeutic exception" requirement, which ethically and legally justifies withholding the truth from C. M. When a patient is likely to suffer a significant and imminent medical harm from a disclosure, the anticipated harms may be a good enough reason to delay or withhold communication. A likely irreversible serious deterioration, heart attack, stroke, or suicide attempt would constitute therapeutic exceptions, but, as Roger Higgs explained, these exceptions to the rule of veracity are extraordinarily rare, and each requires a justification.[61]

Trust and respect for autonomy explain the duty of truth-telling. In this case, C. M.'s paranoia about doctors turns the consideration of trust on its head. She is also incapable of making autonomous decisions about doctors and drugs in particular. Because respect for autonomy cannot be an issue when autonomy is absent, concern for C. M.'s interests should direct Dr. Williams to withhold the information. This conclusion illustrates that there are legitimate exceptions to the truth-telling duty.

Case 5

S. D. is a 49-year-old lawyer and mother of three adolescent children. After two gallbladder attacks, S. D.'s primary care doctor recommended surgical removal of her gallbladder. The experienced laparoscopic surgeon explained the alternative surgical options, and S. D. elected to have a laparoscopic cholecystectomy because it would involve less postoperative pain and allow for a faster return to her normal routine.

During the procedure, the surgeon noticed that he had nicked the bowel and repaired the perforation with a stitch. When he had explained the risks and benefits of the surgery and their likelihood to S. D. in his office and elicited her informed consent, he had mentioned the possibility of damage to her intestine, bowel, or blood vessels among the other risks. He had also assured S. D. that laparoscopic cholecystectomy was a safe procedure.

---

[61] Higgs, "On Telling Patients."

Whether or not this injury is technically considered an error, the surgeon who performed the procedure is likely to feel responsible for what happened and, therefore, inclined to do whatever can be done to set the matter right. In such situations, surgeons often prescribe octreotide, an expensive drug that is intended to help in management of a fistula by reducing secretions in the gastrointestinal tract and inhibiting motility, even though its efficacy in healing intestinal fistulas is unproven. In this case, the nicked bowel might not be considered a fistula. This pattern of behavior suggests the depth of the typical surgeon's emotional reaction to errors and relatively small untoward surgery-related outcomes.

At the same time, the surgeon knows that the patient and her family are likely to regard the injury as an error. Regardless of how well patients are informed about possible complications prior to surgery, patients and their families often expect a perfect result. When something goes wrong, people are quick to identify someone to blame. Anticipating the blame and accompanying anger, this case raises the generic question of how a doctor should respond to an error or even a minor problem that was repaired and is unlikely to involve any negative consequences.

A doctor who commits an error is likely to experience two natural reactions. Envisioning the sadness, anger, and recriminations of the patient and family following the error's revelation, the doctor can be expected to want to avoid the disclosure and even avoid interacting with the patient and family entirely. The other natural response to an anticipated hostile attack is to assume a combative defensive posture. Both of these instinctual reactions would be counterproductive and unprofessional. Avoidance will only give the message that something shameful is being hidden, and defensive aggression will confirm that the doctor's culpable behavior made him vulnerable and in need of defense. And, again, if the information about the nicked bowel is withheld, secrets have a way of coming out, and people who have been misled are often furious when they learn of the deception.

Considering an appropriate response from the safe distance of a hypothetical case allows us to develop an ethically appropriate and useful strategy. A doctor's focus should always be directed at benefiting the patient. Engaging his empathic imagination to envision the patient's condition and needs clarifies the goals for the upcoming interaction. An accurate description of what occurred coupled with a clear and honest prognosis conveys that the doctor is honest and trustworthy. In this case, the surgeon can explain that because he noticed the injury and repaired it during the surgery, he believes that no problems will arise. He should also inform S. D. that a leak could develop and apprise her of the possible symptoms that could indicate a problem so that she can report them promptly. He should also assure the patient that he will follow her carefully to monitor the situation and then be especially attentive until he is confident that there are no negative results from the bowel injury.

When more serious errors occur, they can leave patients living with a significant, enduring, and life-altering result. In such a circumstance, the emotions of the doctor, the patient, and the family will be intense, but the ethical response should be guided by the same considerations. The focus should be on what will benefit the patient and trying to help the patient accept the new situation and adjust to it. A forthright report of what occurred, a clear explanation of the physical cause of the ensuing problems, and an honest prognosis convey that the doctor is still trustworthy.

Also, a caring doctor will appreciate that any patient who has a bad outcome from bad luck or an error experiences a loss. People who experience loss and sadness need to be consoled. This insight should direct the physician to attend to the patient's grief and share the patient's sadness. The surgeon's presence and compassion can be a significant benefit under the circumstances. Frequent visits demonstrate caring concern and a sincere effort to achieve the best possible outcome. And the doctor's knowledge of possible resources and interventions that may be of use (e.g., occupational therapy) and information about the resulting condition can help the patient understand and come to grips with what lies ahead.

That said, the temptation for a doctor to run away and avoid interaction with the patient and family in the aftermath of an untoward outcome can be powerful, particularly when it is reasonable to expect that the emotions of the patient and relatives will be extreme. It is natural to want to avoid exposure to their profound sorrow and the experience of being berated, threatened, and despised. Again, it is useful to understand the psychological forces in play. Patients may feel some guilt and anger for having made the choices that they did. Family members may feel guilt for having encouraged their loved one to accept the treatment or guilt for not having done more to protect their relative from harm, even if there was nothing that they could have done. Relatives will want to do whatever they can to make things right, even though there may nothing useful that they can do. The most that a doctor can do in response to their emotional reactions is to allow them to express their anger and misery and to accept the burden of their outbursts in hopes that it may lighten theirs.

In sum, professionalism directs the same course for responding to errors and bad outcomes that may appear to be errors and even errors that are not likely to be noticed by the patient. The recommendation amounts to providing clear and honest information, spending time with the patient, expressing regrets at the outcome, showing compassion, and trying to help the patient achieve the best outcome possible under the circumstance. In spite of hostility during the initial encounters, patients and family members who are treated with caring and respect are likely to recognize that as much as doctors try to avoid errors, they do occur. Also, with attentive interaction, patients and families tend to calm down and come to appreciate their doctor's concern and attention.[62]

Physicians are also morally obligated and legally advised to be honest and frank about errors.[63,64] This duty extends even to circumstances where litigation might result. Patients who have been harmed by medical errors may be left with medical needs and disabilities that require ongoing care. They may also be left with conditions that interfere with their ability to continue to work or in need of assistance with the tasks of daily living. Such patients are entitled to compensation. And to uphold the trustworthiness of the profession, physicians have to be trusted to tell the truth.

Truth-Telling: Broader Implications

Honesty and truthfulness are explicitly mentioned or alluded to in almost every code of medical ethics. These commitments are the bedrock requirement for being trusted and being trustworthy. That is why truthfulness is a

[62] Worries about malpractice lawsuits are common in medicine. In light of those concerns, it is important to recognize that most states have made physician statements about errors immune to litigation. This minimizes legal exposure and largely eliminates legal justifications for withholding or distorting information related to a medical error. It is also important to realize that malpractice lawyers' advice is consistent with the recommendations presented in this chapter. Furthermore, it is useful to note that medical malpractice lawsuits are typically financed on a contingency basis. Unless the harm to a patient is significant and enduring and can be expected to bring a huge settlement, it is unlikely that a lawyer will accept a case.

[63] Gallagher TH, Studdert D, and Levinson W, "Disclosing Harmful Medical Errors to Patients," *New England Journal of Medicine* 356 (2007, June 28): 2713–2719.

[64] Wisenberg BD, "The Best Response to Medical Errors? Transparency," *AAMCNEWS* January 16, 2018. Accessed August 28, 2018, at https://news.aamc.org/patient-care/article/best-response-medical-errors-transparency/

duty for physicians and why doctors must regard their commitment to honesty with reverence as an essential element of a doctorly character. Without truth and honesty, the profession would not be able to maintain society's trust. Doctors need to recognize that it is critically important for doctors and the medical profession to be believed, and doctors need to be aware that every revelation involving a failure in truthfulness or honesty undermines society's trust in doctors and the profession.

Society needs to be able to rely on the truth of doctors' reports in personal matters, such as documenting and justifying absences from work or school, missing airplane flights, or patient needs for special indulgences like using the elevator because of an injury. Doctors' statements are also the basis for insurance, workman's compensation, and malpractice claims. It is important for both claimants and those who ultimately have to pay the bills to be able to trust the words of physicians.

Society also needs to be able to trust the reports of medical professionals in matters that affect the public health, drug development, and biomedical research. Society wants to be able to depend on medical statements concerning hazards such as air or water pollution and health risks associated with behaviors such as smoking. Society also needs to be able to rely on professional claims about the safety of medical interventions like vaccines and the importance of drinking water, brushing teeth, and getting exercise. And in the face of contagious disease threats, society has to be able to accept quarantine directives from medical professionals as well as assurances about when quarantine is unnecessary. Without trust in the honesty and truthfulness of doctors and the medical profession, society would be deprived of its ability to rely on the expertise that medicine can provide, and we all would be worse off for that loss of trust.

Lying and Withholding Information and Other Actions and Omissions in Medicine

This discussion of truth-telling provides an opportunity to shed some light on the ubiquitous and difficult question of how the ethics of decisions not to act should be analyzed. To understand the matter, it is useful to consider an array of other circumstances in clinical medicine where it arises. Aside from decisions about lying and withholding information, the action/omission distinction may appear to make an ethical difference in a broad array of clinical situations involving pain management, responding to patient needs, withholding and withdrawing treatment, responding to peer requests, and so on. Truth-telling is only one instance where the distinction between doing something and not doing anything may appear to be morally significant, but the seeming difference is ethically irrelevant. Allow me to explain.

Truth-telling has been and continues to be a vexing issue in medicine, and the controversy over withholding or disclosing important information to patients is still not entirely resolved. But whatever it is that makes one choice right and the other wrong does not turn on whether the doctor's mouth moves or remains muzzled. When a doctor chooses to perpetuate or promote a false belief by lying or remaining silent, the rightness or wrongness of that decision will not turn on whether it involved an action or an omission.

Responding to patient needs is a constant feature of medicine. Some patients pose risks to physicians, others are difficult to treat, and sometimes attending to a patient's needs can be inconvenient. Although it is perfectly reasonable for a doctor to want to avoid contracting an infectious disease, avoid a threatening patient (think Tony Soprano), or pass up an opportunity to attend the US Open finals, the decision to bow out of treating a patient or transfer a patient may look like doing nothing, but in fact it could be imposing risks and burdens on the patient and colleagues. There are certainly limits to professional responsibility, and risk exposure and even personal life (e.g., a daughter's wedding) can be a relevant consideration. But the rightness or wrongness of the choice will not turn on whether a doctor acts or is inactive, but the facts of the situation.

Pain management is another telling example where the difference between action and inaction my seem relevant but is not. Doctors should make decisions on whether and how to treat pain by assessing the risks and benefits. Unless there is a powerful reason to withhold pain relief, the pain of patients should be treated. But when a doctor fears that opioids could suppress respiration and cause the death of a patient who otherwise would be likely to survive, the doctor should withhold the drug or find another means for pain relief. Again, the moral assessment of what is to be done does not turn on whether the doctor's response involves action or inaction, but the circumstances of the patient who is experiencing pain.

In two recent articles, Lars Oystein Ursin[65] argued with Dominic Wilkinson, Ella Butcherine, and Julian Savulescu[66] over this issue. Wilkinson

---

[65] Ursin LO, "Withholding and Withdrawing Life-Sustaining Treatment: Ethically Equivalent? *The American Journal of Bioethics*, 19, 3 (2019): 10–20.

[66] Wilkinson D, Butcherine E, and Savulescu J, "Withdrawal Aversion and the Equivalence Test," *The American Journal of Bioethics* 19, 3 (2019): 21–28.

et al. maintained that withholding and withdrawing life sustaining treatment are morally equivalent while Ursin noted differences in how withholding and withdrawing treatment are experienced. Ursin emphasized study findings that showed medical professionals and family members' experience of withholding and withdrawing treatment to be markedly different and their regard of these alternatives as having a significantly different moral valence. He concluded that those reactions should be counted as important ethical elements for distinguishing actions and omissions.

Reactions to allocation decisions involving scarce resources, however, demonstrate that other factors may be in play. In transplant organ allocation, transplant teams regularly make decisions to remove patients who devlop infections from the transplant list or classify them as "inactive," which makes the patient ineligible for receiving a transplant organ while they have that status. Transplant teams make those decisions without apparent moral distress, and patients and their family members accept those verdicts as reasonable. Similarly, decisions to discontinue extracorporeal membrane oxygenation (ECMO) are made by medical staff and accepted by family members. These decisions can be regarded as withdrawing patients from eligibility for transplantation or withdrawing a life-prolonging intervention. Yet, these withdrawal decisions are well tolerated by staff and families, suggesting that the reaction is not inherently psychological. In these examples, the withdrawal of eligibility and treatment are governed by formal policies and procedures that are justified, documented, published, transparent, applied to every similarly situated patient, and clearly communicated.

Decisions on which patients to refuse admission to intensive care units (ICUs) are also usually accepted by medical personnel and families who are informed that a patient does not meet the eligibility criteria for similar reasons. Yet, decisions to discharge patients from ICUs when it is likely that their lives could be prolonged, but not improved, by remaining in the ICU encounter the kind of resistance that Ursin described. It strikes me that the difference resides in the failure to establish appropriate policies and procedures rather than human psychology. Wilkinson et al.'s article highlighted this difference. In other words, what Ursin identified as a psychological factor may instead be the result of institutional leaders who are reluctant to institute the necessary policies. Efforts to slip by ICU discharge decisions under a misnomer like "nonbeneficial care" invite dissention and call for challenge.

In sum, I take a deflationary view of the action/omission distinction. As I see it, there may be instances in which a particular action is morally equivalent to inaction; yet, the distinction between actions and omissions per se is not a morally significant matter. In American parlance, it doesn't amount to a hill of beans in any ethical calculus. There are a host of other considerations that account for the rightness or wrongness of action. For the most part, neither the name that we use to identify the action (e.g., lying or withholding information) nor the fact that a person's choice involves moving or remaining still are the deciding factors in our moral analysis. The factors that are morally telling include knowledge,[67] wherewithal, responsibility, and the details of the situation.[68] In every choice about whether to act or not to act, doctors should try to do the right thing.

Much more can be said about the issue of actions and omissions. I elaborate further in my discussion of the interrelated obligations of peer responsiveness, peer communication, and peer scrutiny in Chapter 8, Physicians' Commitments to Fellow Professionals.

[67] I take a broad and inclusive view of knowledge. I count the foreseeable consequences of action and their likelihood among the kinds of knowledge that are relevant to choices about action and inaction.

[68] I am deliberately omitting "intention" from this list. I understand that authors who work on the trolley problem or endorse the principle of double effect consider it morally relevant. I disagree. That is an argument to be sorted out at another time.

8

Commitments to Fellow Professionals

In everyday life, when someone poses the nongendered question, "Am I my brother's keeper?" the expected answer is, "No, I am not." When the question is asked of a physician, however, the answer should be, "Yes, I am." In fact, a physician should recognize that she is her brother's helper, partner, and keeper. That is because physicians' ability to satisfy their responsibilities to society and patients involves satisfying the duties that one medical professional owes to another. These duties include the interrelated obligations of peer responsiveness, peer communication, and peer scrutiny, and they all derive from the commitment to make the profession worthy of society's trust and the commitment to serve the interests of patients and society. Even though these obligations get no attention in either the World Medical Association Declaration of Geneva[1] or the World Medical Association International Code of Medical Ethics[2] and little mention in national medical association codes of ethics, they are recognized by most physicians. Nevertheless, their omission from formal declarations of physician responsibilities and from the standard accounts of medical ethics leaves some doctors unaware that these are important professional duties. That lacuna suggests that these duties must be spelled out and explained to make it clear that they are essential professional responsibilities for physicians.

Peer Responsiveness

The thirteenth duty of medical ethics is peer responsiveness.
Poets and painters can do their work on their own, and they may even choose not to work at all. Medicine, however, requires collaboration, cooperation, and performance from doctors of all specialties, nurses, social workers,

[1] World Medical Association. *WMA Declaration of Geneva* (2017). Accessed December 13, 2018, at https://www.wma.net/policies-post/wma-declaration-of-geneva/
[2] World Medical Association. *WMA International Code of Medical Ethics* (2006). Accessed December 13, 2018, at https://www.wma.net/policies-post/wma-international-code-of-medical-ethics/

The Trusted Doctor. Rosamond Rhodes, Oxford University Press (2020). © Oxford University Press.
DOI: 10.1093/oso/9780190859909.001.0001

physical therapists, genetic counselors, pharmacists, bioethicists, and so on. Even though this topic is rarely discussed in the bioethics literature, the duty of peer responsiveness is an essential feature of medical ethics and an important element of trustworthy medical practice.

In everyday life, people feel completely free to ignore requests for help from strangers and also neighbors, particularly when the assistance might be in any way burdensome. Even appeals from family members and friends may be refused when responding is inconvenient or risky. In business, trade secrets may be closely guarded, and there is no moral requirement to aid competitors in their efforts. And in other professions, law for instance, there is no obligation to lend a hand to another practitioner outside of one's own firm. The opposite is true in medicine. Responsiveness is required even when it is inconvenient or burdensome or involves legal and reputational risks and no personal benefit or financial compensation. This is because patients would be put at risk without the professional commitment to mutual support, cooperation, and collaboration. Because a request for help signals that a patient has a need that the requesting doctor cannot meet without assistance, responsiveness is a duty for medical professionals.

Treatment for patients with complicated conditions may involve expertise from a variety of specialties. No single individual physician has all of the requisite knowledge and skill to provide all of the tests and treatments that a patient's care may require. Patients who are seriously ill need daily around-the-clock care. Physically, no single individual physician can meet that need. Because the profession has the broad responsibility for meeting the medical needs of patients, because each medical professional has a fiduciary responsibility to her patients, and because no medical professional can do the job alone, each medical professional has the responsibility to do her share in assisting colleagues to meet their patients' needs so that the profession's responsibilities may be met. This requires responding to requests from other medical professionals for assistance (e.g., a consult, collaboration in a surgery) and being generous to peers with advice, explanations, education, feedback, and training. When one doctor phones another at an institution across the country with a question about a case report that might be similar to a current patient situation, the doctor at the other end takes the call and provides all of the information and advice that has been learned from the previous experience. Even though the physician who responds is uncompensated and not obliged by any business relationship, the duty of responsiveness is widely acknowledged. I expect that physicians who respond to their peers' requests for assistance are aware that they would expect a similar response to their own requests for help. In other words, they regard responding to a fellow physician's request to be something that no informed and experienced physician will be able to reasonably reject as being a duty of medical ethics. And the widespread awareness of responsiveness as a duty shows itself in the automated telephone systems that provide a special way (typically, press 1) for doctors who are calling to speak with another doctor to identify themselves as a fellow physician.

Choosing not to respond to a request is not doing nothing; it is failing in a duty to a patient and to colleagues.[3] Medical needs are often time sensitive; thus, delaying a response until it can no longer serve its intended purpose is also a failure to fulfill an obligation to both the patient and the colleague who made the request. The consequences of choosing not to respond to a call for assistance can be as disastrous as any terrible medical error. For that reason, a doctor who chooses to ignore a request for help can be ethically culpable for the outcome.

In his famous 1975 article, "Active and Passive Euthanasia," James Rachels argued that there is no moral difference between killing and letting die per se. To make his case, Rachels asked readers to consider a pair of cases:

In the first, Smith stands to gain a large inheritance if anything should happen to his six-year-old cousin. One evening while the child is taking his bath, Smith sneaks into the bathroom and drowns the child, and then arranges things so that it will look like an accident.

In the second, Jones also stands to gain if anything should happen to his six-year-old cousin. Like Smith, Jones sneaks in planning to drown the child in his bath. However, just as he enters the bathroom Jones sees the child slip and hit his head, and fall face down in the water. Jones is delighted; he stands by, ready to push the child's head back under if it is necessary, but it is not necessary. With only a little thrashing about, the child drowns all by himself, "accidentally," as Jones watches and does nothing.[4]

Rachels noted that we would consider both Smith and Jones to be despicable, and we would not excuse Jones from moral condemnation if he were to plead, "After all, I didn't do anything except just stand there and watch the child drown. I didn't kill him; I only let him die." Rachels's argument demonstrates

---

[3] The broad issue of whether the distinction between actions and omissions should in itself make a moral difference is discussed more fully in Chapter 7.

[4] Rachels J, "Active and Passive Euthanasia," *The New England Journal of Medicine* 292, 2 (1975): 78–80.

that there is no moral difference between withholding life-preserving treatment and allowing a patient to die and actively ending the life. Rachels was addressing the topic of euthanasia, and he was arguing that when it is wrong to end life with active measures, it is also wrong to allow death to occur by doing nothing. He is also arguing that when it is right to allow death to occur, it may also be permissible to end life with active measures, and when active measures minimize suffering, active measures may be more humane than letting death occur without intervention.

His argument, however, makes a more general point. It establishes that when the consequences of action and inaction are the same, if it is wrong to bring about the result with active measures, it may be just as wrong to bring about the result by allowing nature to take its course. I use Rachels's example to demonstrate that inaction can be morally blameworthy. This is particularly true in medicine and particularly relevant to the duty of peer responsiveness.

Case 1

F. M., a 92-year-old woman consults her geriatrician complaining of pain, nausea, and vomiting. The geriatrician examines the patient, questions her about recent constipation, and then calls for a surgical consult. The on-call surgeon wonders if he really needs to respond. He realizes that the patient may have a bowel obstruction and require a bowel resection. Believing that such a major surgery in a 92-year-old is likely to be an exercise in futility, he wonders whether he must respond to the request.

The duty of peer responsiveness provides a clear answer to his uncertainty. The surgeon is obliged to respond to his colleague's request because he was asked for help, and because this could be a surgical emergency, he actually has to respond in a timely way. Ignoring the request or delaying his response is not doing nothing. In this case, where the patient may have a bowel obstruction that requires urgent attention, failing to respond or deferring his appearance could result in the patient's death. If that should happen, the surgeon who did nothing could be ethically culpable and held responsible for the death.

When the surgeon does see the patient, he may find her to be a remarkably fit and cognitively intact woman with a desire to live and return to her independent life. Or, he may find her to be extremely thin and frail, unable to fully understand her situation, somewhat withdrawn but combative, and demonstrating reluctance to accept any medical intervention. After performing his own examination, he may determine that she was likely to benefit from surgery or that she would be unlikely to survive a surgical procedure or be left respirator dependent. Once he has made his assessment of the situation, he is free to recommend surgery or conclude that this patient is not a surgical candidate, but the surgeon must respond.

Whatever the nature of the consult (e.g., dental, dermatological, hematological, transplantation, critical care) and regardless of how irrelevant it may seem, a doctor must respond to a colleague's request for assistance with patient care. When a doctor recalls the situations in which he needed the assistance of a colleague or imagines a situation in which he might feel the need for a colleague's aid in the future, it is easy for a physician to appreciate that peer responsiveness is a doctor's categorical duty. If a physician would want colleagues to respond to his requests for help, the physician should treat requests from them with the same sort of dedicated responsive attention.

Peer Communication

The fourteenth duty of medical ethics is peer communication.
In everyday life, communicating is an effective means for making one's wishes known or advancing one's interests. But while there may be a right to free speech, there is no duty to speak. People who undertake vows of silence do nothing wrong, and people who choose to limit their communication are free to do so unless they have assumed a special obligation that requires them to communicate. Physicians' obligations require that they communicate.

Although numerous authors have discussed the importance of doctor-patient communication,[5-9] communication between medical peers is at least

[5] Makoul G, "Essential Elements of Communication in Medical Encounters: The Kalamazoo Consensus Statement," *Academic Medicine* 76, 4 (2001): 390–393.

[6] Ha JF and Longnecker N, "Doctor-Patient Communication: A Review," *The Ochsner Journal* 10, 1 (2010): 38–43.

[7] Brown JB, Boles M, Mullooly JP, and Levinson W, "Effect of Clinician Communication Skills Training on Patient Satisfaction: A Randomized, Controlled Trial," *Annals of Internal Medicine* 131, 11 (1999): 822–829.

[8] Suarez-Almazor ME, "Patient-Physician Communication," *Current Opinions: Rheumatology* 16, 2 (2004): 91–95.

[9] Duffy FD, Gordon GH, Whelan G, et al., "Assessing Competence in Communication and Interpersonal Skills: The Kalamazoo II Report," *Academic Medicine* 79, 6 (2004): 495–507.

as important,[10,11] and it should be counted as a moral duty. Frequently, several doctors are involved in the care of a patient. Often enough, each of them needs to be informed of what the other knows or learns about a patient who they share. This makes peer communication a duty of medical ethics that is closely related to the fourth duty, to provide care.

Peer communications is certainly an obligation for a physician who requests the help of a colleague. To be able to provide useful assistance, the consulted professional has to be told the kind of specific help the requester needs. For example, when a doctor calls for a consult from liaison psychiatry, the psychiatrist should be informed about whether the requesting doctor wants the patient to be evaluated for decisional capacity globally, for the capacity to make a specific treatment decision, for having depression, or for the treatment of depression. Each of these would require a different response from the responding liaison psychiatrist, and without communication the psychiatrist could only be left to guess what she was supposed to do. Communication is needed to enable the consulted professional to provide the patient and colleague with what is needed and also to avoid repeated calls and interventions and their associated frustrations.

Every doctor has responsibilities to provide appropriate care for their patient, so all of the physicians who are charged with the care of a patient need access to the tools that will enable them to fulfill their duties. Sometimes the tools are instruments, drugs, or access to needed facilities. Sometimes what is needed is information. Clinical findings (e.g., test results) and treatment plans all have to be communicated fully and accurately in order for other professionals to be able to do their jobs.

Each doctor who has some measure of responsibility for the care of a patient needs to have a full understanding of their patient's overall health and be alert to developing problems. That information can help a doctor avoid initiating treatments that might be contraindicated and avoid unnecessary duplication of tests. This means that a gynecologist who orders mammography has the results communicated to the patient's primary care doctor and vice versa. It means that the oncologist who is expert in managing a particular kind of cancer communicates with the primary care physician about

---

[10] Luetsch K and Rowett D, "Interprofessional Communication Training: Benefits to Practicing Pharmacists," *International Journal of Clinical Pharmacy* 37, 5 (2015): 857–864.

[11] Leonard M, Graham S, and Bonacum D, "The Human Factor: The Critical Importance of Effective Teamwork and Communication in Providing Safe Care," *Quality and Safety in Health Care* 13, Suppl 1 (2004): i85–i90.

their shared patient's vulnerabilities to infection, anemia, or impaired kidney function. It also means that the primary care physician communicates developing problems to the oncologist.

The duty of peer communication becomes especially important when doctors are providing care for hospitalized patients.[12-15] The care of seriously ill patients can be complicated, and their condition may change rapidly. Mistakes can happen when a doctor makes decisions without critical information or with misinformation, and the doctor who has the responsibility for making a decision may not be in a position to know whether or not he is missing some key finding at the point when a decision has to be made.

When shifts change, the doctor who is taking up the passed torch of responsibility for a hospitalized patient needs to understand the patient's condition, immediate concerns, treatment plans, test results, studies that need to be ordered, and so forth. Incomplete or inadequate communication, as well as miscommunication, introduces the possibility of serious harm to a patient.[16] When an intervention is started or discontinued, when a test or procedure is ordered, or when a dosage is changed, others on the treatment team need to know what was done and why it was done. And no doctor wants to cause harm to a patient because of a failure in his communication with peers. Communicating what other medical professionals need to know when it is their turn to take over the care of a patient is therefore a duty that doctors have to their fellow physicians and other medical professionals.

A study of Australian hospitals found that communication problems associated with handoffs were responsible for 11% of adverse outcomes. The problems of inadequate communication when staff members change shifts included failures in patient follow-up, test results not being communicated, and wrong drug combinations being prescribed. The potential

[12] Zinn C, "14,000 Preventable Deaths in Australian Hospitals," *British Medical Journal* 310 (1995 June 10): 1487.

[13] Greenberg CC, Regenbogen SE, Studdert DM, et al., "Patterns of Communication Breakdowns Resulting in Injury to Surgical Patients," *Journal of the American College of Surgeons* 204, 4 (2007): 533–540.

[14] Wiegmann DA, ElBardissi AW, Dearani JA, Daly RC, and Sundt TM 34d, "Disruptions in Surgical Flow and Their Relationship to Surgical Errors: An Exploratory Investigation," *Surgery* 142, 5 (2007): 658–665.

[15] Lingard L, Espin S, Whyte S, et al. "Communication Failures in the Operating Room: An Observational Classification of Recurrent Types and Effects," *Quality and Safety in Health Care* 13, 5 (2004): 330–334.

[16] World Health Organization. *The Conceptual Framework for the International Classification for Patient Safety (ICPS)* (2010). https://www.who.int/patientsafety/implementation/taxonomy/ICPS-report/en/

for devastating patient outcomes related to shift changes has led medical organizations to formalize how this difficult duty may be accomplished, and that form of attention from the profession implicitly demonstrates that peer communication is a professional duty. Noting that "the consequences of substandard hand-offs may include delay in treatment, inappropriate treatment, adverse events, omission of care, increased hospital length of stay, avoidable readmissions, increased costs, inefficiency from re-work, and other minor or major patient harm," the Joint Commission on Transforming Healthcare has developed the SHARE plan to standardize successful handoffs of patient responsibility: Standardize critical content; Hardwire new methods into the system; Allow opportunity to ask questions; Reinforce quality and measurement; Educate and coach.[17] The Joint Commission, the World Health Organization, and several authors also recommended that doctors employ team strategies and a standardized communication tool that has been used in other high-risk organizations to improve communication by providing a template to make the reporting consistent. It has been assumed that using such a standardized approach would promote accurate information communication, encourage dia-logue, and increase patient safety.[18,19] SBAR directs the person going off duty to provide a report on the **situation**, review the **background**, provide a full **assessment** of the patient, and provide **recommendations** for how to proceed in the coming shift.

McCulloch, Rathbone, and Catchpole performed a systematic literature review of 14 studies on the effects of teamwork training for clinical staff. Unfortunately, they found that "the evidence for technical or clinical benefit from teamwork training in medicine is weak."[20] Electronic medical records have been suggested as another useful tool in the effort to protect patients

[17] Joint Commission Center announces handoff communication solutions. *Patient Safety Monitor Insider*, October 27, 2010. http://www.hcpro.com/QPS-258250%E2%80%93873/Joint-Commission-Center-announces-handoff-communication-solutions.html

[18] Randmaa M, Mårtensson G, Leo Swenne C, and Engström M, "SBAR Improves Communication and Safety Climate and Decreases Incident Reports Due to Communication Errors in an Anaesthetic Clinic: A Prospective Intervention Study," *British Medical Journal Open* 4, 1 (2014): e004268.

[19] World Health Organization. *Communication During Patient Hand-overs.* WHO Patient Safety Solutions, volume 1, solution 3 (May 2007). https://www.who.int/patientsafety/solutions/patientsafety/PS-Solution3.pdf

[20] McCulloch P, Rathbone J, and Catchpole K, "Interventions to Improve Teamwork and Communications Among Healthcare Staff," *British Journal of Surgery* 98, 4 (2011): 469–479, 479.

from errors caused by inadequate communication.[21] They may facilitate communication by overcoming some communication problems. They can also add new kinds of communication hazards, for example, when inaccurate information is repeatedly cut from one note and pasted into the next, thus immortalizing an error and making it difficult for physicians who read the notes and rely on them to recognize the mistake.

Patient transfers between different hospital units or services, transfers to other institutions, and discharges back to the oversight of a primary care physician create additional opportunities for communication failures. The receiving doctor or team needs to obtain the medical orders for a transferred patient and understand the reasons for those specific orders. Understanding is necessary for avoiding errors and also for grasping which signs and symptoms need to be monitored. Members of the new treatment team also need the information so that they are prepared to explain what is being done to the patient and the patient's family and answer questions that may arise.

Unusual or controversial treatment decisions introduce additional needs for peer communication. The rationale for the decision has to be explained to members of the treatment team, and discussion should be invited. Medical professionals should not be left in the difficult position of having to cooperate with a plan that appears either to violate good clinical practice or to override the orders of a colleague. Controversial decisions require conversation so that all of those who will have to cooperate have an opportunity to raise their questions, offer reasons for their positions, and achieve a team consensus on what should be done. Further dialogue may also be needed to develop the details of how to proceed in implementing the treatment plan.

Fulfilling the duty to communicate adequately with peers requires conveying the message in a way that is effective. When orders are written, they must be legible; when voice mail messages are left, they must be audible; and when details such as names, phone numbers, or record numbers are given, they must be spoken clearly and slowly enough for the hearer to get the message. The responsibilities of peer communication can be discharged in face-to-face conversation, by phone, by relaying the information through other members of a team, or in some printed or electronic form. But the duty is not discharged until the message has been received, correctly understood, and the implications of the information are adequately appreciated.

---

[21] Flemming D and Hubner U, "How to Improve Change of Shift Handovers and Collaborative Grounding and What Role Does The Electronic Patient Record System Play? Results of a Systematic Literature Review," *International Journal of Medical Informatics* 82, 7 (2013): 580–592.

A complicated case that required a good deal of communication at multiple levels demonstrates the importance of communication among all of those who are responsible for the care of a patient.

Case 2

R. T. is a 43-year-old man who is HIV positive and has a history of schizophrenia, chronic hepatitis C, and systolic heart failure. He was admitted to the neurology service with deteriorating neurologic function and symptoms of seizure. He was evaluated for hydrocephaly and seizure disorder and treated for an opportunistic infection. Over the next 6-week course of R. T.'s hospitalization, after he suffered hypoxic respiratory failure secondary to pneumonia and gastrointestinal bleeding, he was transferred to the medicine service, where he has been persistently noninteractive or responsive to voice, but he does respond to painful stimuli. He is ventilator supported with a tracheostomy collar, and he has had a percutaneous endoscopic gastrostomy tube placed to provide him with nutrition, resulting in repeated aspiration events. He has also had repeated infections that required antibiotic therapy.

In spite of maximally aggressive treatment, R. T. has had no improvement in his mental status. He has been receiving transfusions for low hemoglobin of unclear etiology that is not improving. He is severely malnourished and contracted, and he has multiple pressure wounds.

Social workers identified two of R. T.'s relatives. Neither has had any contact with R. T. for the past 20 years, and they do not want to see him or participate in making his medical decisions. R. T. did complete a detailed advance directive on a previous admission. In it he expressed his desire for aggressive treatment, including a full-code resuscitation following a cardiac arrest. The directive also stipulates that, if necessary, he would want a trial on a ventilator but not to be maintained indefinitely with intubation.

At this point, the primary medical treatment team believes that R. T. has no chance of recovery and that he is dying. They have asked for advice from the Ethics Committee on how to proceed.

After a lengthy discussion, the committee members agreed that because artificial nutrition puts R. T. at risk for aspiration and is no longer effective in meeting nutritional goals, it should be discontinued. The committee also recommended that the transfusions and blood draws should be discontinued because they were ineffective and only caused pain. The team was content with those recommendations.

The issue of ventilator support remained problematic. Based on R. T.'s previous wishes, it would be acceptable to remove the ventilator because the trial was not leading to a recovery. In the same advance directive, however, RT had also expressed his wish for a resuscitation attempt following a cardiac arrest. Members of the committee and the treatment team recognized that removing the ventilator would lead to a cardiac arrest. They were troubled by the inconsistency between disconnecting the ventilator and an attempt to resuscitate after the arrest: One action allowed death to occur, whereas the other would be an effort to prevent death.

Because there is no definitive point at which a "trial of ventilator support" ends, the committee allowed ventilator support to be discontinued if the team agreed that doing so was appropriate. The justification for the committee's permission to discontinue the ventilator was legal and ethical: It was consistent with state law and consistent with the patient's previous wishes. The justification for the committee's strong recommendation to attempt resuscitation after a cardiac arrest (without reintroducing ventilator support if it had been removed) was also legal and ethical for the same reasons. In New York State, there is no legal requirement directing which measures must be employed in resuscitation or for how long, but the effort must be sincere and vigorous and employ the means that might be successful and acceptable to the patient. Explaining the rationale for the committee's recommendations required discussion of why it was important to abide by state law and honor the patient's wishes. The conversation also addressed details of how and when the discontinuation of ventilator support might be implemented and the point that the resuscitation need not be prolonged. In the end, the team accepted the legal and ethical arguments that justified abiding by the patient's desire to have a last ditch effort at resuscitation even though no one expected that it would be successful. The comparison of the legal and ethical benefits with the brief duration of the burdens ultimately made sense to everyone in the room.

The need for additional communication then became the focus of discussion. Because the team had originally been so uncomfortable with the situation, it was obvious that the rationale for the Ethics Committee's recommendations needed to be discussed with all of the medical professionals involved, including the nurses, the social workers, and the personnel on the night shift. Everyone involved needed to understand the plan and agree on how to proceed. Because R. T.'s death was imminent regardless of what was done, the issue of discontinuing the ventilator support was left open for the entire treating team to discuss and decide.

Peer Scrutiny

The fifteenth duty of medical ethics is peer scrutiny.
When a patient comes to see a doctor, he typically has inadequate information for trusting and allowing the license that he does. A patient is seldom in a position to make competent judgments about a physicians' knowledge, skills, or character, and, in many medical situations, there is no appreciable opportunity for choice (e.g., there is only whoever is on staff in the intensive care unit, only one pediatric neurologist in the city). Patients need to and do trust their doctors, but when the trust is undermined by unscrupulous, irresponsible, or unprofessional behavior, the profession's ability to deliver good care is impaired.

Patients are not in a position to be able to distinguish competent from incompetent physicians or virtuous, composed, and rational ones from those who are not. They don't know enough about medicine to be able to recognize poor judgment, and they have no opportunities to sufficiently discern a pattern of behavior that might give them pause. Only colleagues with similar training and medical professionals with adequate understanding of their professional commitments are in a position to formulate accurate judgments about a colleague's professional competence.

So, for the profession to be able to continue to do its good work, medical professionals have to ensure that their colleagues are trustworthy. That is to say, doctors have to take up the duty to be their brothers' keepers and keep their brothers to the profession's lofty standards as a serious professional obligation. Peer scrutiny, peer criticism, and peer discipline are therefore required of individuals and the profession. As the New Zealand Medical Association Code of Ethics affirms,

> Doctors have a responsibility to assist colleagues who are unwell or under stress. Doctors have a general responsibility for the safety of patients and should therefore take appropriate steps to ensure unsafe or unethical

practices on the part of colleagues are curtailed and/or reported to relevant authorities.[22]

This conclusion is also explicitly expressed in official statements on professional responsibility from the American Medical Association (AMA), the Charter on Medical Professionalism, and the European Federation of Internal Medicine.[23] Their joint declaration states that physicians have an ethical obligation to report incompetent or unethical behavior, and that doctors are expected to participate in the process of self-regulation. Also, the second principle of the AMA Code of Medical Ethics affirms the following:

> II. A physician shall uphold the standards of professionalism, be honest in all professional interactions, and strive to report physicians deficient in character or competence, or engaging in fraud or deception, to appropriate entities.[24]

Peer reporting and self-reporting have been the primary mechanisms for identifying physicians who are impaired, incompetent, or unethical. Data suggest, however, that the rate of reporting is low.[25–29] Physicians are reluctant to report their peers,[30] and the profession has shied away from

[22] New Zealand Medical Association. *Code of Ethics for the New Zealand Medical Profession* (2014), recommendation 34. Accessed October 28, 2018, at https://www.nzma.org.nz/publications/code-of-ethics

[23] ABIM Foundation, ACP-ASIM Foundation, and European Federation of Internal Medicine, "Medical Professionalism in the New Millennium: A Physician Charter," *Annals of Internal Medicine* 136, 3 (2002): 243–246.

[24] American Medical Association. *American Medical Association Code of Medical Ethics*. ttps://www.ama-assn.org/sites/default/files/media-browser/principles-of-medical-ethics.pdf

[25] DesRoches CM, Rao SR, Fromson JA, et al., "Physicians' Perceptions, Preparedness for Reporting, and Experiences Related to Impaired and Incompetent Colleagues," *Journal of the American Medical Association* 304, 2 (2010): 187–193.

[26] Perry W and Crean RD, "A Retrospective Review of the Neuropsychological Test Performance of Physicians Referred for Medical Infractions," *Archives of Clinical Neuropsychology* 20, 2 (2005): 161–170.

[27] Turnbull J, Cunnington J, Unsal A, Norman G, and Ferguson B. "Competence and Cognitive Difficulty in Physicians: A Follow-up Study," *Academic Medicine* 81, 10 (2006): 915–918.

[28] Kataria N, Brown N, McAvoy P, Majeed A, and Rhodes M, "A Retrospective Study of Cognitive Function in Doctors and Dentists With Suspected Performance Problems: An Unsuspected But Significant Concern," *JRSM Open* 5, 5 (2014): 2042533313517687.

[29] Mansbach WE, Mace RA, Tanner MA, and Schindler F, "Verbal Test of Practical Judgment (VPJ): A New Test of Judgment That Predicts Functional Skills for Older Adults," *Aging and Mental Health* (2018 March 23): 1–9.

[30] Rothstein L, "Impaired Physicians and the ADA," *Journal of the American Medical Association* 313, 22 (2015): 2219–2220.

demanding more oversight[31] or imposing standards for profession-wide self-regulation.[32] National surveys of physicians have shown that about 36% of physicians do not even recognize that reporting instances of significantly impaired or incompetent colleagues is something that they should do.[33,34]

At the same time, a number of recent articles in the medical literature have remarked about the importance of protecting patients from harm by ensuring that physicians are fit to work as doctors.[35-38] A 1999 Australian study found that "cognitive impairment in physicians is responsible for 63% of all the cases of medical adverse events, and most were determined to be preventable."[39] Other articles identified physical and psychological impairments that can make a physician unable to practice. These impairments can be caused by physical disease, sensory deficits, or mental illness, including depression, post-traumatic stress disorder (PTSD), as well as alcoholism and substance abuse. Any of these problems may affect cognitive function and behavior. Authors also identified problems associated with incompetence related to lack of knowledge or skill and immorality involving deliberate transgression of professional duties, particularly duties to patients.[40]

Studies of doctors who have been disciplined for problematic behavior have found that about one-third of these physicians had cognitive impairments that were sufficient to explain their incompetence and account for why their behavior did not improve with remediation. In one study, 148 physicians who had committed various medical errors or infractions were referred for psychological and neuropsychological evaluation by the California Medical Board.[41] This cohort of physicians was found to perform

[31] Benatar S, "Professional competence and professional misconduct in South Africa," South African Medical Journal 104, 7 (2014): 480–482.

[32] Bauchner H, Fontanarosa PB, and Thompson AE, "Professionalism, Governance, and Self-Regulation of Medicine," Journal of the American Medical Association 313, 18 (2015): 1831–1836.

[33] Campbell EG, Regan S, Gruen RL, et al. "Professionalism in Medicine: Results of a National Survey of Physicians," Annals of Internal Medicine 147, 11 (2007): 795–802.

[34] DesRoches et al., "Physicians' Perceptions."

[35] Harrison J, "Doctors' Health and Fitness to Practise: The Need for a Bespoke Model of Assessment," Occupational Medicine 58, 5 (2008): 323–327.

[36] Pitkanen M, Hurn J, and Kopelman MD, "Doctors' Health and Fitness to Practise: Performance Problems in Doctors and Cognitive Impairments," Occupational Medicine 58, 5 (2008): 328–333.

[37] Harrison J, "Illness in Doctors and Dentists and Their Fitness For Work—Are the Cobbler's Children Getting Their Shoes at Last?" Occupational Medicine 56, 2 (2006): 75–76.

[38] Turnbull J, Carbotte R, Hanna E, et al., "Cognitive Difficulty in Physicians," Academic Medicine 75, 2 (2000): 177–181.

[39] Wilson RM, Harrison BT, Gibberd RW, and Hamilton JD, "An Analysis of the Causes of Adverse Events From the Quality in Australian Health Care Study," Medical Journal of Australia 170 (1999): 411–415.

[40] Morreim EH, "Am I My Brother's Warden? Responding to the Unethical or Incompetent Colleague," Hastings Center Report 23, 3 (1993): 19–27.

[41] Perry and Crean, "Retrospective Review."

at a lower level than expected on tests of intellectual and neuropsychological functioning. In another study, 12 of 31 (38%) of physicians who had been reported for problematic behavior were found to have moderate or severe cognitive impairment that could explain their poor performance. And in another study of physicians who had been referred for evaluation for clinical difficulties or behavioral or safety issues, 14 of 88 (15%) were found to have cognitive impairment.[42] These assessments focused on psychiatric and neurological examinations using validated reliable tools that allowed the investigators to quantify and analyze cognitive impairments.[43] The studies demonstrated the potential of neuropsychiatric and neuropsychological assessment and identification of physician impairment.

To protect airline passengers, the US Federal Aviation Administration set an age limit for pilots engaged in certain operations.[44] That was in 1959. There are now also age-based requirements for periodic testing or retirement for judges, air traffic controllers, Federal Bureau of Investigation employees, and firefighters.[45] Patient safety is obviously an issue in medicine, but there are no similar requirements for physician retirement or testing even though the potential for age-related impairment is a growing danger in the United States.[46–48] The number of practicing physicians older than 65 years in the United States has increased dramatically since 1975, and 23% of practicing physicians in 2015 were 65 years or older.

Several studies have explored the relationship between physicians' age and their cognitive and sensory abilities. When the research findings were reviewed by the AMA Council on Medical Education, they concluded that several aging-associated problems impacted clinical performance: decreased information-processing ability and speed, ability to complete complex

[42] Kataria et al., "Retrospective Study."

[43] Turnbull et al., "Cognitive Difficulty in Physicians"; Turnbull et al., "Competence and Cognitive Difficulty."

[44] Ripple GP, *Mandatory Retirement Age for Pilots Is Not Age Discrimination* (Washington, DC: National Business Aviation Association, 2014). https://nbaa.org/flight-department-administration/personnel/age-65/federal-court-mandatory-retirement-age-for-pilots-is-not-age-discrimination/

[45] Dellinger EP, Pellegrini CA, and Gallagher TH, "The Aging Physician and the Medical Profession: A Review," *JAMA Surgery* 152, 10 (2017): 967–971.

[46] Blasier RB, "The Problem of the Aging Surgeon: When Surgeon Age Becomes a Surgical Risk Factor," *Clinical Orthopaedics and Related Research* 467, 2 (2009): 402–411.

[47] California Public Protection and Physician Health. *Assessing Late Career Practitioners: Policies and Procedures for Age-Based Screening: California Public Protection and Physician Health, Inc.* (2015; updated August 11, 2015: 1–40). https://cppphdotorg.files.wordpress.com/2011/02/assessing-late-career-practitioners-adopted-by-cppph-changes-6-10-151.pdf

[48] Beekman ATF, "Aging Affects Us All: Aging Physicians and Screening for Impaired Professional Proficiency," *American Journal of Geriatric Psychiatry* 26, 6 (2018): 641–642.

tasks, difficulty in sorting out irrelevant information, diminished hearing and visual acuity, decreased manual dexterity, and diminished visuospatial ability. While there is significant person-to-person variability in aging declines, studies showed that mean cognitive ability deteriorated by more than 20% between ages 40 and 75. Even though the issue has been noted by leaders of the profession, and even though there is mounting evidence that as physicians age their risk of impaired functioning increases without their noticing their own decline in cognitive ability or function, measures have not been put in place to protect patients in the United States. If omissions were any less ethically relevant than actions, this situation would not be problematic. Inadequate policing of the profession is a problem because of the risks to patients that failure to take action allows.

The AMA defined an impairment as "physical or mental health conditions that interfere with a physician's ability to engage safely in professional activities."[49] Substance abuse may be an especially significant danger because of the availability of drugs in the medical environment and because work pressures can put physicians at risk of depression, burnout, PTSD, and suicide. Self-medication can be a tempting solution for these sorts of problems, and doctors who succumb to substance abuse or alcoholism certainly put their patients at risk of harm. Once a physician with a substance abuse problem is self-identified or identified by others, there are measures that can be taken to help. Physicians who comply with treatment can overcome their problems and then continue to practice medicine in a trustworthy way.

Physical or verbal physician behavior that negatively affects patient care or interferes with other medical professionals' ability to fulfill their duties also needs to be corrected or reported. Potentially problematic behavior includes verbal outbursts, physical threats, refusing to perform tasks, exhibiting an uncooperative attitude, and so on. Disruptive physician behavior has been recognized by both by the Joint Commission and the AMA as a significant problem with negative implications that pose a threat to the safety of patients and others in the medical environment.

In addition to the problems of impaired function, substance abuse, and disruptive physician behavior, there are some incompetent and unethical physicians. As philosopher and attorney Haavi Morreim recognized, people

---

[49] Physician Responsibilities to Impaired Colleagues. *Code of Medical Ethics Opinion 9.3.2.* https://www.ama-assn.org/delivering-care/ethics/physician-responsibilities-impaired-colleagues Accessed 12/11/2019.

in the medical community are likely to feel sympathy for colleagues who are impaired in one way or another and want to help them in whatever ways they can with whatever means that may be effective. The incompetent or unethical physician is regarded differently and does not elicit such charitable responses. Regrettably, there are some doctors who lack the necessary knowledge and skills or fail to keep abreast of the continuously and rapidly developing field. Unfortunately, there are also doctors who act in bad faith, who yield to temptations, and who come to the conclusions that they want to believe in spite of all the evidence to the contrary. Deplorably, there are even some doctors who are immoral, who knowingly and willfully put their own interests before those of their patients and subject their patients to unacceptable risks.[50,51]

Nevertheless, the strong social norms of common morality make doctors reluctant to report other physicians' unprofessional behavior, except in the most egregious cases. From childhood on, we learn not to be a tattletale and to stand by our buddies. In medicine, protecting the trustworthiness of the profession is, however, a moral duty. The residue of common morality leaves doctors feeling the familiar pulls of reluctance to report colleague impairment and the incompetent or unethical behavior of a fellow physician. For that reason, the radical difference between the common morality "don't snitch" mentality and the medical ethics commitment to uphold the trustworthiness of the profession and act in the interest of patients has to be made an explicit feature of medical professionalism and inculcated as part of the ethos of being a physician.

There are, however, additional social factors that work against reporting problematic physician behavior. One additional consideration is that to condemn someone else is to invite scrutiny of oneself. A further consideration is the well-known social phenomenon of punishing the whistle-blower. This is a particular problem in medicine because negative publicity is likely to disrupt referral patterns and have serious financial repercussions on a practice or hospital admissions. This is why institutions often prefer to sweep reports of bad behavior under a rug. Perhaps the greatest worry is that the criticism will be ignored while the whistle-blowing colleague is shunned so that no benefit is achieved while the personal costs are significant.

---

[50] Sanfey H, DaRosa DA, Hickson GB, et al., "Pursuing Professional Accountability: An Evidence-Based Approach to Addressing Residents With Behavioral Problems," *Archives of Surgery* 147, 7 (2012): 642–647.

[51] Khaliq AA, Dimassi H, Huang C-Y, Narine L, and Smego RA, "Disciplinary Action Against Physicians: Who Is Likely to Get Disciplined?" *The American Journal of Medicine* 118, 7 (2005): 773–777.

All of these factors that make physicians reluctant to report raise the question of what measures should be taken to enable physicians to meet their duty of peer scrutiny. Because the profession accepts peer scrutiny as a duty, medical groups at various levels actually take significant steps to fulfill the profession's responsibility. Regularly scheduled clinical conferences and periodic morbidity and mortality rounds provide a venue for offering critical comments that aim at helping fellow physicians improve performance. Some institutions have implemented near-miss programs to identify and address potential individual and systems problems. Some medical specialty boards require periodic recertification to assess whether doctors continue to meet their standards, and other boards are planning to develop their own recertification mechanisms. State medical boards review complaints about physician performance and behavior, and they can impose disciplinary actions, require remediation, and revoke or suspend medical licenses. Many hospitals employ credentialing standards to ensure that clinicians meet standards of professional competency.[52] In addition, in the United States the Health Care Quality Improvement Act (HCQIA) of 1986 established a National Practitioner Data Bank that compiles a database of complaints and punitive actions related to physician practice, ranging from malpractice awards and state licensure actions to adverse judgments rendered by hospitals and medical societies. To ensure that hospitals monitor staff physicians' performance, hospitals are required to check the databank before granting or renewing staff physicians' credentials.

Most physicians support the professional commitment to report all instances of impaired or incompetent colleagues in their medical practice to a relevant authority, but it is often hard to know whether an error is actually an instance of impairment or incompetence. So, when individual physicians actually confront a situation that requires an intervention or reporting, many do nothing because reporting is uncomfortable, hard to do, potentially time consuming, and risky. It is easier for a doctor either to imagine that what appeared to be unacceptable behavior would actually be appropriate if only he knew all of the facts or to interpret the situation as the kind of human mistake that any physician could make. All of this adds up to the fact that reports from peers are an inadequate safeguard[53] for protecting the trustworthiness

---

[52] Additional measures that are in place to ensure physician competence are discussed in Chapter 3, The Commitment to Medicine's Core Responsibilities.

[53] DesRoches et al., "Physicians' Perceptions."

of the profession, and that leaves impaired physicians at risk of causing harm and their patients at risk for suffering harm.

Whether problematic behavior is caused by impairment, such as a neurocognitive or psychiatric disorder, a substance abuse problem, professional or external life stress, inadequate training, personality issues, or serious character flaws, it remains difficult to identify by relying on self- or peer-reports.[54,55] Using Stanford University and Canada as instructive examples, several authors have suggested addressing the problem proactively.[56,57] They recommended that hospitals, healthcare organizations, and states implement mandatory periodic proactive neuropsychological testing programs[58-60] and routine drug testing.[61] A serial assessment program can potentially identify deficiencies in physicians whose clinical competence is impaired. Standard testing of every physician coupled with age-based mandatory testing starting at a certain age would increase the early detection of competency problems and thereby prevent patient harm.[62,63]

In addition, as Dellinger, Pellegrini, and Gallagher noted, starting at age 40, pilots undergo routine physical examinations and accept that work requirement as part of the job." Similarly, athletes accept routine drug testing as part of their sport's routine. Making mandatory testing of physicians a routine and regular feature of medical life throughout a doctor's career would have the advantage of eliminating the stigma associated with testing as well as the reliance on peer reporting for detecting competency impairment.

---

[54] DesRoches et al., "Physicians' Perceptions."

[55] Wynia MK, "The Role of Professionalism and Self-Regulation in Detecting Impaired or Incompetent Physicians," *Journal of the American Medical Association* 304, 2 (2010): 210–212.

[56] Dellinger et al., "The Aging Physician."

[57] Naylor CD, Gerace R, and Redelmeier DA, "Maintaining Physician Competence and Professionalism: Canada's Fine Balance," *Journal of the American Medical Association* 304, 2 (2010): 210–212.

[58] Dellinger et al., "The Aging Physician."

[59] Soonsawat A, Tanaka G, Lammando MA, Ahmed I, and Ellison JM, "Cognitively Impaired Physicians: How Do We Detect Them? How Do We Assist Them?" *American Journal of Geriatric Psychiatry* 26, 6 (2018): 631–640.

[60] Turnbull et al., "Cognitive Difficulty in Physicians."

[61] Pham JC, Pronovost PJ, and Skipper GE, "Identification of Physician Impairment," *Journal of the American Medical Association* 309, 20 (2013): 2101–210.

[62] Levey NN, "Medical Professionalism and the Future of Public Trust in Physicians," *Journal of the American Medical Association* 313, 18 (2015): 1827–1828.

[63] American Board of Internal Medicine Foundation, American Board of Internal Medicine; ACP-ASIM Foundation, American College of Physicians—American Society of Internal Medicine; European Federation of Internal Medicine. "Medical Professionalism in the New Millennium: A Physician Charter," *Annals of Internal Medicine* 136, 3 (2002): 243–246.

In arguing for more routine drug testing Pham, Pronovost, and Skipper offered a similar suggestion. They pointed out that

> When a critical event occurs in most high-risk industries (such as airlines, nuclear power, or railways), a detailed investigation examines a variety of system and individual factors (such as fatigue and substance abuse) that caused or contributed to the event. Directly involved individuals are commonly tested for alcohol and other drugs. Airplane pilots and truck drivers are tested following crashes and near misses. Some law enforcement officers are tested following fatal shooting incidents.[64]

Again, making the investigation of egregious errors and sentinel events that lead to patient death mandatory would make patients safer and the profession more trustworthy. Also, making a physical examination and drug and neuropsychological testing of those involved routine would normalize the response and diminish the stigma that might otherwise be associated with an inquiry. If the investigation were to be regarded as appropriate follow-up, the procedure would detect system problems as well as individual problems without imposing reporting burdens on other physicians, who would otherwise have to blow the whistle on a colleague.

To the extent the routine physician assessments and routine sentinel event examinations can address the bulk of the problems of physician impairment and incompetence, reliance on self- and peer-reporting is minimized. The remaining issues will largely concern patterns of errors that appear to reflect carelessness or poor judgment and the significant matters of problematic personality and bad character. For those serious troubles, the profession has to rely on reports from other physicians to identify what is happening.

Combining three different approaches might overcome the problem of relying on peer reports: professionalism education, psychology, and political change. As a matter of professionalism education, making the duty of doctors to be their brothers' keeper explicit and nurturing medical trainees to take that responsibility seriously can overcome the problem of doctors being unaware that reporting serious problematic physician behavior is a professional obligation. That education can be reinforced by senior physicians and institutional leaders making it a priority. They will need to explain the responsibility repeatedly on occasions such as medical conferences and morbidity and mortality

---

[64] Pham et al., "Identification of Physician Impairment."

rounds. They will also have to explain what the institutional reporting mechanism is and assure possible reporters that their reports will be kept confidential and that they will protected from any untoward consequences.

Psychological benefits can be expected to derive from that educational effort. The Hawthorne effect, also called the observer effect, is said to improve people's performance when they believe that they are being watched. In the case of physicians who are inclined to behave badly when they feel immune to having their poor behavior revealed, the repeated calls for reporting unprofessional behavior will serve to inform the would be wrongdoers that they are being observed. As we all know, there are things that we may do when we believe that we are unobserved that we would not do when we believe that we can be seen. That psychological difference from feeling that others are taking note of what you do can have a significant impact on the behavior of someone who might otherwise be careless or tend to ignore professional duties. The Pygmalion effect, a related psychological phenomenon, can also come into play. This involves higher expectations leading to better results. Clear statements from medical leaders that doctors are expected to uphold the standards of professional behavior are therefore likely to encourage behavior on a higher level.

Policy-level changes are most likely to be effective, but they may be the most difficult to implement. This sort of reform would make institutions responsible for the professionalism of the physicians they employ. We see similar measures in place in animal and human subject research. In both cases, medical institutions are held responsible for the ethical conduct of research, and institutions are vulnerable to serious penalties for the infractions of investigators in their employ. That arrangement aligns the institution's interests with ethical behavior, and it has the important consequence of transforming the whistle-blower from a threat to the institution's reputation into a valued ally and protector of the institution. The institutional requirement to check the HCQIA databank before granting or renewing staff physicians' credentials is a step in that direction, but more is needed.

The numerous recent calls from medical leaders for greater focus on medical professionalism[65-68] needs to include attention to the responsibilities

[65] Byyny RL, Paauw DS, Papadakis M, and Pfeil S, editors, *Medical Professionalism Best Practices: Professionalism in the Modern Era* (Aurora, CO: Alpha Omega Alpha Honor Medical Society, 2017).

[66] Levinson W, Ginsburg S, Hafferty F, and Lucey C, *Understanding Medical Professionalism* (New York: McGraw Hill, 2014).
[67] Cruess RL, Cruess SR, and Steinert Y, editors. *Teaching Medical Professionalism: Supporting the Development of a Professional Identity*, 2nd edition (Cambridge: Cambridge University Press, 2016).
[68] American Board of Internal Medicine Foundation et al., "Medical Professionalism."

that physicians have to one another. Fulfilling these duties are essential elements in upholding the trustworthiness of the profession and critical factors in meeting the obligations that the profession has to patient welfare. Making these duties explicit is therefore a critical element in that agenda. Attending to the interrelated obligations of peer responsiveness, peer communication, and peer scrutiny would be important steps in the evolution of our understanding of what is entailed by medical professionalism.

9

Why Trustworthy Stewardship
Requires Justice

The sixteenth duty of medical ethics is medical justice.
Doctors make decisions about allocating medical resources every day. They decide on the order in which patients will be seen and how much time will be spent with each patient. They determine which patients will have access to which resources, when, why, and for how long. All of these allocation decisions require justice. Even though the amount of resources available (e.g., funding decisions, numbers of intensive care unit [ICU] beds) is often determined at a public policy level, a tremendous number of choices about how to apportion the resources at their disposal are left to physicians.[1] Society trusts the medical community to make those decisions justly, and for the most part the profession makes trustworthy and just allocations.

That said, those who make decisions about the distribution of medical resources in the clinical setting register little awareness of the fact that justice is involved. Justice is the least discussed of Beauchamp and Childress's four principles,[2] and codes of ethics afford the concept no more than a wave in its direction using vague and uninformative language. For example, the World Medical Association International Code of Medical Ethics declares that "a physician should strive to use health care resources in the best way to benefit patients and their community."[3] And the American Medical Association Principles of Medical Ethics, Principle IX, holds that "a physician shall support access to medical care for all people."[4] And the Canadian Medical

---

[1] In this chapter, I focus narrowly on allocation issues that arise for medical professionals and medical institutions within the practice of medicine. I pointedly avoid the allocation issues that arise for health insurance companies and government that involve related but different issues.

[2] Beauchamp TL and Childress JF, *Principles of Biomedical Ethics*, 7th edition (New York: Oxford University Press, 2013).

[3] World Medical Association. *WMA International Code of Medical Ethics* (2006). Accessed December 13, 2018, at https://www.wma.net/policies-post/wma-international-code-of-medical-ethics/

[4] American Medical Association. *AMA Code of Medical Ethics: AMA Principles of Medical Ethics* (2001). Accessed October 28, 2018, at https://www.ama-assn.org/sites/default/files/media-browser/principles-of-medical-ethics.pdf

The Trusted Doctor. Rosamond Rhodes, Oxford University Press (2020). © Oxford University Press.
DOI: 10.1093/oso/9780190859909.001.0001

Association Code of Ethics directs its members to "recognize the responsibility of physicians to promote equitable access to health care resources."[5]

Part of the problem of not recognizing issues of justice as what they are comes from the inadequate accounts that philosophy has provided of justice and medical justice in particular. Most approaches to the ethics of medicine endorse a principle of justice, but they fail to explain the concept and fail to appreciate the complexity of justice. They also fail to notice how the allocations of medical resources in clinical settings are different from the allocation of other commodities or social goods. In fact, most authors who write broadly about justice treat it as a monolithic ethical concept. Theorists each put forward their view of a singular principle of justice as if it was applicable across the board. In their presentations, they typically argue for the acceptance of their principle and against the singular concepts proposed by others. This lengthy chapter aims at providing the needed explanation, elaboration, and clarification.

With prescient insight, Aristotle acknowledged the complexity and contextuality of justice. In his lengthy discussion of justice in Book 5 of the *Nicomachean Ethics*, Aristotle equated justice to the entirety of interpersonal virtue, and he defined justice as giving each his due and treating similarly situated individuals similarly.[6] Yet, he discerned the difficulty involved in determining which features of a situation should be taken into account in deciding that individuals are similarly situated and which of the generally important factors should be given priority in a particular situation. According to Aristotle, justice requires equality in the treatment of equals. Yet, many incommensurable factors, such as relationship, history, consequences, and feasibility, may or may not be relevant considerations in determining which claimants should be held as equal. Justice requires the moral discernment to identify which sorts of factors are significant and how they should be compared in order to make a just allocation in a certain type of circumstance or in some particular situation.

[5] Canadian Medical Association. *CMA Code of Ethics (Update 2004)* (2004), responsibility 43. Accessed October 28, 2018, at http://www.cpsa.ca/wp-content/uploads/2019/01/CMA_Policy_Code_of_ethics_of_the_Canadian_Medical_Association_Update_2004_PD04-06-e.pdf

[6] Aristotle enumerated three types of justice: distributive, retributive, and equity. The discussion of justice in this chapter is primarily concerned with distributive justice, that is, how the limited supply of medical resources should be distributed. Retributive justice is principally concerned with punishments, a topic that is beyond the scope of this project. Taking seriously Aristotle's claim that justice is virtue entire (Aristotle: 1130a9), the rest of this book can be seen as a discussion of what equity requires from medical professionals. Aristotle, *The Nichomachean Ethics of Aristotle*, translated by WD Ross (London: Oxford University Press, 1971).

Although some contemporary philosophers follow Aristotle's insights and recommend an account of justice that draws on an array of reasons,[7] those who write on issues of justice and health care appear to prefer a more Platonic approach. Most typically, they articulate a singular essentialist conception as the comprehensive account of justice. To illustrate the prevailing approach, I briefly sketch the views of a few of the most important philosophers who write about justice and the most prominent competing contemporary accounts of justice that enter discussions of medicine and public health. In this brief overview, of course, I omit many details and lump together approaches that the authors themselves may regard as distinguishing their own view and making it better than other similar positions.

Theories of Justice

In the bioethics literature, the most prominent theories of justice are utilitarianism and accounts that are derived from the work of John Rawls. The latter include Norman Daniels's fair equality of opportunity discussion of justice in healthcare and positions that have been called prioritarianism or egalitarianism.

Utilitarianism

Utilitarianism has a long history in ethics, tracing back to the writings of Jeremy Bentham and John Stuart Mill. It is the view that policies are just when they produce the best outcomes in terms of a single designated measurable outcome. For example, Bentham argued that pleasure was the only thing that all people value; hence, justice should aim at maximizing pleasure.[8] Similarly, Mill adopted happiness as his singular value and argued that justice should aim at maximizing happiness.[9]

Utilitarians thus identify an objective standard for calculating outcomes, and employ that single standard in determining policies and making policy

---

[7] I count contractarian constructivists, such as T. M. Scanlon, in this camp. Scanlon TM, *What We Owe to Each Other* (Cambridge, MA: Belknap Press of Harvard University Press, 1998).

[8] Bentham J, *An Introduction to the Principles of Morals and Legislation*, edited by JH Burns and HLA Hart (London: Methuen, 1982). (Original work published 1789)

[9] Mill JS, *Utilitarianism*, edited by G Sher (Indianapolis, IN: Hacket, 1979). (Original work published 1861)

decisions. Utilitarian allocations aim at maximizing their singular outcome over an entire population. A utilitarian conception of justice is committed to treating people as equals and deliberately ignoring relational and relative differences between individuals. Utilitarians compute the positive and negative consequences of implementing a proposed policy and select a policy to implement based on the aggregate of the desired results for the entire population governed by that policy. On utilitarian grounds, a policy is just when it is efficacious, that is, when it provides the greatest aggregate amount of the specified end.

When addressing decisions about the allocation of healthcare resources, utilitarians focus on measurements of health or life span. A cost-benefit analysis in terms of the one factor that counts is employed to determine the policy for a population. Nothing else is considered because, for utilitarians, justice is defined only in terms of the end that is to be maximized. Who will get the benefit and who will not, how they will use the benefit, and what will happen to those who don't get the benefit are all regarded as irrelevant factors that are deliberately ignored.

Today, utilitarianism appears to be the dominant approach to justice in medical and public health policy. It is popular because the utilitarian calculus makes ethical decisions appear simple, and it allows policymakers to focus on some things that people do value. Utilitarianism provides a metric that allows for numerical calculations and therein offers a method for evaluating all decisions in the same way. For example, some utilitarian policies employ a metric of quality-adjusted life years (QALYs), others employ disability-adjusted life years (DALYs), and others employ disability-adjusted life expectations (DALEs). These approaches are all utilitarian, and they produce allocations that at least seem fair in that they evaluate every allocation decision according to the same singular standard.

John Rawls

Since 1971, many of the positions on justice espoused by philosopher John Rawls, first in *A Theory of Justice*[10] and later in *Political Liberalism*[11] and other works, have come to play a significant role in the philosophical discussion

---

[10] Rawls J, *A Theory of Justice* (Cambridge, MA: Harvard University Press, 1971).
[11] Rawls J, *Political Liberalism* (New York: Columbia University Press, 1993).

of nonutilitarian criteria for the just allocation of social resources. Rawls famously advanced two principles of justice. According to Rawls's first principle, justice requires a liberal democratic political regime to ensure that its citizens' basic needs for primary goods are met, and that citizens have the means to make effective use of their liberties and opportunities. Rawls's second principle regulates the basic institutions of a just state to ensure citizens fair equality of opportunity. The first principle has priority over the second in that it requires political institutions to provide for citizens whatever they must have in order to understand and exercise their rights and liberties. According to Rawls, his two principles taken together ensure basic political rights and liberties, such as liberty of conscience, freedom of association, freedom of speech, voting, running for office, freedom of movement, and free choice of occupation. They also guarantee the political value of fair equality of opportunity in the face of inevitable social and economic inequalities.[12] Both principles therefore express a commitment to the equality of political liberties and opportunities.

These two principles of justice express Rawls's view of the basic commitments that a liberal political society should endorse. Rawls's principles are intended as "guidelines for how basic [political] institutions are to realize the values of liberty and equality" and ensure all citizens "adequate all-purpose means to make effective use of their liberties and opportunities."[13] Together, these principles specify certain basic rights, liberties, and opportunities and assign them priority against claims of those who advocate for the general good or the promotion of perfectionism (i.e., the best possible society).

In Rawls's account, the difference principle is the second condition of the second principle of justice. Recognizing that economic and social inequalities are an unavoidable feature of any ongoing social arrangement, Rawls established his second principle to express the limits on unequal distributions. He held that equal access to opportunities is a necessary feature of a just society, and then, to compensate for eventual disparities and to maintain equality of opportunity, he called for corrective distribution measures through the application of the difference principle. According to Rawls, the difference principle requires that "social and economic inequalities . . . are to be to the greatest benefit of the least advantaged members of society."[14]

[12] Rawls, *Political Liberalism*, 228–229.
[13] Rawls, *Political Liberalism*, 326.
[14] Rawls, *Political Liberalism*, 6.

In other words, governmental policies that distribute goods among citizens must be designed to rectify inequality by first advancing the interests of those who are otherwise less well off than their fellow citizens.

Rawls himself did not explain how to extend his principles of justice to policies involving health and medical care. In fact, he specifically maintained that "variations in physical capacities and skills, including the effects of illness and accident on natural abilities" are not unfair, and they do not give rise to injustice so long as the principles of justice are satisfied.[15] Yet, several prominent authors who write about justice and medicine have seen the relevance of extending Rawls's principles to the allocation of healthcare. They discuss medical allocations by invoking Rawls's principles, and they extend Rawlsian concepts to the allocation of medical resources. One Rawlsian concept that has received especially broad endorsement in the medical ethics literature is his commitment to what he called "fair equality of opportunity." The other concept that has been widely supported in this literature is the "difference principle," and people who have embraced some version of that principle now refer to such views as "prioritarian" or "egalitarian."

Norman Daniels and Fair Equality of Opportunity

Norman Daniels has used the Rawlsian concept of fair equality of opportunity to argue that healthcare should be treated as a basic need. He maintained that "health care is of special moral importance because it helps to preserve our status as fully functioning citizens."[16], Daniels wants us to count at least some medical services as "primary goods" so that they are treated as claims to special needs.[17] From Daniels's point of view, therefore, the allocation of healthcare resources should be aimed at equalizing social opportunity.

Daniels expected his claim to lead to the conclusion that a just society should provide its members with universal healthcare, including public health and preventive measures. Yet, recognizing that a society will limit the amount of healthcare it provides, Daniels proposed "normal species function" as the benchmark for deciding which care to provide. He held that healthcare that will restore or maintain normal species function should be

---

[15] Rawls, *Political Liberalism*, 184.

[16] Daniels N, "Justice, Health, and Health Care," in Rhodes R, Battin MP, and Silvers A, editors, *Medicine and Social Justice: Essays on the Distribution of Health Care*, 2nd edition (New York: Oxford University Press, 2012: 20–33).

[17] Daniels, "Justice, Health, and Health Care."

provided. Nothing has to be provided, however, for those who are already within the normal range of species-typical functioning. Furthermore, in his more recent writing, Daniels pointed to the many social determinants of health inequalities and invoked Rawls's difference principle to claim that a just society should provide the most healthcare to those who are most disadvantaged with respect to health. In Daniels's view, a society should also address socially determined health disparities by attending to the needs of those who fall below the normal level of human function in order to allow those disadvantaged individuals to have equal access to social opportunities.

In sum, Daniels's standard for the design of healthcare systems is providing fair equality of opportunity. For him, the total amount of life years produced, feasibility, or any other factor is not a relevant consideration.[18]

Prioritarianism

Prioritarian views build on Rawls's difference principle rather than his principle of fair equal opportunity and oppose utilitarian approaches to the distribution of scarce resources. Whereas utilitarian allocations aim at maximizing an outcome over a population while deliberately ignoring the relational and relative differences between individuals, prioritarian allocations aim at identifying unwanted inequalities and then distributing resources to compensate for or correct them. Prioritarian allocations reflect a concern for how individuals fare in relation to each other and attempt to advantage those whose position is worse than others', in a sense, to make people roughly equal. For that reason, the position in its more extreme form is also called *egalitarianism*.

Numerous articles in the bioethics literature have addressed medical resource allocations from a prioritarian perspective. For instance, Dan Brock,[19] Frances Kamm,[20] and David Wasserman[21] argued the merits of one

[18] Daniels's "relevance condition" appears to capture this aspect of policy setting. Daniels, "Justice, Health, and Health Care," 26.

[19] Brock DW, "Priority to the Worse Off in Health-Care Resource Prioritization," in Rhodes R, Battin MP, and Silvers A, editors, *Medicine and Social Justice: Essays on the Distribution of Health Care*, 2nd edition (New York: Oxford University Press, 2012: 155–164).

[20] Kamm FM, "Whether to Discontinue Nonfutile Use of a Scarce Resource," in Rhodes R, Battin MP, and Silvers A, editors, *Medicine and Social Justice: Essays on the Distribution of Health Care*, 2nd edition (New York: Oxford University Press, 2012: 165–177).

[21] Wasserman D, "Aggregation and the Moral Relevance of Context in Health-Care Decision Making," in Rhodes R, Battin MP, and Silvers A, editors, *Medicine and Social Justice: Essays on the Distribution of Health Care*, 2nd edition (New York: Oxford University Press, 2012: 79–89).

approach over the other in a variety of vexing cases. They reflected on the difference between policies that will save the lives of a few people or save an arm for several other people. They are concerned with whether public policies should provide a greater advantage to some who are already well off (e.g., save the lives of the able bodied) or provide a smaller advantage to some who are worse off (e.g., save the use of an arm for those with some other preexisting disability). These discussions of "tragic choices" aim at discovering a principled basis for determining who is worse off and for making trade-off decisions. Some focused on identifiable individuals, and some addressed trade-offs of future significant harms against present small harms or more certain imminent harms against more hypothetical distant harms. Typically, these discussions favor policies that will allocate resources to immediate needs over future needs and benefits to identifiable individuals over benefits to those who cannot be currently identified.

Regardless of these differences, prioritarian views maintain a singular focus on the idea that justice requires advantaging those who are worse off than others. As with Daniels, the total number of life years produced, feasibility, or any other reason is not considered relevant.

Challenging Monolithic Conceptions of Justice

In opposition to these reigning views of justice, we actually employ different principles of justice for the allocation of limited resources in different sorts of life activities. For instance, every lottery ticket purchased has an equal chance to win the big prize, and the winner takes all. When it comes to allocating tickets for a blockbuster movie, we rely on the first come, first served principle of distribution. Honors are distributed according to past achievements. Respect is often accorded to the aged and protection to the young. Places on the Olympic team as well as research grants are awarded to those who promise the greatest future contribution. Invitations to our holiday dinners go to our favorite people, family members, and close friends. Family vacation plans can be made by considering which venue is likely to produce the overall greatest amount of happiness for all family members vacationing together. Although these different allocation principles may each be just in particular contexts, two points should be noted. First, these different allocations involve different principles. Second, acting in accordance with a specific principle may be just in certain circumstances, but it may be unjust in others. Furthermore, only a distinctive few principles of justice are acceptable for the allocation of medical care. This means that some principles that are consistent with justice in nonmedical circumstances may not be consistent with justice in medical circumstance. Also, as I explain further in this chapter, different principles of justice are relevant in different contexts of medical practice.

Each of the theoretical conceptions of justice discussed previously reflects a consideration that is important for guiding some allocation policies and some decisions about the distribution of medical resources. The problem with each of these theories is that the claims made in their favor are too sweeping. Because these ideas about justice and medicine are typically discussed singly, in artificially isolated contexts, and with a focus on carefully selected or fabricated examples, it is hard to notice when and how the concepts clash with reality. As philosopher Ronald Green has noted in his criticism of Daniels, the "mistake . . . is trying to decide such matters by reference to a single consideration—and not necessarily the most important one."[22] No single conception of justice provides guidance that is suitable to every circumstance.

This point is easy to miss when authors consider a narrow range of examples. So, I offer an array of especially well-known examples to serve as a challenge to the assumption that a consensus supports a single principle of justice in medicine and public health. Here I appeal to examples from medicine, public health, and public health research that have received attention in the media and were widely discussed. Some relatively recent events that required allocations of medical and public health resources occurred within a short span of time. They received a lot of national attention, and, in each case, the discussions that ensued led to a broad consensus on what justice required. Taken together, they provide vivid examples that show the variety of considerations that can make an allocation of medical and public health resources just: the attack on the World Trade Center in New York City in September 2001, the anthrax attacks in October 2001, the flu vaccine shortage in fall 2004, and Hurricane Katrina in September 2005. Those catastrophes and what unfolded in their wake provide a starting point for appreciating the complexity and contextuality of justice.

[22] Green RM, "Access to Healthcare: Going Beyond Fair Equality of Opportunity," *American Journal of Bioethics* 1, 2 (Spring 2001): 22–23.

Although there has been some debate about strategy (e.g., responding to an actual terrorist smallpox disease attack with universal vaccination) and about the allocation of resources (e.g., which victims to benefit and how much, whether to allocate resources for planning and to which plan, whether to allocate resources for research and what to study), the principles that underlie the decisions made during these crises have been assumed with relatively little contention. Implicit in this silent agreement are the presumptions that (1) everyone knows *the* guiding principle of justice and (2) *the* principle has the solid endorsement of a broad majority of the population.

I question both presumptions. Examining these vivid and challenging examples sheds light on our general approach to the just allocation of a society's limited medical and public health resources. Comparing the commonly invoked principles with the policies that were actually implemented reveals that there is no single principle that supports all of the choices that we consider to be just policies. This discovery, that no single conception of justice explains the array of broadly endorsed medical and public health policies, suggests that there is no single and authoritative conception of justice. No simple formula can tell us what justice requires in all circumstances. Rather, investigation and examination of the situation, reflection on the array of problems involved, the consequences of choosing one path or another, and consideration of whether a policy will promote or undermine society's trust lead to a conclusion about what justice requires in the specific context.

Consider two illuminating examples of medical and public health policies that were implemented in the fall of 2001 immediately after the attack on the World Trade Center.

Medical Emergencies

Triage is the broadly endorsed approach for responding to medical emergencies. It is the approach that had previously been accepted for disaster responses in New York City and rehearsed for implementation at medical facilities throughout New York State. On September 11, 2001, triage was immediately adopted by medical professionals for dealing with the medical needs that were expected once the Twin Towers of the World Trade Center collapsed, and its suitability has not been challenged in any of the literature that I have encountered since then. Allocation by triage acknowledges the seriousness of widespread medical needs and at least the temporary inadequacy of the human and material resources to fully respond to all needs. Triage requires medical professionals to make judgments about the likely survival of patients who need medical treatment. Recognizing that some people have urgent needs (i.e., they will die or suffer significant harm if not treated very soon) and that the resources available are inadequate relative to the need (e.g., supplies, facilities, trained personnel), patients are sorted into groups, and they are either treated or asked to wait according to their group classification. In the most extreme circumstances, those who are not likely to survive are deprived of treatment so that the available resources can be used to save the lives of those who are more likely to live. Those who are likely to die without treatment but who are likely to live if treated promptly are treated first. Those who are in need of treatment but can wait longer without dying are treated after those who are urgently ill.

On the morning of 9/11, the disaster plan that had been previously developed and practiced was implemented at hospitals in the New York City vicinity. Initially, when medical professionals anticipated huge numbers of patients with medical needs, many beds in ICUs were emptied, elective surgeries were canceled, and patients who could have been sent home were discharged. Collection activities in blood banks went into high gear, but the blood banks were only accepting O-negative donors.

We need to recognize which of the principles of justice are and are not reflected in these allocations. In medical emergencies, medical professionals deliberately disregard the concepts of giving everyone a fair equal opportunity to receive medical treatment, and they pointedly ignore relative differences in economic and social standing. Instead, they focus exclusively on the medical factors of urgency of need and likelihood of survival. No one presumes to measure whether or not each patient has previously received a fair or equal share of available resources, and no one stops to assess who has been more or less advantaged. No one sorts out the small differences between individuals that would provide somewhat greater utility in one allocation rather than another. And no one criticizes medicine for not attending to those differences.

In fact, the long tradition of medical ethics, dating back at least to the Hippocratic tradition, requires physicians to provide treatment based on need. Hence, the ethics of medicine appears to require physicians to commit themselves to unequal treatment (since need is unequal) and also to the nonjudgmental regard of any patient's worthiness. These long-standing expectations have not changed over the centuries since Hippocrates or in the years following the tragedies of September 11. These commitments remain intact irrespective of recent writing on the just allocation of medical resources, and they have been neither eroded nor transformed by reflection on the events of the autumn of 2001 and our responses to them.

Emergency triage provides neither equal shares of care nor equal opportunity for future social participation. On the contrary, the distribution of resources under triage aims at avoiding the most deaths. Triage provides everyone a better chance for survival than could be had by an equal distribution of resources.

Consequentialist considerations of efficacy and equality support the well-accepted views on emergency triage. When the time constraints of an emergency and the need for medical resources significantly outstrip the available resources, responses should be based on efficacy and treating everyone with similar medical needs similarly. Yet, it is worth noting that the sweeping exclusions of triage do not mesh with the utilitarian aim of maximizing the greatest utility, particularly when utility might require fine-grained sorting and ranking to distinguish those with the very best chance of survival from those with a good, but less optimal, chance, and those who are likely to live the longest from those with a somewhat shorter life expectancy. Triage, or avoid the worst outcome, is therefore a consequentialist approach, in that it focuses on outcomes, but it is not utilitarian in that it does not aim at maximizing the chosen outcome.

Triage is also not consistent with either fair equality of opportunity or prioritarianism, which take a person's standing relative to others into account. Those considerations are deliberately ignored by medical triage. Clearly, if these different principles of justice (i.e., avoid the worst outcome, maximize utility, fair equality of opportunity, prioritarianism) were applied to the same issues, they would lead to very different decisions. Intuitions that support prioritizing the disadvantaged or providing the greatest benefit to the least advantaged are undermined by the strong sense that nonmedical relative differences (e.g., in previous opportunities or disadvantages) should not come into play in decisions about emergency responses to terrorism and other urgent needs. Emergency triage allocates resources by taking everyone's prognosis and expected outcome into account. When an emergency triage policy is applied, individuals certainly receive unequal lots, and no priority is allowed to those who are more generally worse off in relation to prior medical or non-medical opportunities, advantages, capabilities or the like. Thus, questioning the commitment to fair equality of opportunity in medical triage also invites questions about what the appropriate framework for medical policy decisions should be.

Public Health Measures and Research

In the aftermath of the attack on the World Trade Center and the mail-disseminated anthrax attacks and smallpox scares that followed soon after, public health measures and research were initiated. Public health policies and biomedical research typically focus on populations. Biomedical research attempts to disconfirm hypotheses about predicted outcomes and thereby develop facts about the response of organisms. With respect to human subject research, groups of people are selected for study because of some relevant biological or environmental similarities. Any knowledge gained from the process is useful to the extent that it is applicable to all of those who share the common condition.

Public health policies are also designed to have an impact either on everyone or on only those individuals who are similarly impacted by a particular disease or a health-related condition. The goals of public health and biomedical research are pointedly directed at everyone in the group who might benefit from them. In deliberately focusing on the affected group, public health and biomedical research policies typically provide benefits only to that target group. By looking toward the future, public health officials attempt to develop a generalizable approach to the prevention, reduction, or treatment of biological or psychological problems. By looking back at outcomes, researchers attempt to develop knowledge about biological or psychological reactions. And, as with medical triage in the emergency setting, public health and biomedical research have not been criticized for holding to these agendas.

Whereas public health policies sometimes meet the standard of promoting utility, fair equality of opportunity, or priority for the worse off, sometimes they do not. In some cases (e.g., anthrax, smallpox), interventions are advocated because they are likely to save more lives than some alternative plan. The tremendous amount of resources devoted to decontamination of post offices and office buildings after the mail-disseminated anthrax attacks was widely accepted. But the cleanup policy had only a hypothetical and distant possible benefit.

Public health research sometimes has no impact on the social participation, health, or longevity of the entire population. If it turns out that we never have another disaster similar to what occurred on September 11 or if we never again experience a catastrophe that creates enormous amounts of pulverized concrete and incinerated computers and office furniture, research on their effects may never promote the social participation or health of anyone. In addition, if the burdens of the interventions that the studies support turn out to be prohibitively costly (e.g., give up skyscrapers and computers), they will not be adopted, and no one's fair equality of opportunity will be advanced. Public health research involves a quest for information that may or may not be useful. It also sometimes directs resources to the needs of a relatively few affected individuals. So, the standards of promoting fair equality of opportunity or maximizing health may, at least sometimes, be incompatible with those views of justice. Many other uses of the resources devoted to public health research could be more likely to promote fair equality of opportunity or maximize health in the population. If considerations of fair equality of opportunity were the only factor to be taken into account, projects that promoted it should have preference over public health research, for example. Yet, the consensus in favor of public health research suggests that other reasons support the broad endorsement it receives.

The Flu Vaccine Shortage and Hurricane Katrina

Next, recall the flu vaccine shortage in the fall of 2004 and Hurricane Katrina in the fall of 2005 and consider the actions that were taken in response. In 2004, when it became clear that there would not be enough flu vaccine to meet the expected demand, people recognized that it was important to find a better way to allocate the limited supply of flu vaccine than to allow it to go to the aggressive, the lucky, and those with good connections. Communities around the country, and then, finally, the US Centers for Disease Control and Prevention (CDC), promulgated distribution policies that allotted vaccine to those who were likely to die or suffer serious harm if they contracted the disease and then implemented schemes to restrict distribution accordingly. The supply was therefore directed to the immunocompromised, the very young, pregnant women, the elderly, first responders, and medical care providers who would be called on to treat flu-infected individuals.

These policies were very broadly endorsed and supported with excellent compliance. The almost total absence of debate over their implementation was evidence of the extent of the consensus on how the allocation should be handled. Aside from the advocates for children and the elderly, who each argued that their constituent group should have even more priority over others in the vaccine target group, the US population accepted the plans that were implemented.

The principle supporting flu vaccine allocation was not utilitarian in that utility would have disqualified the elderly and the immunocompromised because their vaccination could be expected to provide relatively few life years, a small QALY payoff. The policy took into account neither previous injustices nor disadvantages, and it did not try to equalize opportunities in some wider sense. The principle inherent in the vaccine distribution policy was "avoid the worst outcome," which, in that context, was taken to mean avoid the most serious illnesses and deaths. The consensus of support and the lack of opposition speak to how the importance of one particular goal can be obvious to experts who take seriously their duty to uphold society's trust. It also reflects how the justice of what was done can be apparent to the public.

Reaction to what happened before, during, and after Hurricane Katrina illustrates a broad consensus at the other end of the spectrum. In the case of Katrina, there was general agreement that the US government had failed to adequately prepare for the disaster, failed to warn and protect Gulf Coast residents, failed in its attempts at rescue and meeting the tremendous needs of affected communities in the aftermath, and failed in providing honest and timely communication about the formaldehyde risk of the trailers that were later provided to shelter some who had been left homeless. These realizations point us to the broad agreement on the importance of investment in disaster preparedness, meeting the urgent needs of all citizens, making leadership appointments based on qualifications rather than cronyism and politics, and timely and honest communication. Again, this consensus on values is not a matter of chance or coincidence. Rather, it reflects society's trust in the profession's stewardship of medical resources and confidence that the medical community will take the lead in planning and acting to protect the public and promote the importance of critical human concerns.

Justice in Allocations for Medicine and Public Health

We all are vulnerable to death, pain, illness, and disability, and we all want to avoid those consequences for our loved ones and ourselves. We also all have to acknowledge that there are not enough resources to provide for every medical need and public health project that we might like to support. Although some Rawlsians and other scholars characterize this problem by distinguishing ideal from nonideal theory, I'm inclined to see scarcity in Hobbesian terms as an inevitable feature of human life in the real world.[23] Thus, we have to prioritize our values and sacrifice some of what we might want so that we can be more likely to secure those things that are more important to us. Because the achievement of certain goals is essential to our enjoying others, because certain hardships are more enduring and painful than others, and because this is so for almost everyone almost always, in the situations that arise people tend to agree on the primacy of some important concerns. These features of our shared human nature make the concordance on some matters of medical and public health justice not contingent and coincidental, but genuine agreement that expresses the human importance of some significant feature of a situation. This natural consensus provides us with an array of principles of justice that are relevant to allocations in medicine and public health.

Triage may be the appropriate guiding conception of justice for policies that respond to large-scale emergency situations. The justification for triage is that it is the policy most likely to avoid the worst outcome and save the greatest number of lives. When medical professionals explain it well, the public can acknowledge that triage-based allocations of resources are just. Reasonable people would want to survive a disaster, and they would want their loved ones to survive. Forgoing treatment for those who are least likely to survive, to provide the best chance of survival for the most people, yields the result that rational and reasonable people want most. No one who considers the matter in advance, before the heat of the crisis, could reasonably reject it.[24] As long as the same criteria for providing treatment are applied to everyone, the loved ones of those from whom treatment is withheld would not have grounds for complaining of injustice. A triage allocation of emergency services is, therefore, likely to be accepted as a just and trustworthy allocation of resources in emergency circumstances.

Disaster preparedness requires the allocation of communal resources for research, training, and equipment. Policies to allocate resources for preparedness and research are justified because the ability to respond **efficiently**

---

[23] Hobbes T, *Hobbes's Leviathan* (Oxford, UK: Clarendon Press, 1965). (Reprint from original work published 1651)

[24] In this analysis, I draw freely on T. M. Scanlon's conception of justice (Scanlon, *What We Owe*).

could crucially depend on preparedness and the information learned from scientific studies. The benefits that can be had from preparation would not be available without the prior contribution from a common pool. Hence, it is just for institutions and agencies led by medical professions to advocate for providing resources for preparedness and research to help improve the tools at their disposal and increase the chance for a good outcome and, at the same time, minimize the chance for the worst outcome (i.e., **maximin**). The salience and importance of these supporting reasons make these policies just and trustworthy.

Public health measures are often justified by the **public good** of protection against disease that they provide. In the face of a credible risk of biological warfare, mandatory vaccination against a serious contagious disease is a just policy when a reasonably safe and effective vaccine is available. Medical leaders will need to explain that required vaccination provides protection from disease, that is, something that everyone values. They will also need to explain that those who might refuse to comply with recommended vaccination would be free-riders who treat others unjustly. They expect to benefit from herd immunity by taking advantage of those who act from goodwill and a sense of communal responsibility while not shouldering their fair share of burdens. Mandatory vaccination that would require everyone to shoulder a fair share of the burden of safety would be supported by the **anti–free-rider principle**. And when it comes to actually dispensing vaccine in the face of a credible risk, because the relative differences between individuals may not be significant enough to justify treating any groups in some special way, a distribution scheme based on **efficacy** or **equality**, such as a lottery, may be in order.

Furthermore, there may be good reasons for allowing a few to be exempt from mandatory vaccination. Those with impaired immune systems would be particularly vulnerable to any associated vaccine risks and bear more than the typical burden of being vaccinated. If everyone else in the society were vaccinated, exempting those few who would otherwise bear an **undue burden** would not significantly increase the risk for others. Trusted medical professionals are able to recognize such relevant differences, and they should be empowered to implement the appropriate responses that instantiate justice.

The public health concerns after September 11 and Hurricane Katrina reflect three different principles of justice. Clean air, clean water, and sewage treatment are the kinds of public benefits that everyone needs constantly.

Their **vital and constant importance** to well-being is a justification for policies to provide and protect those public goods. In many settings, clean air, clean water, and sewage treatment are also the kinds of benefits that no one can have unless everyone has them. Thus, making them available or unavailable at all makes them available or unavailable to everyone in the society. In many situations, these are also services that can be provided with greatest **efficacy** by providing them for everyone.

Interventions that provide for everyone's **vital and constant needs** are also likely to make the greatest difference in health and well-being for the economically and socially least advantaged. The well-to-do could leave town for the clean air of the country or purchase gas masks to protect themselves from air pollution. They would also have the wherewithal to purchase bottled water, dig private wells, and install private sewage systems. The well-to-do would be better off with the general availability of clean air, clean water, and sewage treatment. Yet, the underlying interrelation between poverty and disease and the consequent disparity between the well-to-do and the poor with respect to health status and life expectancy[25,26] suggest that the economically and socially disadvantaged would enjoy an even greater benefit from policies that made these benefits generally available.[27] In addition to vital importance and efficacy, the **difference principle** is a further reason for providing these services. This example illustrates how multiple principles of justice can converge in support of a public health policy.

The Complexity of Justice

The incongruity between any simple conception of justice on the one hand and policy consensus on the other suggests that searching for *the* simple essential meaning of justice is a wild goose chase. It also suggests an alternative view of justice. When we stop to examine our own thinking about these issues, we notice that we actually invoke different reasons to support different principles and different rankings of considerations in different contexts. That

---

[25] Daniels, "Justice, Health, and Health Care."

[26] Smith P, "Justice, Health, and the Price of Poverty," in Rhodes R, Battin MP, and Silvers A, editors, *Medicine and Social Justice: Essays on the Distribution of Health Care*, 2nd edition (New York: Oxford University Press, 2012: 255–263).

[27] Furthermore, the continuous lack of such basic goods as clean air, clean water, and sewage treatment for some, while others enjoy them as private resources, is likely to enrage those who are deprived and therefore promote social instability.

insight suggests that there is no single principle that defines justice. With sensitivity to the complexity of human values and the different contexts of medical needs, we can appreciate that a variety of reasons are involved in justifying different medical and public health resource allocations. Even though a contextual approach to determining the just distribution of resources will sometimes favor one principle and at other times prioritize another, good allocation decisions will express widely shared views about the primacy of some considerations over others and reflect reasons that no one can reasonably reject for guiding decisions in such circumstances. In this sense, a contextual view of justice is not random and not idiosyncratically subjective. Rather, it expresses deep human similarities, common human concerns, and shared priorities that relate to our human mortality and vulnerability.

An Overview of Justice in Medical Practice

Appreciating that justice in different domains can be informed by different principles, we can move on to distinguishing a variety of appropriate and compelling principles to govern resource allocations in different areas of medical practice. To the extent that we can identify appropriate reasons for determining medical resource allocations within a specific kind of medical context, we can say that justice in that domain of medicine is determined by those principles. To the extent that we can rule out reasons that are inappropriate, we can say that those principles should have low priority in that sort of medical context and that implementing policies for promoting such goals would be unjust. The just allocation of medical and public health resources is and should be governed by a variety of reasons that physicians recognize and endorse for their saliency. And when those reasons are explained with appropriate examples, reasonable people will be able to appreciate the justice of those decisions.[28]

Several principles of justice have a legitimate place in medical and public health allocations. To achieve justice in resolving the practical problems of resource allocation that arise within medicine and public health, medical professionals' decisions should focus on mutually supported and compelling reasons. These broadly endorsed overarching reasons are the principles of

---

[28] Daniels N and Sabin JE, "Limits to Health Care: Fair Procedures, Democratic Deliberation, and the Legitimacy Problem for Insurers," *Philosophy and Public Affairs* 26, 4 (1997): 303–350.

medical justice. They include **the anti–free-rider principle, avoiding undue burdens, avoiding the worst outcome, the difference principle, efficacy, equality, maximin, providing public goods,** and **attending to the vital and constant importance to well-being.**[29,30] To the extent that the scarcity of resources makes it impossible to fulfill all legitimate claims, some principle(s) will have to be sacrificed, and some medical interventions that are supported by compelling reasons will have to be scaled down from an ideal level, delayed, or abandoned. When these hard choices have to be made, medical professionals are trusted to make decisions for good reasons that reasonable people would support.[31]

Philosopher Leonard Fleck's view on the complexity of justice is similar to mine in that he also appreciates that numerous different considerations have to be taken into account and prioritized in making specific medical allocation decisions and providing a distribution plan that is just.[32] There is, however, one significant difference in our positions. I see the solution to allocation questions in the consensus of medical professionals. Fleck argued instead for turning to democratic deliberation, that is, focused conversations with groups of lay citizens led by an unbiased moderator, as the way to identify just allocations of medical resources. Fleck was skeptical of the possibility of achieving consensus on these issues and regarded democratic deliberation in public meetings as the best means to achieve a reasonable ordering of our medical priorities.

I see merit in the search for consensus, but I worry that relying on democratic deliberation for medical policy decisions introduces two problems. (1) Whereas medical ethics provides a set of shared commitments as a starting point for deliberation among medical professionals, people from the general public who happen to be involved in a democratic deliberation are likely to have radically different personal values that may be inconsistent with each others' and inconsistent with the ethics of medicine. The results of a democratic deliberation can therefore turn on who the participants happen to be, how widely their values are shared, and what sorts of reasons inform

---

[29] I am not arguing that this list is a full elaboration of the relevant considerations for justice in medicine and public health.

[30] Examples of allocation principles that are most typically excluded from the list of principles of medical justice include winner takes all; first come, first served; previous social contributions; respect for the aged; protection of the young; promise of future social contributions; favorite people.

[31] Daniels's "relevance condition" appears to capture this aspect of policy setting. Daniels, 2012: 16.

[32] Fleck LM, *Just Caring: Health Care Rationing and Democratic Deliberation* (New York: Oxford University Press, 2009).

their values. (2) The leader of a democratic deliberation will select the salient examples for presentation to the audience and explain the issues for their deliberation. As any experienced teacher knows, the choice of examples and framing the question are likely to have a huge impact on the result. This could make the resolution of a democratic deliberation more the result of the leader's position than the result of the public's assessment. An assembly of medical professionals would have the background to offer different kinds of examples during the deliberative process and the experience and confidence to suggest ways to reframe the issue. That would make the emerging consensus less likely to reflect the influence of the deliberation leader.

At the clinical level, it strikes me that the direct personal experience of physicians is critical for informing justice in resource allocations. Having witnessed medical professionals achieve consensus on reasonable plans for the allocation of medical resources and numerous other controversial medical issues, I am optimistic about their ability to identify just policies for allocation of medical resources. I believe that this occurs because there is broad background agreement among doctors and other medical professionals on the duties of medical ethics. This eliminates many possible sources of conflict and provides a solid starting point for their deliberations. In a sense that background agreement amounts to what Rawls referred to as "an overlapping consensus" that goes a long way in mitigating "the burdens of judgment."[33] In my experience, the process works most of the time, that is, as long as the conversations are not hijacked by politics, bullying, misleading language, or concepts from common morality.

In making difficult choices about the ranking of projects and priorities and the design of policies, different considerations will have different importance in different kinds of situations. There is no obvious reason to presume that one priority will always trump the others. When the priority of a principle reflects the endorsement of an overlapping consensus of medical professionals and can muster society's endorsement, we have good reason to consider the policy to be just.[34] When large groups of people rank the competing considerations differently, a significant consensus on the principles that are irrelevant may emerge, and that consensus can serve as the basis for designing a just policy. To the extent that flexibility can be supported by the

---

[33] Rawls, *Political Liberalism*. Rawls's philosophy has been an important touchstone for proponents of democratic deliberation, such as Joshua Cohen and Amy Gutmann.

[34] In *Political Liberalism*, John Rawls used the term *overlapping consensus* to describe the agreement of "reasonable and rational" people.

available resources, policies should show tolerance for different priorities. And when extreme scarcity and urgency limit the options, the public tends to trust expert physicians to make the allocation decision.

Thus far, I have offered criticisms of various monolithic views of justice and tried to justify the relevance of several principles of medical justice. I now turn to explaining what justice requires in the practice of medicine. Without claiming to offer a complete account that covers every sort of medical activity, I sketch what justice requires in four of the most notable medical domains: (1) nonacute care, (2) acute care, (3) critical scarce resources, and (4) public health.[35] By addressing allocation issues that arise in each of these medical domains, I try to avoid the pitfall of cherry-picking examples to exemplify my view. As you should expect at this point, I argue for the saliency of a number of different principles of justice in each domain.

Justice in Nonacute Care

Nonacute care includes several different patient care venues. These groupings are not mutually exclusive. Some patients actually receive care in several venues, some all at once, and some at different times over the course of an illness or over their lives. It is important to attend to how different principles of justice function in each.

Chronic Care
Many people live with illness. Most of the time, they do not require acute care, and they manage their condition(s) largely on their own with periodic doctor visits. The range of chronic conditions includes, for example, asthma, diabetes, kidney failure, high blood pressure, colitis, HIV, lupus, and cancer. The medical needs of people with chronic illness may be serious or mild, but all of these patients should receive whatever medical care they require. Allocation of medical resources to meet their medical needs is supported by the principle that requires clinicians to **attend to the vital and constant importance to well-being**. Patients should receive what they require to maintain or restore their well-being.

---

[35] There is a fifth domain: justice in the allocation of resources for biomedical research. A great deal can be said about which research projects to prioritize. Should financing and effort go only to clinically relevant projects, or should basic science be given equal weight? Among worthy scientific projects, which should receive the most resources? I set those issues aside for another day.

As in every treatment decision, choosing the specific treatment for an individual patient to receive should involve consideration of maximizing the desired results while minimizing burdensome side effects. That is, treatment decisions should be governed by the **maximin** principle. The more serious the anticipated consequences of forgoing treatment, the greater the tolerance for treatment-related side effects should be: The less serious the consequences of forgoing treatment, the lower the tolerance for burdensome side effects. This means that justice always requires physicians to compare risks and benefits when they are selecting a treatment plan that serves a patient's interests.

To the extent that well-being is important to everyone, patients with similar medical needs should be provided with comparable treatment in accordance with the principle of **equality**. And to the extent that the available resources are limited, **efficacy** should guide the use of medical interventions. When an inexpensive option is appropriate, it should be tried first, and when expensive interventions are likely to provide little benefit, it is legitimate for them to be withheld.

The **difference principle** should also play a significant role in the just provision of chronic medical care. The difference principle reflects a broadly shared commitment to the idea that some people need more help than others, and because of their need, they should receive more help than others do. People who are poor, work several jobs, and have a hard time making ends meet; people who care for several children with little social supports; people who live in environments that present special health challenges (e.g., pollution, violence, contamination)[36,37]; people with mental or physical disabilities[38,39]; people who are old and frail[40]; people who are distrustful of medical professionals[41]; and people with limited medical literacy are likely

---

[36] Wolff J, "Health Risk and Health Security," in Rhodes R, Battin MP, and Silvers A, editors, *Medicine and Social Justice: Essays on the Distribution of Health Care* (New York: Oxford University Press, 2012: 71–78).

[37] Smith, "Justice, Health, and the Price of Poverty."

[38] Silvers A, "Health Care Justice for the Chronically Ill and Disabled: A Deficiency in Justice Theory and How to Cure It," in Rhodes R, Battin MP, and Silvers A, editors, *Medicine and Social Justice: Essays on the Distribution of Health Care*, 2nd edition (New York: Oxford University Press, 2012: 299–312).

[39] Ozar D and Sabin J, "Oral and Mental Health Services," in Rhodes R, Battin MP, and Silvers A, editors, *Medicine and Social Justice: Essays on the Distribution of Health Care*, 2nd edition (New York: Oxford University Press, 2012: 401–411).

[40] Francis L, "Age Rationing Under Conditions of Injustice," in Rhodes R, Battin MP, and Silvers A, editors, *Medicine and Social Justice: Essays on the Distribution of Health Care*, 2nd edition (New York: Oxford University Press, 2012: 355–362).

[41] McGary H, "Racial Groups, Distrust, and the Distribution of Health Care," in Rhodes R, Battin MP, and Silvers A, editors, *Medicine and Social Justice: Essays on the Distribution of Health Care*, 2nd edition (New York: Oxford University Press, 2012: 265–277).

to need more resources than others with similar medical conditions who are more able to manage on their own without extra supports.

The Black Report on the health outcomes of people in Britain who have access to the very same National Health System demonstrated that merely providing equal medical care still leaves the less well-off with significant health disparities.[42,43] Similarly, research in the United States identified numerous factors that contribute to heath disparities.[44] This evidence suggests that to compensate for social disadvantages, justice requires greater investment of medical resources to help people who are worse off in some respect(s) to achieve health outcomes that are comparable to others'. Different sorts of interventions will be required depending on the individual's needs and what is likely to be useful. Strategies can include more frequent checkups than standardly allowed, accessible clinic locations, longer than standard clinic hours, educational interventions, and even home visits.

Well-Patient Care

Many people who are well still want and need medical care. These patients include people who have no illness as well as people who seek medical attention for issues that are not per se disease related. This fact is frequently overlooked, but today's medicine includes well-patient services across the spectrum from well-baby care to aid in dying.

In this light, it is important to recognize that the medical profession is a social artifact created by giving control over a set of knowledge, skills, powers, privileges, and immunities exclusively to a select few who are entrusted to provide their services in response to the community's needs and to use their distinctive tools for the good of patients and society. As I explained in Chapter 2, medicine is very much like other fields in this respect. Consider that firefighters are called to rescue cats and children from tall trees, and we rely on police to return lost children and call on them to subdue an escaped tiger (as happened once in New Jersey) even when no fire or law enforcement issues are involved. Firefighters and police have the wherewithal, so they get

---

[42] Gray AM, "Inequalities in Health. The Black Report: A Summary and Comment," *International Journal of Health Services* 12, 3 (1982): 349–380.

[43] Berridge V, "The Black Report: Reinterpretting History," in Cook HJ, Bhattacharya S, and Hardy A, eds. *The History of the Social Determinants of Health* (Andhra Pradesh, India: Orient Blackswan, 2010).

[44] Office of Disease Prevention and Health Promotion, Healthy People 2020. *Disparities*. Accessed August 30, 2018, at https://www.healthypeople.gov/2020/about/foundation-health-measures/Disparities

the job. Similarly, the special knowledge, powers, privileges, and immunities of medicine explain why the role of medical professionals extends beyond the boundaries of health and disease. Doctors have the wherewithal, so they get the jobs that involve using their distinctive knowledge and exercising their special powers, privileges, and immunities to fulfill their duties of **attending to the vital and constant well-being** of their patients.

In the bioethics literature, numerous authors make a project of defining *the* goal of health care or *the* scope of medicine. They typically define the goal in terms of a biological consideration like health, disease, or normal species function. These approaches are appealing because they allow their proponents to employ seemingly objective standards in drawing neat lines between services that should be covered by health programs and services that should not, typically excluding services such as plastic surgery and assisted reproduction. Unfortunately, distinguishing legitimate claims for medical services from those that are not is not that simple, and employing biological definitions to stand in for ethical considerations creates problems of injustice.

Norman Daniels, for example, employed normal species function as his standard for determining which patients should be allocated medical treatment and which should not.[45] His paradigm case involved the provision of growth hormone treatment for children who would have short stature. Daniels was willing to support the treatment for those children who were growth hormone deficient, but not for children who would benefit equally, but whose short stature was related to their having short parents and growth hormone levels within the normal range.

Daniels's use of the normal species function criterion occurred within the context of his broader view of justice in healthcare, but introducing the biological standard of normal species function within his theory actually created an internal conflict. The problem begins with his framing the issue in terms of the biologically based concept of "healthcare" rather than the profession-based concept of "medical care." Then Daniels argued for the importance of providing healthcare as a basic human need and framed his argument in terms of Rawlsian principles of justice. He seemed to overlook the fact that the ability to enjoy fair equality of opportunity and participate in the social and political sphere without unfair disadvantage is a social standard for achieving justice, not a biological one. Daniels's acceptance of

---

[45] Daniels, "Justice, Health, and Health Care."

Rawls's social standard implies that social barriers to fair competition have to be taken into account in the just allocation of medical resources, even when those factors do not involve deviations from normal species function. Thus, all children with expected short stature should equally have access to growth hormone therapy because short stature is a detriment in our social world, and it is likely to impede their future opportunities.

Furthermore, access to primary goods, which is required by Rawls's first principle of justice, is not circumscribed by biology. Primary goods not only include food and healthcare, as Daniels would acknowledge, but also include social elements. Thus, factors that might interfere with being treated with respect within the social domain (e.g., looking old) and factors that frustrate the ability to participate in the social life that members of our society aspire to share (e.g., missing or discolored teeth) could merit medical resources based on Rawlsian principles.

Another factor supporting well-patient care is that some of it, such as periodic monitoring of low-risk pregnancies, well-baby visits, and annual checkups, has a preventive justification. They provide comfort and support and therein help to establish and maintain an ongoing and trusted physician-patient relationship. Other well-patient care is actually focused on helping patients achieve social goals. Healthy male and female patients may want medical assistance for purposes of birth control because, at various stages in their lives, procreation is not consistent with their other social goals. A female patient who is over age 35 and has species-typical low fertility may want medical intervention for assisted reproduction. For her, the desire to be a mother, raise a biologically related child, and share in the parenting experiences of her peers may be a significant element in her achieving happiness and well-being. The 70-year-old male patient with normal virility may want medical assistance for sexual activity to enhance his well-being with physical intimacy. And a patient with a large hemangioma on her face that does not impede any biological function may want treatment that will shrink it away so that her appearance will no longer impede her social interactions.

These examples challenge the definitions of medicine that characterize the field in terms of health and disease and dispute accounts that would constrict the legitimate goals of medicine to a demarcated sphere of abnormal human functioning. Instead, we need to think of medicine more broadly. For instance, in the twenty-first century, we have come to regard homosexuality as a normal condition. We also accept gender dysphoria as a medical condition and see that transgender identity is real. From today's perspective, we acknowledge the merits of hormonal therapy, surgery, and other supportive interventions for transgender people. When a mature transgender patient experiences social difficulty because the patient's facial features do not match the chosen gender and prevent social acceptance as a person of that gender, facial reconstructive surgery may be important for improving the patient's well-being.

At a certain point, some patients are left with diseases that have no cure. There is nothing that medicine can do to improve their health or extend their lives. They may be dying, and they may be experiencing pain that is normally associated with their condition. Pain management that does nothing to address the underlying cause of the pain or prolong life may, nevertheless, be an important benefit that medicine can provide and thereby advance well-being.

And then there is aid in dying, physician-assisted suicide, and euthanasia. When life is burdensome, as life sometimes is, it can be important to be able to share one's thoughts about ending it all with one's doctor.[46] Access to aid in dying may also be important, especially for people who value their independence and control over their lives: They may need to feel as if they have the power to end their lives. Doctors have unique roles to play in these decisions. Because of their experience, they can appreciate when an elderly patient with no underlying illness has irremediably lost the will to eat and live and can help support that patient's choice of hospice care. They can also appreciate the burdens of disease-related deterioration and provide the desired assistance to make continued living worthwhile. They can assess when the wish to die is the effect of a treatable depression and provide the intervention to help the patient heal. And when a patients sees life as no longer worth living and nothing can be done to improve the situation, a caring trusted doctor can help to bring the patient's suffering to an end.

Because only medicine has the wherewithal to address these needs, these are all legitimate uses of medical resources. Patients should be entitled to these needed interventions, and physicians should be paid for their time and effort. Allocation of medical resources to meet the social goals of patients should be supported because these services are **important to well-being**. Every patient with similar needs should be treated similarly in accordance with the principle of **equality**.

---

[46] Muller D, "Physician-Assisted Death Is Illegal in Most States, So My Patient Made Another Choice," *Health Affairs* 31, 10 (2012): 2343–2346.

Preventive Medicine

Although we often think of medicine as curing disease or ameliorating its effects, many medical measures aim at protecting, promoting, and maintaining health and preventing disease, disability, and death. Some of these efforts involve offering education; others involve advocating for community-wide interventions to prevent disease (e.g., fluoridating drinking water, controlling the mosquito population); and some involve individual interventions (e.g., vaccination). Such efforts are justified by several principles. **Providing public goods** is relevant because the benefit will accrue to everyone. The **anti–free-rider** principle is relevant because, to the extent that disease is communicable, everyone should do a fair share in preventing transmission. For example, everyone should cover their mouth when coughing to help stop the spread of germs. **Avoiding undue burdens** is important because some preventive measures that are minimally burdensome to most people may involve serious risks of harm for others. **Equality** is an important consideration because we are all vulnerable to disease, and everyone prefers to avoid it and remain healthy. Preventive measures are also justified by the **efficacy** and **maximin** principles because preventing disease is often far more clinically effective, cost effective, and less burdensome than treating disease after it develops. Screening and testing individual patients for disease (e.g., annual physicals, newborn screening, mammography, Pap smears, reproductive genetic screening and testing) are also justified by the **efficacy** and **maximin** principles. Furthermore, some types of screening provide individuals with the opportunity for taking measures that could avert serious conditions or impede future life choices (e.g., testing for ovarian reserve).

The **difference principle** also has a role in the just allocation of preventive medicine benefits. Beliefs, fears, culture, inertia, and the overwhelming demands of life can all amount to barriers that preventive medicine initiatives have to overcome. Some individuals and groups may have particularly difficult hurdles to surmount in order to receive medical care. In some cases, incentives for accepting testing might be in order.[47] In other cases, extra time and effort to garner trust may be what is needed.

For example, African Americans often harbor residual feelings of distrust toward medicine derived from a long history of abuse. People from that

[47] Rhodes R, "Perspectives: Incentives for Healthy Behavior," *Hastings Center Report* 45, 3 (2015): Inside back cover.

community, which also has a high incidence of sickle cell disease, may regard screening for the sickle cell trait as a genocidal plot. Helping African American patients to make informed decisions about screening may therefore require extra time, education, and conversation.[48] The **difference principle** would support such efforts as a matter of justice.

Domiciliary Care

A good portion of home care, nursing home care, and hospice care is primarily housing and feeding. Nevertheless, in the United States the cost of this care is typically included in the healthcare budget because it does involve some medical services provided by medical professionals. Often, the patients who are recipients of this care are not expected to be cured of their disease, and these residential facilities are frequently expected to be the patients' domicile until death.

Justice requires medicine to provide the care that will keep these patients clean, safe, fed, hydrated, and free of pain because as members of our society we have a duty to **attend to the vital and constant importance of their well-being.** No reasonable person would be willing to forgo these benefits for themselves or their loved ones. And, as trusted guardians of their patients' welfare, physicians are required to ensure that these needs are met.

Justice in Acute Care

Consider again the emergency room and the allocation of hospital beds and facilities. There, in the apportioning of limited medical resources, need matters and urgency matters because they play an important role in **avoiding the worst outcome.** Patients with significant medical needs can only receive the care that they require in an acute care facility: The level of technology and expertise are available nowhere else. Also, those with urgent needs, that is, those who will die soon or imminently without medical attention suffer serious harm from delays in treatment. They should be treated first, before others who may have arrived earlier but who could wait for treatment without serious untoward consequences. Beyond that, for those who are similarly situated with respect to need and urgency, patients should be treated similarly, that is, the principle of **equality** should govern medical allocations.

---

[48] McGary H, "Racial Groups, Distrust."

Although distributing the same size slice to everyone who pays for a slice of pizza would be just, giving the exact same medical treatment to each patient is obviously not the rule in medicine because patients' bodies and medical needs are different from one another in numerous ways. **Equality** in this sense requires giving similar treatment to patients with similar needs. All patients who are having a stroke should be provided with similar interventions, and all patients with a myocardial infarction should be provided with similar interventions, but those interventions will not be the same. Differences in the treatment are justified by physical differences that call for different clinical responses, such as the type of intervention, the amount of drug adjusted to the weight of the patient, or the time of symptom onset.

In the allocation of acute medical care, other considerations like age, past contribution to society, promise of future contribution, or personal attachment, which may be appropriate for the distribution of honors and opportunities, should play no part. Hence, allocations in the emergency room and the rest of the hospital should be governed by a narrow set of considerations (i.e., urgency, need). It may sometimes be politically difficult to ask a colleague, celebrity, or relative of an important donor who is in need of care for a sprained ankle to wait for treatment, but justice requires that urgent needs be attended first. Allocations of medical resources in the acute care setting should only be governed by principles of medical justice.

Justice in the Allocation of Critically Scarce Resources

Although all medical resources are limited, some resources are critically scarce. Some, such as beds in an ICU, are scarce by design because governments sometimes limit the number of ICU beds that each institution may have as a cost containment measure. Other resources, such as transplant organs, are limited because of individual reluctance to donate the organs of a deceased relative, because of natural scarcity, or because of legal structures (e.g., required request for organ procurement rather than presumed consent to govern). Other critically scarce resources are limited by the rarity of ingredients; manufacturing difficulty; or the tremendous cost of production of, for example, an extremely rare and expensive clotting factor or cancer drug; or a robotic suit that is worn as an exoskeleton to help a disabled person walk.

Triage should be the guiding principle in the allocation of these critically scarce resources. When there is not enough for everyone with similar medical needs to receive the benefit, the scarce supply should be withheld from those who are most likely to die soon regardless of treatment so that the resources can instead be allotted to those who can be expected to receive an objectively measured significantly greater benefit from them (e.g., more years of interactive life). In such circumstances, **triage** can be expected to help avoid the most avoidable deaths or other catastrophic outcomes.[49]

Sometimes the patient with the greatest or most urgent medical need should be passed over so that a patient with lesser need or urgency may receive the resource. In this way, the worst outcome is averted. As illustration, imagine a patient with organ failure with metastatic cancer and a life expectancy of less than 6 months. Even though that patient may have the greatest need, the organ should instead be allocated to another patient on the transplant list with an excellent chance of surviving for at least 5 years with a transplant. Two deaths within a few months is a worse outcome than one death and one long life.[50] This is not to say that one life is worth more than another, but a remark about justice. It is just to take the likelihood of significant differences in the duration of benefit into account in the assignment of scarce transplant organs. This justification can be explained to the public, and it is likely to receive their broad endorsement. Similarly, it is just to remove a critically ill patient who is comatose and unresponsive to treatment from the ICU so that some other patient with an acute medical need for ICU care and a good likelihood of return to normal function will survive. In such a case, the significant difference between restoring consciousness and the ability to interact as compared with merely extending life in a permanently unconscious state is a difference that most people can appreciate and support as a basis for decision making.

For those waiting in line to purchase a movie ticket, first come, first served matters, but in the allocation of scarce medical resources factors such as who had a place in the unit first is irrelevant. Likewise, the surgery of a patient

[49] Engelhardt HT and Rie MA, "Intensive Care Units, Scarce Resources, and Conflicting Principles of Justice," *Journal of the American Medical Association* 255, 9 (1986): 1159–1164. Engelhardt and Rie endorsed a triage approach similar to mine and suggested employing "an *ICU treatment entitlement index* (ICU-EI)" that balances the probability of benefit, length of survival, and quality of success to set "criteria for admission to, and continued treatment in and discharge from an ICU (1162).
[50] Schiano TD, Bourgoise T, and Rhodes R, "High Risk Liver Transplant Candidates: An Ethical Proposal on Where to Draw the Line," *Liver Transplantation* 21, 5 (2015): 607–611.

waiting for a scheduled procedure should have to wait when the operating room is needed for a patient with a surgical emergency.

The allotment of scarce drugs should be treated similarly, but sometimes the contextual complexity means that more factors have to be taken into account in the allocation decision. Some drugs are used for several different purposes. When the limited supply of a drug is inadequate, the **triage** principle should govern the distribution, but its interpretation may have to be more nuanced. As a general rule, when some patients need the drug as a life-saving therapy, they should get preference over those who need it to address some less urgent need. When some patients need the drug to address a potentially fatal medical problem that has no alternative treatment, their need should be prioritized over other needs that can be addressed with different interventions that are nearly as effective. And when the shortage affects patients with a similar condition, to the extent that physicians are able to distinguish patients who are likely to reap a significant benefit from those who are not, **triage** dictates that treatment should be withheld from patients who are significantly less likely to benefit.

Decisions concerning expensive treatments should be governed by similar considerations, but the issues that they raise may seem different. Some medical treatments are relatively inexpensive, but others are resource intensive and costly. When does a treatment cost too much? This is a question that can only be answered within the context of the politics and the wherewithal of a particular society. The answer turns on the needs of the people, the wealth of the society, and how much of its wealth the society is willing to allocate to medical care. Some societies decide that they can afford to pay for kidney dialysis treatment and organ transplantation. Others cannot or do not.

Equality requires that the payout threshold within a society should be the same across the board. This means that the same financial limit to maximum expenditure should be applied to an expensive cancer drug and organ transplantation, ICU care, exoskeletons, and so on. **Efficacy** requires that payout be tied to outcomes. In some systems, such as the British National Health Service, calibrating the QALYs provided by each medical intervention has been used as a means for allocating its limited supply of medical resources. Applying the same metric across the board to all treatments ensures that different medical needs are treated similarly and that biases against diseases (e.g., HIV) or patient groups (e.g., alcoholics) do not lead to unjust denials of treatment. This is rationing. Rationing is most acceptable, and therefore just, when the standards for disallowing some medical interventions, and the procedure for reaching those decisions, are transparent and based on limits that are accepted as fair.

Objections to Medical Triage . Rationing is controversial and so are some of the other resource allocation implications that I have argued are required by justice. A number of these positions have been vigorously opposed in the bioethics literature, and authors who would disagree are likely to raise concerns about first come, first served; identifiable others, killing, the right to life, the rule of rescue, and other issues.

One objection to removing some specific life-preserving treatment or removing a patient from an ICU invokes the concept of first come, first served. Although giving priority to those who are first in the queue may be a just procedure in allocating seats for a movie or even in determining which of several patients with relatively minor medical needs will be treated next, it should not be the standard for distributing more critical services. Policymakers in medical institutions typically recognize that critical and urgent needs should be treated differently from other needs. As I already noted, patients with urgent needs for surgery are moved to the top of the list for an operating room (i.e., pink slipped), and the next patient in line with a less urgent need is bumped down in the queue. The same reasoning justifies prioritizing patients with critical or urgent needs and removing patients from critical care or discontinuing the treatment of patients with a scarce drug. In other words, first come, first served should not be a factor in rationing scarce but critical medical resources.

Another objection comes from authors who see a moral justification in distinguishing identifiable patients from future patients who have yet to be identified. They might accept a decision to remove a patient from the ICU when there is a patient with a critical need actually in the emergency room who is likely to die without immediately receiving ICU care. They would not, however, accept the removal based only on confidence that there will be another patient with such an urgent need arriving very soon. The two circumstances could be experienced psychologically as being very different, but ethically they are not. Either the likelihood of deriving a significant benefit justifies further critical care or the low likelihood of deriving a significant benefit justifies removal from the critical care unit when those resources are scarce in the community. Low likelihood of deriving a significant benefit is the relevant consideration.

Decisions to remove transplant candidates from the organ recipient list because of their low likelihood of deriving significant benefit (e.g., related to metastatic disease) or making patients inactive on the list (e.g., related to sepsis, a blood infection that might be effectively treated) reflect policies that deny identifiable patients transplant organs. At the same time, the recipient of the next organ is not yet identified because the ultimate organ allocation decision is the result of applying the same formula to all of the patients on the organ recipient waiting list when the next transplant organ in the region becomes available.

Organ transplantation practices that have been developed over decades by physicians who are involved with the care of transplant patients can teach us important lessons for making decisions that involve the removal or withholding of resources. Patients who are listed for a transplant organ are explained the rules that will govern their eligibility. Patients and their family members, as well as every member of the transplant team, have a clear understanding that a serious deterioration will end a transplant candidate's eligibility for a transplant. A similar practice of clearly communicating the criteria for continued eligibility for critical care, including the use of extracorporeal membrane oxygenation (ECMO) to provide both cardiac and respiratory support for patients whose heart and lungs are unable to sustain life, should be incorporated into critical care practice. The rules should be posted outside of each unit, and on admission patients or their surrogates should be provided with a printed copy of the eligibility rules for that level of care.

The most serious objection to removal of patients from critical care, the transplant list, or revoking access to a scarce drug is the claim that doing so amounts to killing, or stated more dramatically, killing an innocent person who has the right to life. The question, however, is not about what to call the action, but about what is the right thing to do. When the same principles of justice are applied to all similarly situated patients, the patient who is denied access to the intervention has no right to it even when continued access to the intervention would prolong life. Again, as I see it, **triage** is the principle of justice that should govern these decisions. Either the likelihood of deriving a significant benefit justifies the allocation of the scarce medical resource or the low likelihood of deriving significant benefit justifies terminating eligibility for the intervention.

In making these life-and-death decisions, the issue should be which reason, or principle of justice, would trustworthy medical professionals agree on as right for governing such decisions. The issue is not whether to call the decision "killing" or "letting the patient die."[51] The justice of the policy

---

[51] Rachels J, "Active and Passive Euthanasia," *The New England Journal of Medicine* 292, 2 (1975): 78–80.

or the actions do not turn on whether the death of the patient is foreseen as inevitable or even intended.[52] It is justified to withdraw or withhold[53] an intervention when doing so conforms with justice, in this case, when it would **avoid the worst outcome.** No one has an unlimited right to all of the medical resources needed to keep that individual alive: We are each entitled to only a fair share of resources in keeping with the widely accepted governing principles of justice.

Justice in Public Health

Public health measures have contributed dramatically to reducing the death rate and increasing life expectancy in populations. Because of their success, their value is broadly acknowledged, at least in public discussion. Nevertheless, claims for the allocation of societal funds to public health projects are always in competition with claims for projects of other sorts. Ideally, considerations of justice should determine how a society's funds are allocated among the important needs for expenditures on social goods such as public health, education, defense, safety, transportation, law enforcement, the arts, and clinical medicine. Yet, the issues of justice persist even when we focus solely on a single domain.

Within public health we are challenged to decide how limited resources should be allocated: Which projects should be addressed first? How much of the resources in the common pool should be apportioned to which efforts? What sorts of considerations should be taken into account, and which factors should be ignored? Should all of the funds be directed at providing immediate benefits, or should some resources be allotted to prepare for future possible public health needs or public health research? In times of urgency and need, how should limited supplies be distributed? Which populations should be rescued when not all can be? How should the multitude of competing claims be prioritized? This domain is especially complicated because all of the reasons that are appropriate in other sorts of medical decisions are relevant principles of justice within public health. Therefore, public health officials have the challenging task of establishing principled priorities for

[52] Kamm FM, *Morality, Mortality Vol. I: Death and Who to Save From* It (New York: Oxford University Press, 1993).
[53] Issues involving action and omission or withdrawing and withholding treatment are discussed in more detail in Chapters 7 and 8.

each sort of public health activity by justifying why those considerations are particularly important or appropriate factors for such projects.

In the preliminary sections of this chapter, I said a good deal about justice in public health. Here let me add just a few further points. When public health resources are distributed justly, the allocation decisions are likely to have society's support. When justice is not achieved, the decisions are likely to be criticized. Both sorts of experiences can be instructive. Two more recent public health predicaments in the United States present contrasting stories of how public health responses can be just or unjust. One is largely a tale of justice being done. The other is a tale of justice being ignored and grave injustice being perpetrated on some of the least advantaged people in our society. Together they offer valuable lessons about justice in public health.

Ebola in the United States

The 2014 outbreak of the Ebola virus was concentrated in three small West African countries: Guinea, Liberia, and Sierra Leone. Ebola is a highly contagious hemorrhagic fever that is spread through contact with an infected person's bodily fluids. The virus incubation period can be 2 days to 3 weeks. Symptoms include fever, joint and muscle pain, and internal and external bleeding. The fatality rate for infected people in Africa was estimated to be 60%.[54] According to the World Health Organization, as of February 10, 2016, a total of 28,603 suspected cases had occurred in the hot spot African countries, including 15,217 laboratory-confirmed cases and a total of 11,301 Ebola deaths.[55]

As early as July 28, 2014, the CDC started posting briefings about the Ebola virus on the CDC website to inform the public as well as medical and public health officials who needed the information. The communications included updates on what was happening in the United States and around the world, recommendations for prevention, and guidance for health departments and medical institutions on treatment and containment of the disease. By the end of December 2014, there were more than 120 communications posted there. In addition, CDC officials, including Dr. Tom Frieden, the CDC director, periodically tweeted critical information, for example, "Ebola is contagious

---

[54] Centers for Disease Control and Prevention. *Ebola (Ebola Virus Disease): Case Counts.* Accessed February 15, 2016, at http://www.cdc.gov/vhf/ebola/outbreaks/2014-west-africa/case-counts.html

[55] Centers for Disease Control and Prevention. *CDC Ebola (Ebola Virus Disease): 2014–2016 Ebola Outbreak in West Africa.* Accessed February 14, 2016, at https://www.cdc.gov/vhf/ebola/history/2014-2016-outbreak/index.html

only if person is experiencing active symptoms. Incubation period for symptoms is 2–21 days/average 8–10 days."

On September 30, 2014, Eric Duncan was diagnosed with Ebola at Texas Health Presbyterian Hospital Dallas. He was the first person to be diagnosed with the disease in the United States. He died there on October 8th. His was one of only two Ebola-related deaths in the United States. Ultimately, eleven cases of Ebola were reported in the United States, including nine people who had contracted the disease outside the United States (seven of them had been medically evacuated from other countries).

Throughout the period from September through December 2014, state and local health departments and hospitals, particularly in gateway cities like New York, worked closely with the CDC in coordinating their responses to the disease. Specific institutions were designated as receiving centers for possibly infected patients, and they prepared biocontainment units to provide treatment while also developing and practicing procedures for protecting caregivers. Medical professionals received extensive training and practice in using protective gear and conducted weeks of drills. President Obama also announced the formation of rapid response teams that were to travel to hospitals with newly diagnosed patients.

President Obama and the public health experts who advised him, however, refused to institute a travel ban on Ebola-endemic areas because that would have been ineffective in preventing the spread of the disease and because the restriction would have worsened the situation by interfering with efforts to contain the disease in Africa. Starting in October 2014, they did initiate a program to screen passengers for disease symptoms at the five airports where most passengers arrive from the three most affected countries. Also, the New York City health department committed 500 staffers to tracking the approximately 300 persons from West African affected countries who arrive in the city every day and to tracing and monitoring people who had contact with people who had developed the disease.

Most of these public health measures should be seen as acts of medical justice in response to the threat of a deadly and readily communicable infectious disease. The public health officials involved identified appropriate goals for the initiatives that they instituted. They recognized that it was critical to contain the spread of the infectious disease, to limit the number of people exposed to Ebola, and to prevent these individuals from spreading the disease to others. In that respect, the policies that were adopted expressed the principles of **avoiding the worst outcome** and **providing public goods**.

The medical community also facilitated measures to provide treatment for those who became infected and protection for those who provided their care. Those efforts reflected concern for the **vital and constant importance to well-being**. The reliance on available data and science demonstrated the commitment to **efficacy**, whereas the refusal to institute counterproductive measures merely for political posturing reflected commitments to the principle **avoid undue burdens**. In sum, the response to the crisis shows how public health policies can be just and effective. The clear and honest communication about Ebola in the United States also prevented unwarranted fear and encouraged citizens to trust the directions that they received from their public health officials.

At the same time, politicians in several densely populated states with large numbers of people returning from West Africa instituted 21-day quarantine for those who had been in contact with Ebola-infected individuals. Those actions were hardly justified because the disease is only infectious when exposed individuals develop a fever. The quarantine measures therefore appear to be politically motivated unjust restrictions of liberty.

Water in Flint, Michigan

A vivid example of a failure of justice involved the water supply crisis that erupted in Flint, Michigan.[56] Flint was under control of a state emergency manager when officials were considering a switch to the Flint River as a stopgap drinking water source until a new pipeline was finished. A 2011 study had found that using Flint River water would require extensive treatment to make the river water safe for drinking, including an anticorrosive agent for water pipe treatment at a cost of about $100 a day. On March 26, 2013, as plans for changing the Flint water supply proceeded, Stephen Busch, an official with the Michigan Department of Environmental Quality's drinking water division, informed state officials that the use of the river could lead to multiple problems. He specifically enumerated health risks related to increased exposure to cancer-causing disinfectant byproducts and microbes in the water. Then, just 8 days before the city changed to the Flint River as its water source, a treatment plant supervisor, Mike Glasgow, also warned state regulators of the risks involved. Nevertheless, in April 2014, the state

[56] City of Flint. *City of Flint: Water System Questions & Answers* (2015, January 13). Accessed February 14, 2016, at https://www.cityofflint.com/wp-content/uploads/CoF-Water-System-QA.pdf

changed the water supply arrangements for the city from paying Detroit for Lake Huron water to using water from the Flint River without any payment.

Shortly after the change was implemented, there was a spike of Legionnaires' disease that left nine dead and nearly 80 people ill. Residents noticed that the water looked dirty, smelled bad, and had an odd taste. The river water was subsequently investigated. The Flint River water has not been conclusively linked to the legionnaires' disease outbreak, but it was found to contain high levels of bacteria as well as high levels of corrosive iron and lead. Because the necessary water treatment was neither required nor provided, and because about half of the residential water lines in Flint are made of lead, the pipes began to corrode, and as they did the freed-up lead leached into the home water supply.

For several months, Flint residents, a team of investigators from Virginia Tech, and Dr. Mona Hanna-Attisha, a local pediatrician at Hurley Medical Center, complained to Michigan state officials about the water in Flint. Their complaints were initially dismissed and disparaged as spurious and politically motivated. Eventually, city officials began to investigate and respond. In August 2014, they issued boil water advisories after fecal coliform bacteria were found in the city's water supply. By September 2015 officials issued cautions about drinking the water, and in October 2015, after months of denial and delay, the city reverted to using Detroit's Lake Huron water supply. The change came too late to have an effect on the pipe damage and stop lead from leaching into the household water.

It wasn't until January 2015 that officials informed residents that their water supply was in violation of the Safe Drinking Water Act. The first notices also claimed that Flint water was safe to drink, but warned that infants, the elderly, and those with a severely compromised immune system "may be at increased risk and should seek advice about drinking water from your health care provider."[57] By switching back to the Detroit water system, the city restored its compliance with the Safe Drinking Water Act, but the problem of lead in the water remained.

Experts at the US CDC warn about the risk of lead that gets into the blood of children. The problem is explained on the CDC website. "Protecting children from exposure to lead is important to lifelong good health. Even low levels of lead in blood have been shown to affect IQ, ability to pay

---

[57] Schuch S, *Flint Hospitals Make Adjustments Amid City's Water Problems* (Updated January 17, 2015; posted January 9, 2015. Accessed February 14, 2016, at https://www.mlive.com/news/flint/index.ssf/2015/01/local_health_officials_show_li.html

attention, and academic achievement. And effects of lead exposure cannot be corrected."[58] Children in Flint under the age of 5 have already been found to have high lead levels in their blood.[59]

All of this is a tragedy that could have been averted. At this point, the corroded water pipes in this city of nearly 100,000 have to be replaced. The pipe replacement cost is estimated to be at least $1 billion; the public health costs have yet to be counted. The population of Flint, Michigan, is largely minority and poor, with 40% of its residents living below the poverty line. Because no one living in the richest country in the history of the world should be deprived of safe drinking water, it is obvious that the population was treated unjustly. What was done to the residents of Flint clearly violated central principles of justice: avoiding undue burdens, avoiding the worst outcome, the difference principle, efficacy, equality, maximin, providing public goods, attending to the vital and constant importance to well-being. Thus, it is legitimate to wonder how such an obvious injustice could have occurred. Was it the result of neglect, undervaluing a politically weak population, or putting cost savings before human lives? Were ears turned deaf because of twisted political priorities, or were there serious flaws in the chain of command that prevented warnings from being heard? How can such tragedies be averted in the future?

Our recent experience has also taught us lessons about communication and trust and their importance in the design and implementation of just public health policies. After the fall of the World Trade Center Twin Towers, public health officials from the Environmental Protection Agency and government representatives, including the former head of the Environmental Protection Agency, Christine Todd Whitman[60][62]; former New York City Mayor, Rudi Giuliani[63,64]; and former president, George W. Bush,[65] failed

[58] National Center for Environmental Health, Centers for Disease Control and Prevention, *Blood Lead Levels in Children* (CDC Fact Sheet). Accessed February 14, 2016, at https://www.cdc.gov/nceh/lead/acclpp/lead_levels_in_children_fact_sheet.pdf

[59] National Center for Environmental Health, *Blood Lead Levels in Children*.

[60] DePalma A, "Tracing Lung Ailments That Rose With 9/11 Dust," *The New York Times*, May 13, 2006. Accessed September 4, 2011, at https://www.nytimes.com/2006/05/13/nyregion/13symptoms.html

[61] Sierra Club. *Updated Ground Zero Report Examines Failure of Government to Protect Citizens* (2006). Archived from the original on June 11, 2010.

[62] Neumeister L, "Judge Slams Ex-EPA Chief Over Sept. 11," *San Francisco Chronicle*, February 2, 2006. Associated Press. Archived from the original on May 24, 2008.

[63] DePalma A, "Ground Zero Illnesses Clouding Giuliani's Legacy," *The New York Times*, May 14, 2007.

[64] Smith B, "Rudy's Black Cloud. WTC Health Risks May Hurt Prez Bid," *New York Daily News*, September 18, 2006.

[65] Heilprin J, "White House Edited EPA's 9/11 Reports," *Seattle Post-Intelligencer*, June 23, 2003.

to honestly communicate about the dangerous air quality and need for protection from the toxic environment. For example, in a press release on September 18, 2001, Ms. Whitman announced that, "We are very encouraged that the results from our monitoring of air-quality and drinking-water conditions in both New York and near the Pentagon show that the public in these areas is not being exposed to excessive levels of asbestos or other harmful substances." She also declared that, "Given the scope of the tragedy from last week, I am glad to reassure the people of New York . . . that their air is safe to breathe and the water is safe to drink."[66]

Today, thousands of people who worked at the ground zero site are ill and dying, at least in part because of the failures to provide full and honest disclosure.[67-75] Apparently, those who made the decisions to withhold information and promulgate false reports were more concerned with promoting political ends than with promoting the goal of safety—a truly central human value. Similarly, false and misleading reports before, during, and after Hurricane Katrina cost lives and exacerbated the tragedy. Inaccurate and misleading communications undermined trust in government, in public health pronouncements, and in public health policy. When people believe that they are being deceived and that the reasons for policies are personal or political advantage rather than the public good, they are less inclined to trust and accept the pronouncements and cooperate with the policy.

In contrast, instances of honest communication contributed to cooperation with policy and success in avoiding deaths and serious illness. These examples highlight the need for full, honest communication and education about matters of public health and their importance in promoting justice.[76] This is an important caution for doctors who are involved in public health

[66] Lombardi K, "Death by Dust," *Village Voice*, November 21, 2006.

[67] DePalma A, "Illness Persisting in 9/11 Workers, Big Study Finds," *The New York Times*, September 6, 2006.

[68] "What Was Found in the Dust," *New York Times*, September 5, 2006.

[69] CNN. "New York: 9/11 Toxins Caused Death". CNN. May 24, 2007. Archived from the original on June 18, 2007.

[70] CNN. "New York: 9/11 Toxins Caused Death."

[71] CNN. "New York: 9/11 Toxins Caused Death."

[72] World Trade Center Pregnancy Study, Columbia University, *CCCEH Study of the Effects of 9/11 on Pregnant Women and Newborns* (2006).

[73] Shukman D, "Toxic Dust Legacy of 9/11 Plagues Thousands of People," *BBC News*, September 1, 2011.

[74] Smith S, "9/11 " 'Wall of Heroes' to Include Sick Cops," *CBS News*, April 28, 2008.

[75] Grady D, "Lung Function of 9/11 Rescuers Fell, Study Finds," *New York Times*, April 7, 2010.

[76] The importance of truthful reporting is discussed in greater detail in Chapter 7.

policy. Basing decisions on illegitimate considerations can distort and per-
vert policy and thereby subvert trust.

Conclusion

In this chapter, I have put forward a long and intricate argument opposing
monolithic accounts of justice that strike me as oversimplifying attempts
to reduce the unavoidable complexity of justice into a single and often-
inappropriate principle. In addition to trying to show that these simplistic
views are mistaken, I also identified the kinds of reasons that are most salient
in different arenas of medical practice. In presenting this material, I tried to
show that we need to understand justice as a conclusion from the reasonable
consideration of the relevant factors that are involved in particular kinds of
decisions.

This discussion aimed to provide models for thinking about the most typical circumstances in which physicians and other medical professionals are
unavoidably required to make decisions about the allocation of the scarce resources at their disposal. It also focused on providing guidance for the policy
decisions that every practice area inevitably requires because the many
professionals who interact within the space have to coordinate their actions.

In this chapter, I explicated several principles of justice that should be employed in the allocation of medical resources and identified some factors
that should be considered irrelevant and eschewed. These conclusions are
justified by broadly shared judgments about what is and should be acceptable within medical practice and what should not be. Unfortunately, there
is no simple rule, procedure, or measurement device to rely on in making
these distinctions. We have to turn away from the dazzling appeal of simple
answers and accept the fact that discernment and judgment are needed
for identifying the requirements of justice within medicine's contextual
complexity.

Committees and panels of medical professionals that make allocation
decisions for their specialties and institutions typically demonstrate their personal commitment to justice. Acting from that doctorly virtue, they struggle
to find just solutions and remain alert to ways in which their initial guidance
may be less than ideal. They critique their previous recommendations and
refine and amend them in ongoing efforts to more closely discern and ap-
proximate what justice requires. The commitment to justice and the process

of critique and improvement have allowed the medical profession to advance ethically along with the scientific progress that receives far more public attention.

Although there is still much room for improvement, primarily related to problems in the structure of our medical systems, this discussion has largely supported the standard decision frameworks that have been developed in various domains of medical practice as being informed, appropriate, reasonable, and just. My contribution to this ongoing work has been to make the underlying principles of justice explicit and to show which principles have been categorically rejected for guiding the allocation of medical resources. My hope is that with these tools in hand the profession can continue to make strides toward achieving justice in medical care.

Table 9.1 enumerates the multiple principles of medical justice that are appropriate to allocating medical resources among those who need them. These salient reasons are the principles of medical justice that should be employed in making the contextually complex decisions in the real world of medicine that is far removed from alluring ivory tower simplicity. The table shows the domains in which each principle is a relevant concern and the domains in which some concerns should be considered largely irrelevant. The table makes it vividly clear that some principles are relevant or irrelevant considerations in different medical domains.

For long-standing questions about medical justice, we find guidance in the like-minded judgments made by physicians over the centuries. For new and novel issues, we rely on consensus views expressed in the judgment of medical professionals who aim at seeking trust and making trustworthy decisions that earn the public's endorsement and support. Decisions about allocations of medical resources in new and novel situations will have to be developed as issues emerge, and first drafts will have to be critiqued and refined as insight develops.

Because of my limited imagination, and reasonable limitations on space, this chapter does not provide definitive answers to every allocation issue that arises in medicine. The future is long, new technologies can be expected to create new dilemmas, and novelty continues to create the ethical challenges of life. The models that I have provided are intended to serve as a road map for navigating thorny issues that will inevitably demand decisions about what medical justice requires.

Table 9.1 Justice in Medicine

Domains of medicine	Principles of Medical Justice								
	Anti-Free-Rider	Avoiding Undue Burdens	Triage	The Difference Principle	Efficacy	Equality	Maximin	Providing Public Goods	Promoting Well-Being
Nonacute care									
Chronic care				√	√	√	√		√
Well-patient care				√	√	√			√
Preventive care	√	√		√	√	√	√	√	√
Domiciliary care						√			√
Acute care			√		√	√			
Critically scarce resources			√		√	√			
Public health	√	√	√	√	√	√	√	√	√

10

Why Doctors Must Develop a
Doctorly Character

As I argued in Chapter 2, *the first and fundamental duty of medical ethics is seek trust and be deserving of it.* That core obligation has two elements. The first, "seek trust," directs action; what doctors do should be consistent with what patients and society entrust them to do, and it should not undermine the future trust of the profession. The second element, "and be deserving of it," is intended to direct doctors to develop the special sort of character that being a physician requires. As I have tried to make clear throughout my discussion of sixteen duties of medical ethics, the commitment to fulfill each duty should be enabled and supported with a character that disposes doctors to reliably fulfill their professional duties. This means that physicians need to develop the appropriate inclinations that will support them in meeting their responsibilities.

In that vein, I argued in Chapter 2 that doctors are not only responsible for promoting the welfare of patients and society but they also should genuinely care about their good. I maintained that physicians are duty bound to maintain a nonjudgmental and nonsexual regard of patients and to uphold their patients' confidentiality. They need to be staunch supporters of those duties, feel comfortable in upholding them, and experience discomfort when they notice their own reluctance to do so. They must show respect for patient autonomy and experience doing so as an allegiance. Doctors have to be truthful and honest and regard their own truthfulness and honesty with reverence. Doctors should be responsive as well as effective communicators and their brothers' keepers, and those actions should be approached with a sense of dedication. They must be just in the allocation of the resources at their disposal and uphold that responsibility with a sense of faithful loyalty and without being tempted to advantage favorites or penalize foes. And their duty to base their treatment decisions on the findings of biomedical science must be accompanied with sincere dedication to the advancement of medical science. Altogether, physicians need to develop a doctorly character that

The Trusted Doctor. Rosamond Rhodes, Oxford University Press (2020). © Oxford University Press.
DOI: 10.1093/oso/9780190859909.001.0001

fills them with pleasure and pride, whereas the prospect of failing in their professional duties is associated with inner distress.

In the history of moral philosophy, theorists have advocated different approaches to ethics. Some have regarded ethics as being entirely about rules, principles, and duties. Others have described ethics entirely in terms of virtues and character. And others have argued that both elements have a place in morality. Some ecumenical views of ethics that embrace both duties and virtues do not however explain how they differ, what place these two elements have in morality, and whether they can clash with each other.[1] Recognizing the importance of attending to both duties and virtues is not enough because we must also understand how they work together to constitute a normative framework.

I draw attention to these differences to justify my aim in this chapter. Here I press a case for regarding medical ethics as involving both duty and virtue united in a specific way. For these purposes I use both duty and virtue in a broad sense meant to capture alternative approaches to ethics rather than focusing on particular exemplars of different views. By *duty*, I mean to indicate the deontic rules, principles, and obligations that define right action. By *virtue*, I similarly cast a wide net, without here distinguishing them, to capture the feelings, sentiments, dispositions, inclinations, attitudes, and emotions associated with good character.

In what follows, I align myself with a particular tradition of moral and political philosophers who have appreciated the interconnection of behavior and character. For them, character is the sum total of a person's virtues and vices. Virtues and vices, often called "attitudes" in contemporary bioethics discussions, dispose a person to choose and behave one way rather than another. They are the habitual inclinations to feel a certain way about a sort of object or in a particular context and act a certain way with respect to that object or kind of situation. Moral and political theorists who recognize the importance of these habitual feelings in promoting the behavior that they want from citizens therefore emphasize the necessity of deliberately cultivating civic virtues.[2-4]

[1] Beauchamp TL and Childress JF, *Principles of Biomedical Ethics*, 7th edition (New York: Oxford University Press, 2012).

[2] Aristotle, *The Nicomachean Ethics of Aristotle*, WD Ross, translator (London: Oxford University Press, 1971).

[3] Hobbes T, *Hobbes's Leviathan* (London: Oxford at Clarendon Press, 1965) (Reprint from original work published 1651).

[4] Rawls J, *Political Liberalism* (New York: Columbia University Press, 1993: 262).

Because the ethics of medicine is markedly different from the ethics of everyday life, physicians need to learn what their distinctive duties are.[5–8] In addition to understanding what their professional obligations require them to do, they need to develop the distinctive character of a physician and become the kind of doctor who is likely to fulfill those special duties.[9–13] And because the virtues of a physician are radically different from those of everyday life, the distinctive virtues of physicians have to be identified and nurtured.

When people accept and endorse the duties of the medical profession as the standards for guiding their professional actions, they also commit themselves to fulfill those obligations. To the extent that professional virtues facilitate professional actions, choosing to become a doctor commits physicians to developing the habitual dispositions that will dispose them to fulfill their professional responsibilities.

It is common to think that it is quite enough to do the right thing, but I am claiming that more is required. This claim is likely to strike today's readers as somewhere between quaint, strange, and outlandish largely because the language and discussion of virtue and character are not currently popular.[14] My unconventional assertion requires an argument, so I make the case for why doctors must develop the full array of doctorly virtues by describing what they are and explaining why they are needed.[15]

---

[5] Jones JW, McCullough LB, and Richman BW, *The Ethics of Surgical Practice: Cases, Dilemmas and Resolutions* (New York: Oxford University Press, 2008).

[6] McCammon SD and Brody H, "How Virtue Ethics Informs Medical Professionalism," *HEC Forum* 24, 4 (2012): 257–272.

[7] Brody H and Doukas D, "Professionalism: A Framework to Guide Medical Education," *Medical Education in Review* 48, 10 (2014): 980–987.

[8] Sade RM, editor, *The Ethics of Surgery: Conflicts and Controversies* (New York: Oxford University Press, 2015: 2–3).

[9] Churchill LR, "The American Association for Thoracic Surgery 2016 Ethics Forum: Working Virtues in Surgical Practice," *The Journal of Thoracic and Cardiovascular Surgery* 153, 5 (2017): 214–217.

[10] Pellegrino ED and Thomasma DC, *Virtues in Medical Practice* (New York: Oxford University Press, 1993).

[11] Karches KE and Sulmasy DP, "Justice, Courage, and Truthfulness: Virtues That Medical Trainees Can and Must Learn," *Family Medicine* 48, 7 (2016): 511–516.

[12] Pelligrino ED and Thomasma DC, *The Virtues in Medical Practice.*

[13] Rhodes R and Cohen DS, "Understanding, Being and Doing: Medical Ethics in Medical Education," *Cambridge Quarterly of Healthcare Ethics* 12, 1 (2003): 39–53.

[14] Beauchamp and Childress (*Principles*, 34) have noted that the once-prominent place of virtues in the medical literature and the American Medical Association (AMA) Code of Ethics has largely vanished. Describing the evolution in the AMA code, they pointed out that, "The 1980 version for the first time eliminated all traces of the virtues except for the admonition to expose 'those physicians deficient in character or competence.'"

[15] In addition to those cited, others have discussed the need for physicians to have specific virtues. They each offered their own lists, typically without an explanation for what they have listed or not and

Today, we recognize certain negative emotions as both undesirable and malleable. It has been common to talk as if we should try not to hate and not to feel contempt or jealousy. We should try to rid ourselves of prejudicial feelings toward people based on race, religion, sexual orientation, or nationality. We find those emotions unacceptable in themselves and dangerous because they tend to steer people toward immoral acts. By holding people responsible for their negative emotions, we evidence our belief that those inappropriate feelings are tractable. If people are to some extent educable with respect to their negative emotions, in principle their positive feelings should be equally plastic. The key to moderating our emotions is recognizing that we can change what we feel.

This perspective on feelings asserts that not only is what we do up to us, but, to a significant degree, what we feel is up to us. We make ourselves capable of ethical behavior by using moral principles and skills of analysis to inform our decisions and nurturing the inclinations that we choose to develop or suppressing those that we determine are improper. We can fashion ourselves into emotionally well-tuned instruments so that we can act with freedom in recognizing and performing the actions that advance our chosen ends. Reasoning and feeling are not so much distinct capacities but rather interrelated faculties that reciprocally promote each other and together sculpt a person's moral capacity. In a discussion of beneficence in his *Doctrine of Virtue*, Immanuel Kant provided a sketch of the process. He explained that,

Beneficence is a duty. If someone practices it often and succeeds in realizing his beneficent intention, he eventually comes actually to love the person he has helped. So the saying "you ought to love your neighbor as yourself" does not mean that you ought immediately (first) to love him and (afterwards) by means of this love do good to him. It means rather, do good to your fellow man, and your beneficence will produce love of man in you (as an aptitude of the inclination to beneficence in general).[16]

---

why. In my account, in addition to the virtues associated with each duty of medical ethics, I follow Aristotle's list because it provides an overall rationale for the scope of these additional virtues, and it justifies them by linking them to the specific kinds of invisible inclinations that lead people away from fulfilling their duties.

[16] Kant I, *Doctrine of Virtue*: Intro XII, c:{02. ci. note 21. Guyer, P. *Kant and the Experience of Freedom: Essays on Aesthetics and Morality* (Cambridge: Cambridge University Press, 1993): 366 and 377

The Virtues of Medicine

Aristotle's moral philosophy remains an important touchstone for moral theorists, and his work in ethics is eminent for its thorough and coherent discussion of virtues and their relationship to right action. Aristotle recognized that for an action to be right, it must be right in every respect: The right thing must be done to the right degree, at the right time, to the right people, and in the right way. In other words, he recognized that moral action is complicated because numerous factors have to be considered together. He also appreciated that judgments about each of those multiple considerations has to be on target, and if any element is mistaken, the chosen action could be the wrong thing to do.

Aristotle understood that various unconscious elements influence our decisions, the kinds of factors that we now identify as biases, prejudices, conflicts of interest, and the like. For him, character development was the defense against these unwanted invisible inducements that are likely to influence our choices. Character development involves the cultivation of the various virtues, inclinations to have an appropriate specific kinds of emotion that can effect action, that is, feelings that avoid both the extremes of taking excessive pleasure or excessive pain in some object of desire that may sway us. Virtues are developed through habituation, and the desired virtuous inclinations can be fostered and reinforced either through upbringing or by a person's deliberate effort to make herself into the kind of person that she chooses to be.

Because the kinds of invisible attractions that can influence action are features of human nature and are the same for everyone, I follow Aristotle's classification of the several virtues, using his somewhat inelegant names. He noted their awkwardness and explained that in some cases there was no fitting word for the virtue and in other cases there was no fitting term for the associated vices. That linguistic problem persists in today's English, but the concepts can be made clear, and I discuss the virtues according to his order of presentation. In each case, I explain what the virtue entails, explain its specific role in facilitating exemplary medical practice, and highlight how the virtue promotes physician professionalism. To the extent that a physician already has the desired inclinations, this discussion explains why he should hold fast to them and continue to nurture his virtues. To the extent that a physician notes incompatible personal dispositions that are potential obstacles to fulfilling duties of medical ethics, the discussion should explain why those habitual feelings and attitudes must be transformed and replaced with inclinations that will facilitate professional behavior.

Intellectual Virtues

Physicians not only must be competent, but also must feel a desire to be life-long learners and maintain competence. It is not enough for physicians to make treatment decisions based on the available scientific evidence; they must feel a commitment to science. Doctors should have a love of learning, but not be so focused on abstract intellectual concepts that they lose sight of the practical issues that they must address in the service of their patients. Being discerning, mindful, and analytically astute are all important skills that physicians are obliged to develop, but they must also feel an allegiance to maintaining that approach.

Physicians must also develop the intellectual virtue that Aristotle called "practical wisdom." In medicine, that is the judgment necessary for iden-tifying the benefits, risks, and burdens associated with various medical interventions, assessing them, comparing them, and making treatment decisions that are the most appropriate means for advancing the medical interests of patients. Practical wisdom also entails awareness of the effects of biases and prejudices, and a commitment to focusing on the available evi-dence in order to avoid distortions of judgment.

Doctors also need judgment to recognize when a medical problem exceeds their competence and requires expertise that they do not have. And they need discernment to recognize the skills and limitations of others when they make referrals, recommendations, or level criticisms.

Moral Virtues

Aristotle described each of the moral virtues as "the mean" of feeling, an emo-tional reaction that is neither too intense nor too mild, but one that achieves just the right degree of the specific emotional state relative to the specific sit-uation. Aristotle is aware of the potential criticism that achieving the mean of emotions is impossible to identify or achieve. He remarked that, "It is the mark of an educated man to look for precision in each class of things just so far as the nature of the subject admits; it is evidently equally foolish to accept probable reasoning from a mathematician and to demand from a rhetorician scientific proofs."[17] In other words, he recognized that moral emotions are not the kind of thing that can be specified with exactness. What is important is steering clear of extremes and identifying one's own inappropriate emotions and trying to compensate by guiding one's inclinations in the opposite direction. On this view, virtuous people actually take pleasure in doing what they ought to do, and they find it easy to do the right thing. Neither are they pulled away from doing their duty by conflicting desires nor do they experience moral action as a battle in which they must force themselves to fulfill their duties and do what they ought.[18]

Someone with a virtuous character needs all of the virtues because any sort of excessive desire or aversion can tug a person in the wrong direction and away from duty. For example, a person with an extreme aversion to social interaction will be reluctant to fulfill duties that require some degree of interpersonal face-to-face interaction. Someone lacking a concern for honor may lack the motivation for developing her talents. And an individual who is consumed by accumulating wealth is likely to violate every obligation that offers a possibility for self-enrichment. Because these feelings may arise with any action, a person's feelings associated with each of these objects has to be restricted within the range of moderation. Any emotional attraction that is unduly powerful can tempt a person to violate duty, and often enough, people yield to temptation and fail to do what they ought.

Courage

The virtue of courage is the mean relative to performing any action that might involve fear or confidence. Someone with the virtue of courage feels just the

[17] Aristotle, *Nicomachean Ethics*, I, 3; 1094b.24.

[18] Aristotle and Kant appear to take different stands on this point. Aristotle was clear and consistent in counting the most desirable character to be one that takes pleasure in doing the right thing. He called someone who is tugged away from right action but able to make himself do the right thing in the end "continent." That person's character is less admirable than a virtuous person's because he is always at risk of being incontinent, and therefore, he is less reliable. I am aligning myself with Aristotle on this point because his position is especially relevant to medical ethics, where being trustworthy entails reliably fulfilling one's obligations.

Kant found greater "moral worth" in the person who overcomes temptation to do the right thing rather than the person who experiences no temptation and finds pleasure in doing what she should. At the same time, Kant suggested that a person's ultimate aim should be to develop emotions that are compatible with right action, such as loving ones' neighbor. In other words, Kant's position on this issue may be more compatible with Aristotle's than is generally appreciated.

right amount of fear and confidence for their particular circumstance, which is the mean between the extremes of the incapacitating fear of cowardice and the over confidence of rashness. For example, when drawing blood, a doctor should feel some confidence in her ability to accomplish the task efficiently and some fear of breaking the needle or missing the vein and causing too much pain or bleeding. A novice should feel more fear than someone who has more experience, and the experienced person should feel less fear in performing a blood draw that in performing a Whipple surgical procedure.

Doctors often speak of feeling "comfortable" or "uncomfortable" in performing a task or procedure, but that should not be the standard for physician action because comfort may be merely a report of hubris or insecurity. Comfort should not be mistaken for virtue because some may feel comfortable when they are unprepared, while others may feel uncomfortable when they are amply prepared. Feeling the appropriate level of fear and confidence is the mark of courage, but it is always hard to gauge what that just right amount should be. Is a physician cowardly when she is reluctant to try a new drug for a particular indication because she is experienced in managing the dosing and side effects of the familiar treatment? Or is the one who prescribes the new drug as soon as it is approved for marketing rash? The only measure is the well-developed virtue of courage in its support of the intellectual judgment.

Courage is a critical virtue for doctors because others rely on them and because their actions often put others at risk. We always hope that doctors will benefit patients and society in their employment of medicine's distinctive knowledge, powers, privileges, and immunities, but physicians are always aware that their efforts might end badly. Even when the appropriate treatment is chosen and when it is carefully implemented, a patient may have a bad reaction or some catastrophic accident may occur. It is also possible for a doctor to overlook, underappreciate, or be ignorant of some critical factor in making a medical decision. In full awareness of these possibilities, doctors need courage in making a diagnosis, selecting a treatment plan, and acting on that plan. They also need to muster courage in responding to the unanticipated and unfortunate outcomes of their actions and courage in acknowledging their limitations and calling for help from colleagues when they recognize that it is needed.

Furthermore, doctors need courage in executing all of the social interactions that medical practice entails. Cognizant of the impact of their words, facial expressions, and body language, and how each word or gesture may be riveting and recalled, erased from memory, misunderstood, or misinterpreted, they need courage in order to communicate accurately with patients, family members, and other medical professionals. In communicating with patients and family members, doctors need courage in choosing their words and trying to accurately communicate the critical facts without destroying reasonable hope. Courage is particularly important in communicating an unfortunate prognosis, informing a patient of an error, and using the D word, "dying," when they recognize that death is imminent.[19-21] And courage is required for a conversation about organ donation after death.[22, 23] Doctors need courage in order to rely on their communication with peers for conveying what needs to be done in the care of a patient. Fear that those on the next shift will not adequately understand the treatment plan or the symptoms that should be monitored would prevent a physician from ever leaving the floor.

Because medicine is a profession rather than a freelance individual activity, doctors have the uncomfortable duty of being their brothers' keepers. This means that physicians are responsible for maintaining the trustworthiness of the profession. It gives each doctor obligations for policing the profession and advocating for institutional policies that are consistent with trustworthiness.[24] Courage is needed to have the difficult conversation with a fellow physician about her limited or deteriorating skills, impairment, or inappropriate interactions.[25] Courage is needed for reporting serious problems that could challenge institutional policies or leadership and expose the complaining physician to possible personal social, reputational, or financial risks.

[19] Buchan ML and Tolle SW, "Pain Relief for Dying Persons: Dealing With Physicians' Fears and Concerns," *Journal of Clinical Ethics* 6, 1 (1995): 53–61.

[20] Lo B, Quill T, and Tulsky J, "Discussing Palliative Care With Patients: ACP-ASIM End-of-Life Care Consensus Panel. American College of Physicians-American Society of Internal Medicine," *Annals of Internal Medicine* 130, 9 (1999): 744–749.

[21] Lo B, Snyder L, and Sox HC, "Care at the End of Life: Guiding Practice Where There Are No Easy Answers" [Editorial], *Annals of Internal Medicine*, 130, 9 (1999): 772–774.

[22] Herrin V and Poon P, "Talking About Organ Procurement When One of Your Patients Dies," *ACP-ASIM Observer* (2000 February).

[23] Williams MA, Lipsett PA, Rushton CH, et al., Council on Scientific Affairs, American Medical Association, "The Physician's Role in Discussing Organ Donation With Families," *Critical Care Medicine* 31, 5 (2003): 1568–1573.

[24] This issue is discussed in greater detail in Chapter 8, Physicians' Commitments to Fellow Professionals.

[25] Boisaubin EV and Levine RE, "Identifying and Assisting the Impaired Physician," *American Journal of Medical Science* 322, 1 (2001): 31–36.

Temperance

Everyone enjoys bodily pleasures: food, drink, entertainment, sleep, sex, and so on. Temperance is the virtue that keeps our desires for these pleasures in check. Doctors need to avoid the inclinations for self-indulgence as well as the inclination to insensibility. To maintain their ability to function at a professional level, doctors need an adequate diet and sufficient rest. Too much attention to food, drink, sex, entertainment, and sleep can lead to neglect of duty, whereas too little attention can leave a physician incapable of performing competently. This may mean that a doctor with a much anticipated reservation at a new, highly acclaimed restaurant has to choose between the desired gourmet experience and attending to a patient in need when no colleague is available to cover for him. With the virtue of temperance, his epicurean desires are moderate and within bounds, and he will not experience the decision as a wrenching challenge. He will comfortably choose his patient's welfare over gastronomic delights. Temperance can even protect a doctor from the temptation to forgo clinical responsibilities to see the New York Yankees play in the World Series, play a round of golf with a celebrity, or attend a Billy Joel concert when a patient's welfare is on the line and no one else with the requisite expertise is available to perform the necessary task.

Clinical practice presents unusual temptations and opportunities for abuse that require doctors to cultivate temperance. The stress and physical demands of clinical medicine together with the availability of drugs in an environment where physician behavior is largely unsupervised have led too many doctors to addiction. Also, the intimacy of the doctor-patient relationship, coupled with patients' nakedness and the touching involved in examinations and medically induced impaired patient consciousness, can encourage sexual feelings and tempt doctors to engage in behavior that is inconsistent with the ethical requirement for nonsexual regard.[26] Well-modulated temperate feelings related to bodily pleasures must therefore be an element of a physician's character.

---

[26] Council on Ethical and Judicial Affairs, American Medical Association, "Sexual Misconduct in the Practice of Medicine," *Journal of the American Medical Association* 266, 19 (1991): 2741–2745.

Virtues Concerned With Money

Money and all that it can buy are the chief source of today's concern over conflicts of interests in medicine. Fee-for-service arrangements and physician-owned medical facilities encourage doctors to offer services that are not needed,[27,28] while managed care arrangements and length-of-stay or readmission penalties discourage doctors from providing needed medical care.[29,30] Low levels of compensation from Medicaid and some insurance companies, compounded by high costs for malpractice insurance, impose financial pressure on many practices. In addition, there are patients who are willing to pay for concierge services and treatments that few doctors offer. These situations provide opportunities for doctors to charge whatever the market will bear and accept only self-pay patients,[31,32] and they leave many patients with limited access to medical care.[33] Charging exorbitant fees is also unseemly, and it undermines the public's trust in doctors and the profession.[34]

Regarding one's attitude toward money as a virtue that physicians should nurture makes it clear that doctors should not esteem colleagues for their

[27] Snyder L and Neubauer RL, American College of Physicians Ethics Professionalism and Human Rights Committee, "Pay-for-Performance Principles That Promote Patient-Centered Care: An Ethics Manifesto," *Annals of Internal Medicine* 147, 11 (2007): 792–794.

[28] Council on Ethical and Judicial Affairs, American Medical Association, "Conflicts of Interest. Physician Ownership of Medical Facilities," *Journal of the American Medical Association* 267, 17 (1992): 2366–2369.

[29] LaPuma J, Schiedermayer D, and Seigler M, "Ethical Issues in Managed Care," *Trends in Health Care Law and Ethics* 10 (1995): 73–77.

[30] Sulmasy DP, "Physicians, Cost Control, and Ethics," *Annals of Internal Medicine* 116, 11 (1992): 920–926.

[31] Carnahan SJ, "Concierge Medicine: Legal and Ethical Issues," *Journal of Law Medicine and Ethics* 35, 1 (2007): 211–215.

[32] Jones JW, McCullough LB, and Richman BW, "Ethics of Boutique Medical Practice," *Journal of Vascular Surgery* 39, 6 (2004): 1354–1355.

[33] Doherty R, Medical Practice and Quality Committee of the American College of Physicians, "Assessing the Patient Care Implications of 'Concierge' and Other Direct Patient Contracting Practices: A Policy Position Paper From the American College of Physicians," *Annals of Internal Medicine* 163, 12 (2015): 949–952.

[34] Such practices are completely consistent with Principle VI of the American Medical AMA's Code of Ethics which allows that,
VI. A physician shall, in the provision of appropriate patient care, except in emergencies, be free to choose whom to serve, with whom to associate, and the environment in which to provide medical care.
This is the only principle in the code that grants permission to freely choose what to do rather than dictate physician responsibilities. It is incompatible with the powerful statement in the code's preamble, which declares that, "As a member of this profession, a physician must recognize responsibility to patients first and foremost, as well as to society." It also contradicts AMA Principle IX, which holds that,
IX. A physician shall support access to medical care for all people.

wealth, and they should not use their professional role as a means for becoming wealthy. Physicians' desire for money must be moderated because excessive concern with accumulating wealth is likely to tempt doctors to violate their duty and compromise their commitment to patients and society.[35] For those who indulge their extreme attraction to money, the allure of accumulating wealth has been known to entice doctors to commit fraud and put patients at risk of harm. When that sort of behavior becomes publicized, it seriously tarnishes the reputation of the profession.

Virtues Concerned With Honor

Similar concerns arise over doctors' excessive desire for honor. Physicians certainly should be ambitious in achieving their goals for becoming trustworthy and revered clinicians and researchers. They should take pride in their care of patients and their research. They are entitled to respect, and they should value the esteem of colleagues for their insight, intelligence, skills, creativity, and commitment to patients. Being unduly humble about one's achievements can be problematic in medicine because it may involve a failure to accept important roles in medical leadership and education that sustain the profession.

Doctors need to take pride in their accomplishment, but only the recognition that they deserve. Excessive concern for honors and glory can tempt doctors to overstate their achievements, take credit for work that is not their own, or succumb to fabrication or plagiarism. The need to avoid such liabilities shows that excessive concern for honor is a vice in doctors, and that doctors need to develop an appetite for only merited honor that is within the bounds of moderation.[36]

---

[35] Emanuel EJ, "Enhancing Professionalism Through Management," *Journal of the American Medical Association* 313, 18 (2015): 1799–1800.

[36] Although there is some overlap of my Aristotelian list of virtues and the lists of other authors who discuss the virtues of good doctors, I pointedly omit integrity from my list. Integrity is not a virtue in the traditional sense of the term because it does not pick out a specific object that incites pleasure or pain and it is not a mean between extremes of a feeling. There is also vagueness in what people mean by "integrity." Some people use the term to mean fulfilling duties of honesty, truthfulness, or justice. In that sense, they are referring to duties and misclassifying them as virtue. If they intend to redefine virtue, that requires its own justification. Some use the term *integrity* to indicate a general commitment to fulfilling one's duty. Again, that conflates duty and virtue. And then, there are people who pride themselves for integrity or righteousness. They appear to have an excessive desire for honor or to use the term, rather than argument, to claim the moral high ground and justify their stands on issues. Some display rigidity in clinging to a single ethical consideration while failing

Virtues Concerned With Anger

Medical practice involves interactions with many people in many roles. People in these various roles have numerous responsibilities, and they may have both reasonable and unreasonable expectations of one another. And sometimes somethings go badly, and doctors react to what has occurred. There are times when doctors should be angry or furious with themselves or another for what was done or left undone. There are also times when no one is at fault, and nothing could have or should have been done differently. And there are times when a doctor has to maintain calm in order to effectively manage an emergency or complete a procedure.

An irascible person who is quick to display anger and spew venomous hostility on any occasion should not be a doctor, and neither should a person who holds onto anger and allows it to fester while refusing to be appeased. Because medicine constantly involves interactions with others, doctors need to maintain a productive work environment by tempering their inclinations to anger and developing some degree of tolerance for the things that can go wrong. When hostility is counterproductive, it should be eschewed. When a modicum of dissatisfaction can be effective in communicating that standards of medical practice must be upheld, a fitting amount of anger should be displayed. But in most circumstances, equanimity should be the physician's goal because composure reassures patients and team members and promotes trust.

Virtues of Social Intercourse

Because interaction and communication are integral elements of medical practice, physicians need to master the virtue of social intercourse. This virtue involves being pleasant to those you know well as well as those who you meet for the first time and being able to put them all at ease almost immediately. It involves sincerely conveying warmth and interest without being obsequious or disingenuous. Humor, smiles, expressions of sympathy, and touch can all be aids in social interactions. Physicians with this virtue are not cold, aloof, disinterested, or disdainful. And doctors who develop

---

to appreciate the complexity of moral life. That use of the term should not be counted as a virtue, but perhaps the opposite.

this virtue are able to gain their patient's trust and forge effective working relationships with colleagues and students. Physicians who take pleasure in their interactions express their comfort with social engagement, and that makes others feel comfortable as well.

Australian surgeon Miles Little has noted that presence is a distinctive duty and virtue of surgeons.[37] I agree, but I would extend the point beyond surgeons. I see presence as part of the fiduciary duty of physicians, and I see the associated inclination to be present as an aspect of the virtue of social intercourse. Doctors need to feel comfortable being with their patients and interacting with them because their presence helps to comfort patients. Presence through phone calls, emails, and bedside visits to hospitalized patients reassures them that their doctor is informed, involved, and engaged in directing their care. Doctors who lack this virtue are likely to minimize their interactions and visits. Their absence will be noted and tend to undermine their patients' trust.

A critical part of a physician's job is eliciting information from patients, family members, and colleagues. Doctors' questions must be coherent, effective, and posed with tact even when they concern intimate personal information and when asking would embarrass anyone else. And after posing their questions, physicians have to listen to what is said in answer and observe whatever can be learned from how the information is shared. Answers must be received with nonjudgmental acceptance and without impatience. Importantly, physicians often have a great deal of information that they need to share with patients, their family members, colleagues, and students. Conversations therefore have to be clear and accurate, and the communication has to be efficient because physicians typically have too much to do in too little time.

Physicians who take pleasure in these interactions and feel pride in navigating them efficiently and successfully demonstrate the requisite virtue. Those who find these interactions unpleasant and burdensome need to invest effort in cultivating the virtue.

---

[37] Little M, "The Fivefold Root of an Ethics of Surgery," *Bioethics* 16, 3 (2002): 183–201.

Caring

Aristotle's name for this virtue was "friendship," and he devoted Books VIII and IX of *The Nicomachean Ethics* to it, while the other moral virtues are discussed one after the other in the latter part of Books III and IV. The amount of attention that he devoted to friendship tells us that he saw friendship as more critically important than the other virtues. As I read Aristotle, this is because he regarded friendship as the virtue associated with treating others justly.

Justice wasAristotle's subject for all of Book V. Listing it among the moral virtues, he nevertheless offered no direct reference to its associated feelings. As philosophers J. O. Urmson[38] and also Bernard Williams noticed, "We might, as in the case of the other excellences, expect to be told what the particular emotion involved is and what the two extremes are between which justice is a mean, one exhibiting too much, the other too little, of the relevant emotion. But this we do not get,"[39] at least not explicitly in Book V. Aristotle explained that the distinctive nature of justice is its concern with allocating goods,[40] and it, "alone of the virtues, is thought to be 'another's good', because it is related to our neighbour; for it does what is advantageous to another, either a ruler or a co-partner."[41] All of the other virtues relate to an individual's personal character development. Justice tells us how to treat others, and acting justly is supported and enabled by having the appropriate degree of affection for others.

Justice tells us that there are some things that we owe to everyone, but we frequently owe some people more than we owe others. We ought to do the morally required action toward others, and to do that reliably we are morally required to develop feelings of goodwill, the virtue of caring along with skills of moral analysis. The care imperative commands us to feel and show some caring toward everyone. On a continuum from what philosopher Julia Annas has called "civic friendship"[42] to the magnitude of love one feels for

---

[38] Urmson JO, *Aristotle's Ethics* (Oxford, UK: Blackwell, 1988).

[39] Williams B, "Justice as a Virtue," in Rorty AO, editor, *Essays on Aristotle's Ethics* (Berkeley: University of California Press, 1980: 189–200). In this article, Williams tried to identify the kind of feeling or motive that is characteristic of justice and injustice. He ultimately concluded that, "It is a mistake, one that dogs Aristotle's account, to look for 'a particular motive which the unjust person displays because of his injustice'" (199). For Williams, "There is no one motive characteristic of the unjust person, just as there is no one enemy of just distribution" (198).

[40] Aristotle, *Nicomachean Ethics*, V, 1;1129b1–12.

[41] Aristotle, *Nicomachean Ethics*, V, 1; 1130a5.

[42] Annas J, "Plato and Aristotle on Friendship and Altruism," *Mind* 86, 344 (1977): 532–554.

a best friend, parent, child, or spouse, we ought to feel greater affection for some than others because of the special roles that someone may have or the history of a particular relationship.

The doctor, in relation to his patients, because of his oath, his knowledge and skill, his state license, or the mutual social understandings that accompany his position, has a special role that brings with it the special duty of caring for his patients and acting for their good.[43] A history of interacting with his patients may strengthen that obligation still further. Moreover, the inequalities in medical knowledge and skill, and, for the seriously ill, the inequalities in physical well-being and fear, characterize the doctor-patient relationship with a special need for caring.

To paraphrase Aristotle's remark about rulers, the good doctor should care for his patients as a shepherd does for his sheep, looking out for his patients' interests rather than for his own.[44] In being a good shepherd to his patients, the good doctor not only must be nonjudgmental, truthful, and respectful of their autonomy and act for their good, but also must care a good deal about their welfare. Without special caring feelings, it becomes more likely that he will fail in his other special duties, including his duty to communicate caring.[45] The good doctor not only must be an excellent practitioner with an understanding of what is owed to his patients, but also, as a matter of professional obligation, must be equipped with affection so that he will be able to reliably care for and care about the well-being of his patients. So, to distinguish civic friendship from doctors' affection for their patients, I adopt the term of feminist ethics and call this doctorly virtue *caring* and regard it as a kind of love for patients.

Physicians' duty to care about or love their patients is clearly distinct and different from common morality. In ordinary life, people typically feel free to choose who they love. People typically recognize their duty not to harm others applies to everyone, but that does not translate into a moral

---

[43] In conversation, Joe Fitschen pointed out that legal proceedings may be a parallel situation. The accused is presumed innocent before the law and would therefore be entitled the same concern that was due anyone else before the judge. Furthermore, because the judge has the special obligation of ensuring that the accused is given a fair and just trial, the judge has the special obligation to feel concern for the accused. That is not to say that the judge should deviate from the law to favor the accused. That would show an excess of feeling.

[44] Aristotle, *Nicomachean Ethics*, VII, 1109b5–7.

[45] *A Complicating Factor: Doctor's Feelings as a Factor in Medical Care* (Hohokus, NJ: Transit Media Communications), a film by Dr. Richard Gorlin and staff, Icahn School of Medicine at Mount Sinai, makes this point dramatically.

obligation actually to feel deep affection or love for everyone.[46] In Chapter 2, I discussed a number of cases that demonstrated that doctors actually have a moral responsibility to cultivate sincere caring for each of their patients. Those examples strengthen my case for recognizing that the character of a good doctor is distinct and different from the character of other admirable people and explain why the distinctive inclinations and virtues of a trustworthy doctor must be nurtured. They also show that caring is the virtue that enhances doctors' ability to uphold the second duty of medical ethics, which requires doctors to act for the benefit of patients and society. Furthermore, because the duty to serve the interests of patients and society is universally recognized by physicians and medicine's professional organizations as the core duty of the field, recognizing that the associated virtue of caring is a critical tool in meeting that obligation supports my overall account of medical ethics as distinct and different from common morality.

I use the term *caring* broadly to capture the affection of brotherly love, concern for the other's good, empathy, sympathy, compassion, and sensitivity to the other's situation. Even when people are committed to fulfilling their moral obligations, emotions play a role in what they identify as being required by duty. This factor makes the epistemological problems of identifying and categorizing what we see and how we see it problems in morality. The purely dispassionate stance that has been idealized in some theoretical discussions should be rejected because appropriate emotions are essential moral apparatus for beings whose vision, imagination, and will are hindered or aided by their feelings. Achieving the right amount of emotion is a self-adjusting process of moral self-education. It begins with the existential doubt of recognizing that what we feel may be insufficient or excessive and that emotions can and sometimes should be modified because only well-moderated caring facilitates ethical judgment.[47] Cultivating emotions from the desire to fulfill one's professional responsibilities and acting with the aid of those fostered emotions is the opposite of being dragged around by our feelings. Rather, it is taking responsibility for our feelings just as we take responsibility for our actions.

---

[46] The golden rule requires us to love they neighbor. People typically read that imperative in a minimal way. Here I argue for why doctors must cultivate love for their patients in a robust way.

[47] Curzer HJ, "Is Care a Virtue for Health Care Professionals?" *The Journal of Medicine and Philosophy* 18, 1 (1993): 51–70. Curzer argued that care is a vice. He focused on what I see as an excess of caring, and I agree that such an extreme of feeling is vice. In this discussion, I focus on the mean, not the extreme, and I advocate for well-regulated feelings of goodwill.

Love Thy Patient

My aim in this chapter has been to describe the inclination that should accompany doctors' primary commitment to their patients' well-being and the spectrum of positive emotions (call them caring, concern, friendship, brotherly love, love, etc.) and to argue that physicians ought to feel affection for their patients. The crucial message is that acting from duty alone is an inadequate grounding for ethics, and that is especially true in medicine. Caring provides insight into what is required and motivates doctors to muster the required effort to meet the needs that morally demand their response.

Because ethics must address the reality of human nature, morality does not end with duty. It extends to the feelings that interfere with people recognizing what their duty requires and meeting their obligations. The ethics of medicine therefore has to address feelings as part of its broad aim of making doctors and the medical profession trustworthy. This includes appreciating that feeling appropriate emotions is a necessary tool for enabling doctors to reliably succeed in doing what they ought to do. That in turn makes doctors duty bound to develop fitting feelings. Such well-habituated constant feelings are the virtues of good doctors and an essential element of medical professionalism.

Once a doctor has decided what ought to be done in a situation, she should try to do it. But when doing something else instead is easier, more pleasant, or personally more advantageous, people do not always do their duty. Will weakens. What seemed morally necessary starts to look less important or optional. Competing alternatives begin to appear more plausible. And when the physician acts, she sometimes does what she thought was wrong just a short while before or what she will know was wrong tomorrow.

Beyond its role as a corrective of ethical judgment, caring is something that we also value in itself. Feminist philosophers have pointed out the significance of care in the family and intimate relationships,[48-50] but its value should also be acknowledged in the doctor-patient relationship. For example, patients who receive good medical treatment are often upset or angry when they feel that their doctors do not care about them personally. From the perspective of duty alone, this seems like a peculiar response

[48] Ruddick S, "Injustice in Families: Assault and Domination," in Held V, editor, *Justice and Care: Essential Readings in Feminist Ethics* (Boulder, CO: Westview Press, 1995: 203–223).

[49] Held V, *The Ethics of Care* (New York: Oxford University Press, 2006).

[50] Gilligan C, *In a Different Voice* (Cambridge, MA: Harvard University Press, 1982).

because physicians have done precisely what was supposed to have been done. This patient reaction should, however, inform us that more is required of physicians, even when they are seeing twenty patients a day. When interacting with a patient, a doctor must do the right thing with the feeling of fellow love.

The upset of patients who accurately perceive the absence of affection makes sense when we recall that patients need to trust their doctors. To trust a physician the patient has to sense the physician's goodwill. Without that, the patient is left with the impression that the doctor is not trustworthy, which in turn makes the patient reluctant to accept her treatment recommendations. In other words, to be trustworthy, a good doctor needs to convey her love for her patients. And because acting skills are not standard physician competencies, to successfully impart genuine concern for the patient's well-being, the doctor should feel it sincerely.

A doctor's sincere interest in promoting her patient's well-being is not to be confused with a charming "bedside manner." Physicians sarcastically extol a colleague's ability to charm patients with a suave "bedside manner," but they genuinely esteem a colleague who demonstrates compassionate devotion to patients. Patients want the former, but are sometimes duped by the latter because we all want others to treat us with guileless caring. That susceptibility allows us occasionally to be taken in by deception.

Caring is an effective prophylaxis against the serious moral afflictions of bad faith, limited moral vision, and weak will (i.e., incontinence). Thus, the prescription to love thy patient is good medicine for the good doctor. Because moral judgment and ethical action are imperiled by the absence of feeling and by unsuitable feelings, appropriate caring becomes as much a moral imperative as obedience to duty. Doctors need caring, first to help them know what they ought to do and then to help them do what they believe they should do.

An appropriate level of caring can be a formidable weapon in defending physicians from serious and ubiquitous moral hazards. Those who want to do the right thing need to be able to identify the morally salient features of a situation, and they also need caring feelings to enable them to assess the weight of the various considerations and protect them from self-deception and tilting the balance toward their own advantage. Because having the appropriate caring feelings is often essential for recognizing and doing the right thing, developing such feelings becomes a matter of professional responsibility.

Character development is a process of continuous self-regulation aimed at creating the habitual doctorly disposition to think about action in terms of moral duties and feel as a good doctor should. It is unlikely that someone who lacked the requisite character could consistently do what was ethically required. A doctor who has the virtue of caring is not pulled by feeling either too much or too little caring about their patients or towed about by too much or too little caring for her own interests. The physician with the virtue of caring will feel what she should, to the extent that she should, toward those for whom she should have the feelings. Having these well-tuned emotions will make it easy for her to act virtuously, that is, to consistently fulfill her duties.

Physicians often find it difficult to fulfill their obligations to noncompliant patients who repeatedly ignore their medical advice and engage in self-destructive behavior only to return for time- and energy-consuming medical rescue. Physicians also have trouble tending to hateful patients, the distrustful, combative, demanding, manipulative, litigious, or abusive ones. Some patients' behavior makes it hard to be sympathetic, and the lack of feeling makes it hard to do one's duty. Without the feeling of goodwill toward a patient, only the commitment to duty enables (continent) physicians to overcome their disinclination to be involved with that patient's treatment. Caring about the patient can help to overcome frustration, annoyance, the force of greed, the power of comfort, the fear of danger, and even the repulsion of disgust. In addition, when a doctor actually cares about a patient, doing her job is pleasurable and personally rewarding.

At the other end of the spectrum, extreme concern for a patient's well-being may incline a physician who loves her patient too well to do what she would otherwise have determined was wrong. Excessive caring may incline a physician, who had previously believed that it was immoral to break a research protocol, to actually provide a drug outside of a study to a particular patient who plucked a tender chord in her heart. Caring too much might lead a surgeon to provide a second, third, or fourth transplant organ to a beloved patient who would be denied retransplantation according to the standards of justice in organ distribution that she would otherwise support. Future patients who could benefit from the knowledge gained in a scientifically valid clinical drug trial and the other patients on the organ transplant recipient waiting list who must wait longer (or die) have to be taken into account as a matter of justice. The physician who cares too much about the patient in front of her and too little for those she does not see displays an excess of feeling and is likely to be pulled away from doing what she would otherwise regard as the right thing. Similarly, a physician who cares too much about meeting the needs of patients is likely to neglect her own needs and work herself to exhaustion. Ideally, a physician will care about each patient as she should and thus find it easier to do what justice requires. Striving to achieve that ideal makes approximating it more likely.

This conclusion has important implications for medical practice. It has even more dramatic implications for structuring medical institutions, designing a national system for healthcare delivery, and medical education.

Medical Institutions

Because medical institutions are supposed to embody the commitments of the medical professions, they should strive not only to deliver excellent medical care but also to do so in a way that addresses the complex needs of the people they serve. Medical institutions that are not caring in their organization and delivery of patient services fail to meet the standards that have been and should be embraced by the profession. Outpatient clinics that deliver clinically acceptable medical treatment but, by design, regularly keep patients waiting hours for appointments in a crowded, uncomfortable space display a lack of caring. Hospitals that do not respect confidentiality or provide for privacy and comfort as they administer appropriate medical treatment display a lack of caring. Institutions that tolerate the rude and calloused behavior of professional or ancillary staff display a lack of caring. And, because insensitive and unfeeling behavior makes people want to stay away, such design flaws and uncaring behavior fail to meet the medical needs of those they are committed to serving.

Because the medical profession undertakes an obligation to provide for the medical needs of the community through its monopoly on medical practice, the profession should be committed to advocating for policies and mechanisms that would allow the duty to be fulfilled. At the public policy level, a healthcare system that is designed to leave some people suffering without care, or suffering as they wait in line for care, displays a lack of caring. And medical reimbursement systems that are designed to encourage physicians to spend less time with each patient or prioritize personal advantage over their patient's good display an insidious lack of caring.[51]

[51] This seems to be the essence of the AMA's criticism of some managed care plans. Glasson J, Plows CW, Clarke OW, et al., "Ethical Issues in Managed Care," *Journal of the American Medical*

Organizations that represent the profession are obliged to promote a healthcare system that genuinely attends to the medical needs of everyone in addition to promoting medical research and technologically advanced treatment.

Medical Education and Promoting Professionalism

Because becoming a doctor is a process of acquiring knowledge and skills as well as a process of character transformation, it is reasonable to expect a learning curve in virtue formation as well as in other competencies. Whereas everyone accepts that novices have a distance to travel before becoming competent in the clinical skills of a physician, authors who address the behavior and attitudes of medical trainees often remark on their failings and the negative impact of the "hidden curriculum." They see an educational process that dehumanizes noble characters and they find support for their opinions in surveys of medical trainees.[52]

Apparently, these critics do not attend to the uniqueness of medical virtues or the progression that is required for the development of a physician's character. Perhaps the surveys that find novices exemplary and those in the midst of training lacking are searching for the wrong things or looking for the right thing but at some intermediate point in the process of moral development. And, perhaps our educational programs have failed our students by ignoring their responsibility for molding professional character.

Drawing on authors who describe a process of moral development,[53] becoming an ordinary ethically competent moral agent involves a process of moral development. Once we appreciate that training a doctor involves creating a new professional persona, that is, a person with a new and different character, it is not surprising that medical trainees often require a

Association 273, 4 (1995): 330–335. Designing reimbursement plans to encourage ethical behavior has been discussed in the literature, such as Erde E, "Economic Incentives for Ethical and Courteous Behavior in Medicine: A Proposal," *Annals of Internal Medicine*; 113, 10 (1990): 790–793; Arnold RM and Forrow L, "Regarding Medicine: Good Doctors and Good Behavior," *Annals of Internal Medicine* 113, 10 (1990): 794–798; Spicker SF, issue guest editor, "Prospective Payment: DRGs and Ethics," *The Journal of Medicine and Philosophy*, 12, 2 (1987).

[52] Hafferty W, O'Donnell F, Baldwin DC, *The Hidden Curriculum in Health Professional Education* (Hanover, NH: Dartmouth College Press, 2015).
[53] Kohlberg L, *Essays on Moral Development, Vol. I: The Philosophy of Moral Development* (San Francisco: Harper & Row, 1981).

period of learning before becoming the professionals we want them to be. Although some students seem to arrive in medical school with a developed sense of medical professionalism, we see many students who move through a staged pattern of professional character development. Some begin their training very much focused on their own survival and achievements. By the subinternship year and the early stages of residency, some appear to focus largely on being accepted by their team of peers. But by the time they become senior residents and fellows, most trainees seem to have internalized the hallmark medical commitment to patients. That said, medical educators can more reliably produce physicians who model professionalism by making a deliberate effort in that direction.

To be a medical professional, a trainee has to develop from being a decent individual with personal virtues who makes decisions about personal action with reference to personal values and commitments to being a physician who acts from professional virtues and makes professional decisions with reference to medical commitments and professional values. Although we try to carefully select medical trainees, we should expect that the process of medical education involves students' progression from starting off as bright and compassionate individuals, to the students becoming a part of the medical team (something akin to joining a new family), to these same students becoming clinicians who incorporate professional values into sound medical decisions and who also mentor future generations of physicians. In the process, our trainees have to learn how to work collaboratively in a medical team, put their patients' good before their own, convey trustworthiness, and be trustworthy medical professionals.

The challenge for medical education is to make the transformation explicit and to intentionally train students to have the virtues, knowledge, and skills of an exemplary physician and, at the same time, to inhibit the inculcation of counterproductive attitudes and habits. Because virtues are essentially habits of feeling and acting, molding the distinctive habits of a physician requires repetition. Also, because character formation is a process, the judicious cultivation of physicianly virtues must be threaded throughout medical education and treated as a crucial element of medical training. These educational obligations cannot be discharged with a short course tacked onto the beginning of the first year or the end of the final undergraduate year as an irrelevant but decorous appendage; they must be integrated throughout medical education.

Although it is important for medical educators to convey the content and rationale for the distinctive duties of medical ethics, it is also crucial for students to accept the duties of medical ethics as core professional values. Faculty members must make that obligation obvious and nurture the development of a physicianly character. Over the past 45 years or so of bioethics activism, some version of ethics has been included in the standard curriculum of most medical schools. But a medical school that has not taught its graduates to love their patients has failed in preparing physicians for the work they will have to do. Diagnostic and treatment skills and an understanding of the ethical duties of doctors are only part of the mental paraphernalia that physicians need in order to think, speak, and act in accordance with the long-espoused professional standards of medicine. Students must also be guided to develop a doctorly character.

Conclusions

The ethics of medicine should be understood as a commitment to the distinctive duties of the profession and the development of a doctorly character.[54] Doctors need to be sensitive to the complex interrelation of human reason and emotions. They need to understand and accept the scope of their distinctive duties, and they need to make themselves into people who are inclined to fulfill their professional obligations. Those who accomplish both exemplify professionalism, and they are entitled to the trust that patients and society invest in them.

Molding the character of future physicians is too important a matter to leave to chance. The hazards of ignoring the importance of character development and leaving this aspect of medical education by default to the silent or hidden curriculum, and thereby allowing medical trainees to develop unprofessional habits of feeling and acting as matters of luck, should be acknowledged by the profession,. Medical educators need to appreciate that medical education is a transforming activity and not merely the conveyance of a body

[54] Churchill, LR and The American Association for Thorasic Surgery, "Ethics Forum: Working Virtues in Surgical Practice" *The Journal of Thorasic and Cardiovascular Surgery* (2016) 153, 5: 1214–1217, 1217. Philosopher Larry R. Churchill offered a similar insight with a somewhat different list of virtues. He wrote, "I propose an addition to the official AATS Code of Ethics in the form of an oath: Let me cultivate in myself and in my colleagues those elements of character that are most conducive to patient care and professional well-being: trustworthiness, equanimity, empathy, advocacy, compassion, courage, humility, and hope" (Churchill, "The American Association for Thoracic Surgery.")

of knowledge. They have to take seriously their role in nurturing the distinctive character of trustworthy doctors and employ educational programs to teach and inculcate the distinctive duties, virtues, attitudes, and behaviors that physicians need to embrace in order to fulfill their special social role and obligations. Valuing moral development and encouraging mindful attention to the duties of the profession ultimately produces trustworthy physicians and promotes excellence in patient care.

11

Resolving Moral Dilemmas

How to Resolve a Moral Dilemma

For the most part, physicians proceed with their medical practice without any particular awareness of the moral dimension of their actions. A patient asks for medical assistance, and the physician identifies what is needed and provides the assistance that is in order. The ethical dimension of what is being done can be overlooked because the requirements of duty are obvious and the way to proceed is providing good medical care. The simplicity and the clarity come from the consistency with what the duties of medical ethics dictate. A competent doctor cares about the well-being of her patients. She uses her medical knowledge, skills, powers, privileges, and immunities for their benefit and mindfully provides the needed standard of care with non-judgmental and nonsexual regard while upholding her patients' confidentiality, showing respect for their autonomy, and justly allocating the resources at her disposal. The involved significant ethical duties go unnoticed because they all direct the doctor toward the same action.

Occasionally, however, a situation just appears to be a mess. In such baffling circumstances, the source of confusion is typically different duties of medical ethics that call for inconsistent actions. Any moral system that involves more than a single principle, rule, or duty inevitably confronts the problem of moral conflict. Moral conflicts arise when two or more cherished values are relevant considerations in a situation but point to different and incompatible actions. Ethical dilemmas are part of life, and because medical practice involves navigating them in a trustworthy way, doctors need a systematic and reliable approach to guide them to a trustworthy resolution when they find themselves confronting such situations (Table 11.1).

Gert, Clouser, and Culver recommended that decisions in such circumstances need to be justified by referencing their ten rules.[1] Beauchamp

---

[1] Gert B, Culver CM, and Clouser KD, *Bioethics: A Systematic Approach* (New York: Oxford University Press, 2006).

The Trusted Doctor. Rosamond Rhodes, Oxford University Press (2020). © Oxford University Press.
DOI: 10.1093/oso/9780190859909.001.0001

Table 11.1 How to Approach a Clinical Ethical Dilemma

- Collect all relevant data that could help resolve the matter.
- Identify the duties involved and explain how they relate to the case.
- Identify the duties that conflict in the situation.
- Formulate a question of ethics that reflects the conflict.
- Decide which duty should have priority and support that choice with factors relevant to the case OR find an alternative that avoids the dilemma.
- When uncertainty persists, ask, Is there is some missing information that would help to resolve the dilemma? Which information? How will it help to resolve the dilemma?
- Evaluate the decision by asking if it is what a consensus of exemplary doctors would agree is the resolution that would uphold the trustworthiness of the profession.
- Plan the practical steps for implementing the decision, focusing on the details of the case and the foreseeable issues in the near future.

and Childress recommended balancing and specification or engaging Rawlsian reflective equilibrium for resolving ethical dilemmas.[2] For more particular conundrums involving duties clashing in a particular situation, however, neither the approach offered by Gert, Clouser, and Culver nor those suggested by Beauchamp and Childress are efficient enough to actually serve as a useful guide for doctors. They are too abstract, cumbersome, and difficult to apply in the clinical arena. There have been a few other attempts at describing the process of moving from principles, rules, virtues, and facts to action-guiding moral conclusions, but the details have not been articulated clearly enough to be useful in a practical way.[3,4] Physicians who face moral dilemmas need specific guidance that can be used to resolve ethical dilemmas and relatively quickly achieve team consensus on an effective plan for moving forward. Thus, a more detailed template is needed for resolving case-specific dilemmas.

The step-by-step procedure outlined above has been useful in the clinical arena. Unsurprisingly, this clear and replicable structure for resolving ethical

[2] Beauchamp TL and Childress JF, *Principles of Biomedical Ethics*, 7th edition (New York: Oxford University Press, 2012: 381–387). John Rawls acknowledged that reflective equilibrium has limited usefulness and expected it to provide broad agreement only on a few basic principles for the establishment of democratic societies. Perhaps we can consider the broad implicit endorsement from the community of medical professionals of the sixteen duties of medical ethics that I have presented in this book to be something akin to a Rawlsian "overlapping consensus." As I have suggested by employing real and hypothetical examples for deriving the sixteen duties of medical ethics, agreement on those core responsibilities can be achieved through a process of reflective equilibrium.

[3] Lo B, *Resolving Ethical Dilemmas: A Guide for Clinicians* (San Francisco: Lippincott, 2005).

[4] Kaldjian L, Weir R, and Duffy T, "A Clinician's Approach to Clinical Ethical Reasoning," *Journal of General Internal Medicine* 20, 3 (2005): 306–311.

dilemmas is not very different from standard medical thinking that is used to arrive at a diagnosis and a treatment plan. Following this sort of approach for resolving an ethical dilemma can provide clinicians with a resolution of their ethical dilemma, an explanation of why a particular conclusion is appropriate and allow them to feel confidence in making their decision on how to proceed. It is especially useful for medical teams to work through the dilemma together so that they can address everyone's concerns and develop a plan that they all can support. Allow me to explain the procedure one step at a time.

Collect Relevant Data

As in making standard medical decisions, the starting point is collecting all of the relevant data that could help to answer the question of medical ethics. This information will include the medical facts (e.g., diagnosis, prognosis, treatment options); the patient's or family's preferences, priorities, and values; and relevant legal and institutional policies.[5] The tools for gathering the data are the standard apparatus of good clinical practice. A doctor should use examination and history-taking skills, including communication and listening skills, and she needs to display an empathetic attitude while attending to the responses of the patient and family. In addition to medical skills, moral imagination, that is, trying to envision what it is like to be in another's predicament, is an important tool in forming a deep understanding of the experience and needs of the patient and family. Moral imagination can enable a doctor to recognize and appreciate the burdens of being ill and being in the particular situation at hand.

Typically, an assessment of the patient's capacity and the identification of a healthcare proxy are part of the data set that could be important in resolving the dilemma. Details of the social history, including descriptions of the richness or absence of family relationships, baseline mental and physical function, and the home environment should be incorporated into this collection of the background data.

---

[5] Jonsen AR, Siegler M, and Winslade WJ, *Clinical Ethics: A Practical Approach to Ethical Decisions in Clinical Medicine*, 8th edition (New York: McGraw-Hill Education, 2015). This volume features the "four topics method" that is useful for collecting the background data of a specific case.

Table 11.2 The Duties of Medical Ethics

---

1. Seek trust and be deserving of it.
2. Use medical knowledge, skills, powers, privileges, and immunities to promote the interests of patients and society.
3. Develop and maintain professional competence.
4. Provide care based on need.
5. Be mindful in responding to medial needs.
6. Base clinical decisions on scientific evidence.
7. Maintain nonjudgmental regard toward patients.
8. Maintain nonsexual regard toward patients.
9. Maintain the confidentiality of patient information.
10. Respect the autonomy of patients.
11. Assess patients' decisional capacity.
12. Be truthful in your reports.
13. Be responsive to requests from peers.
14. Communicate effectively.
15. Police the profession.
16. Ensure justice in the allocation of medical resources.

Identify the Duties Involved

The next step is identifying the various duties that may be involved in the situation (Table 11.2). Identifying the duties involved allows doctors to appreciate why the case presents a moral dilemma. Explaining just how each duty is relevant to the situation helps to clarify the core concepts and dissect the problem.

Identify the Conflicting Duties

Once the relevant duties are clearly identified and understood, the next step is to identify the duties that are issuing inconsistent direction. This step in the process allows doctors to identify and focus on the source of the problem by recognizing that the situation involves important duties that cannot be satisfied at once. It also allows them to see how the clash between duties gives rise to moral conflict by directing opposing courses of action.

Sometimes, however, this part of the analysis may reveal that the difficulty lies in what a single duty (e.g., promote the patient's interest, provide care based on need) requires in the situation. For example, when a frail elderly patient with dementia has a bowel obstruction the surgeon may be uncertain about what would count as serving this patient's interests.

Would surgery to relieve the obstruction serve the patient's interests or would her interests be better served by deciding against performing the surgery to spare her the complications that are likely to ensue given her overall poor physical condition and her inability to cooperate with her postoperative care.

In order to resolve the ethical dilemma, the particular duties that conflict in the situation, or the ambiguity between the different directions suggested by a single duty, need to be identified.

Formulate a Question That Reflects the Conflict

Some medical questions involve procedures or medications. A question about a procedure may involve a request for information about *how* to proceed. For instance, a student in an orthopedic rotation might ask, "*How* do I reduce a fracture?" A medication question might involve dosing issues. A resident might ask, for instance, "*What* is the correct dosage of this antibiotic?" or "*How frequently* is the antibiotic to be administered?" or "*When* should the antibiotic be administered, before or after the surgery?

A question about ethical action is a question about what an agent *should* or *should not* do. Typically an ethics question that is the focus of a moral dilemma will ask a question about what *should* be done. An ethics question for guiding the resolution of an ethical dilemma will also identify the duties involved and identify the conflict that is at the heart of the conflict.

Formulating a clear question of ethics is analogous to the identification of a chief complaint in clinical medicine: It requires the team to identify the main ethical issue that is the crux of the problem. Once the conflicting duties are identified and discussed, formulating a question is usually rather straightforward. Occasionally, in an especially complex case, just as a patient may have more than one medical problem at a time, two or three dilemmas may be involved. In such a situation, several different questions may have to be formulated. Regardless of how many separate questions are involved, formulation of the question directs further consideration to the target issue(s). Surprisingly, it is often more difficult than it may seem to formulate a useful ethics question. By following the preceding steps, constructing the core question becomes a rather straightforward matter. A clearly formulated question guides the crucial deliberation that follows and keeps the deliberation focused on finding an appropriate resolution.

Decide Which Duty Should Have Priority

Once the dilemma is clearly defined in a focused ethics question, the next step is to present reasons for going one way or another in light of the relevant factors of the case. When the treatment plan involves a number of medical professionals acting in concert to implement the decision, it is often important to have a team or multiteam discussion so that the array of information available can be shared and the factors that different people consider important can be aired and examined. And sometimes it will be critical to involve the patient or the patient's family in the conversation. Considering who should participate in the discussion is often important, and failing to include people who have critical input in what is done can create additional problems. In other words, mindfulness is needed every step of the way.

In all such conversations, participants need to be aware that the people involved may prioritize the obligations involved differently. The participants should try to see their goal as a process of communicating together to find an acceptable course in a difficult and unfolding situation. This perspective is more appropriate than regarding the process of moral deliberation as an exercise in dispute mediation between antagonistic and opposing parties. Mediators take their job to be successfully concluded when everyone involved leaves the mediation feeling somewhat dissatisfied, as if the other side may have gotten a better deal. Medical professionals should have the opposite perspective and try to find a solution that everyone involved can accept and live with as the appropriate course under the circumstances.

In most cases, the patient, the family, and the medical team all want the same thing: whatever serves the patient's interests. There may nevertheless be legitimate disagreement about what that entails. Reaching agreement about what to do requires all of those involved to share their reasons for choosing a particular course. Consensus can only be achieved through a free and open discussion where all of the parties have an opportunity to explain their concerns, ask questions, challenge assumptions, introduce previously overlooked factors, offer suggestions, and consider options.

In the discussion, it is important to recognize that the priorities of the team may be different from the patient's or family's, and that even when everyone shares the same goals, those involved may disagree on how to achieve them. In deciding which of two conflicting duties to uphold and which to sacrifice, the discussants should identify especially important factors that are relevant to the case and tend to support a choice for going one way rather than the other. They should continue to share reasons until they are able to achieve a consensus on how to proceed.

Sometimes, over the course of a discussion, a previously unnoticed alternative emerges. One such circumstance is discussed in detail in Chapter 12. In that situation, the parents of three sons had to decide which of their sons should be the bone marrow donor for their 11-year-old who had sickle cell disease and leukemia and needed a bone marrow transplant. The two involved treatment teams were divided over how to proceed. One team favored using the better matched sibling as the stem cell donor to minimize the effects of graft-versus-host disease. The other team favored using the sibling who was a less perfect match and did not have sickle cell disease because his stem cells might also cure the sickle cell disease. The parents identified a third option of not proceeding with the bone marrow transplantation. Under the circumstances, because the chance of success was low and the psychological and physical risks were significant for all of the family members, everyone agreed that choosing not to proceed with the transplant was an acceptable option. When a new option avoids the dilemma, it may be a way to achieve a successful resolution.

Explaining what makes right acts right in his important book, *The Right and the Good*, Sir William David Ross explicitly stated what any thoughtful person should recognize. He wrote, "It is obvious that any of the acts that we do has countless effects, directly or indirectly, on countless people, and the probability is that any act, however right it may be, will have adverse effects."[6] In the Summary chapter at the end of his second book on moral philosophy, *Foundations of Ethics*, he made the same point. There he explained that

> in deciding what I ought to do, it is evident that I must consider equally *all* the elements, so far as I can foresee them, in the state of affairs I shall be bringing about. If I see that my act is likely to help M, for instance, and to hurt N, I am not justified in ignoring the bad effect, or even treating it as less important than the good effect, merely because it is the good effect and not the bad one that I *wish* to bring about. It is the whole nature of that which I set myself to bring about, not that part of it which I happen to desire, that makes my act right or wrong.[7]

---

[6] Ross WD, *The Right and the Good* (London: Oxford University Press, 1930: 41).
[7] Ross WD, *Foundations of Ethics* (London: Oxford University Press, 1939: 318, italics preserved). This argument can be seen as a powerful rejection of the principle of double effect and the view that there is a significant moral distinction between acts and omissions.

When faced with the difficult task of deciding which of alternative courses is right, the difficulty frequently involves a moral dilemma, a situation in which conflicting obligations point us in opposite directions. In such situations, every choice violates some cherished principle or important obligation and involves some moral sacrifice. As Philippa Foot explained, "The situation may be such that no one can emerge with clean hands whatever he does."[8] Any of the alternative actions will involve wrongdoing in the sense that some duty is violated even when, all things considered, the chosen action is the right thing to do. This plain fact about conflicting obligations has been observed in the ethics literature since Aristotle, and, just in the twentieth century, in addition to Ross and Foot, it was discussed at length by Isaiah Berlin,[9] H. A. Prichard,[10] Bas van Frassen,[11] Bernard Williams,[12] Ruth Barcan Marcus,[13] and Bernard Baumrin and Peter Lupu,[14] among others. The point of all this is to explain that the rightness of any particular action will turn on the reasons supporting it, the reasons that count against it, and their saliency. As Foot explained, "For one for whom moral considerations are reasons to act there are better moral reasons for doing this action than for doing any other."[15]

In any discussion of the dilemmas that physicians must resolve, it is unacceptable to ignore, overlook, or turn a blind eye to any of the relevant considerations, including the duties involved and the kinds of practical factors that Jeremy Bentham directed us to consider, such as the likelihood of having the desired and undesired effects, because these are often the critical considerations that tend to make a choice wrong or right in a specific case.[16]

Occasionally, in spite of sincere efforts to consider and compare all of the relevant factors, uncertainty persists and no obvious solution emerges from a discussion. In such cases, as in situations when a clinical diagnosis is elusive,

---

[8] Foot P, "Moral Realism and Moral Dilemmas," *The Journal of Philosophy* 80, 7 (1983): 379–398, 388.
[9] Berlin I, *Four Essays on Liberty* (London: Oxford University Press, 1969).
[10] Prichard HA, *Moral Obligation and Duty and Interest: Essays and Lectures* (Oxford: Oxford University Press, 1968).
[11] van Fraassen BC, "Values and the Heart's Command," *The Journal of Philosophy* 70, 1 (1973): 5–19.
[12] Williams B, *Problems of the Self* (Cambridge: Cambridge University Press, 1973); Williams B, "Politics and Moral Character," in Hampshire S, editor, *Public and Private Morality* (Cambridge: Cambridge University Press, 1978: 62–64).
[13] Barcan MR, "Moral Dilemma and Consistency," *The Journal of Philosophy* 77, 3 (1980): 121–136.
[14] Baumrin B and Lupu P, A Common Occurrence: Conflicting Duties, *Metaphilosophy* 15, 2 (1984): 77–90.
[15] Foot, "Moral Realism," 385.
[16] Bentham J, *The Principles of Morals and Legislation* (New York: Hafner Press, Macmillan, 1948).

there may be some missing information that would help to resolve the dilemma. When that seems to be the case, it is important to identify which information is needed and how it will help to resolve the dilemma. The group can then agree on a plan to find answers to the open questions.

In another case involving bone marrow transplantation, a dilemma emerged about whether or not a patient with a history of mental illness should be accepted for bone marrow transplantation with an anonymous well-matched (10/10) allogeneic donor. The duty of nonjudgmental regard suggested that a mental illness diagnosis should not prejudice the team against providing needed treatment. The duty to provide care based on need raised questions about whether the patient's inability to cooperate with the demanding procedure would actually meet his needs or harm him. To resolve the dilemma, questions had to be answered about alternatives to bone marrow transplantation, the nature of the patient's mental illness, his ability to understand his situation, his desire to undertake the procedure, the patient's history of compliance with other medical treatment, whether an adequate plan was in place for addressing his mental health needs during his hospitalization, and whether an adequate plan was in place for his postdischarge care.

When all of the information was assembled and shared, it turned out that there were no alternative treatments for the patient's condition. It was reported that the patient understood his life-threatening situation, the details of the procedure, and the anticipated hospital course, and he wanted to live. He had been compliant over many years with treatment for Ewing sarcoma, the medical condition that now left him with a lethal bone marrow failure disorder. His regular psychiatrist had worked with him and the inpatient psychiatric team in preparation for the hospitalization. And a postdischarge plan that appeared adequate was in place. With all of those questions answered, the dilemma was resolved. The team appreciated that he was likely to be a difficult patient to manage on the unit, but they all accepted that it was their duty to provide him with medical care that served his interests.

Evaluate the Decision

Clinicians typically justify their treatment decisions by referring to the standard of care. The same should hold true with the ethical choices that clinicians are required to make. Thus, once a decision is made, those involved should check themselves by considering whether the resolution is one that a consensus of exemplary doctors would agree on as a course that would uphold the trustworthiness of the profession. In other words, this step asks doctors to reflect on how their most esteemed colleagues who were fully informed of the case details would be likely to view their decision. This is an important step in resolving ethical dilemmas in medicine because questions of medical professionalism are not personal decisions. They should not be resolved by individuals consulting their hearts or personal comfort level. Instead, questions of medical professionalism have to be adjudicated by consulting with peers and adhering to the duties of medical ethics. This step is designed to ensure that doctors base their decision on profession-endorsed duties of medical ethics. Physicians who make this question a touchstone of their clinical practice demonstrate their commitment to medical professionalism.

Plan the Practical Steps for Implementing the Decision

A decision on the solution of an ethical dilemma has to be implemented. It is important to appreciate that the right thing has to be done in the right way and recognize that there are innumerable ways for good plans to go wrong. Once a course of action is agreed on, it is time to plan how to proceed. The plan needs to be clear and detailed. Doctors need to envision what is just over the horizon and plan the practical steps that should be taken by focusing on the nuances and details of the case. Forethought and planning for the anticipated eventualities and complications are required. For example, the appointment of a proxy by a patient with a deteriorating medical condition should be addressed, and a patient with a prognosis of imminent death who expresses fear of pain and abandonment should be reassured by her doctor pledging to be there with her every step of the way and promising to provide her with whatever palliation she might feel she needs.

When developing a plan, it is important to keep in mind that creative solutions should reflect the patient's needs and goals. Creativity and resourcefulness are important tools, as is empathic imagination, which can aid the doctor in appreciating the patient's needs in what lies ahead. Plans must also be communicated effectively with the team, the patient, and the family, and this means that the ability to communicate effectively is also an important skill for piloting the patient and the team along the route.

Putting the Model to Work

To illustrate how this model of clinical moral reasoning can be employed in resolving ethical dilemmas, consider a couple of case examples:

Case 1

Mrs. H. T., a 78-year-old, high-functioning woman with congestive heart failure, chronic renal insufficiency, and pressure ulcers was admitted to the hospital because of an exacerbation of her heart failure. She had been living with her sister for the past 30 years. As her illness recently worsened, her sister became her primary caregiver.

The sister is also the patient's healthcare proxy. She was present in the hospital daily and made significant personal efforts to clean her sister's wounds using unsanitary methods. She refused both nurse and physician requests to leave these procedures to the hospital staff, but the patient never objected to her sister's behavior.

The medical team involved with this case was distressed and enraged by the sister's refusal of standard-of-care treatment. Their preference was to have her removed from the hospital and a security guard posted at the door of Mrs. H. T.'s room. When they called for an ethics consult, they wanted endorsement of their position, but they were willing to work through the moral deliberation process. So, we began at the first step.

- *Collect all relevant data that could help with resolving the matter*: The team reported that Mrs. H. T. did not respond to treatment for her heart failure, and her renal insufficiency worsened to the point of uremia requiring dialysis. In spite of maximal medical therapy, her mental status worsened from the uremia, and she developed irreversible multiorgan failure due to her severe progressive cardiac and renal disease. At this point, they described the patient's prognosis as poor.

   As Mrs. H. T. lay in bed obtunded, her sister refused to allow residents to enter the room, although she did allow the attending physician to enter. There are no other family members who can be called on to intercede. The proxy form that had been completed by Mrs. H. T. offered no more specific guidance, but there was a line written in that stated, "My sister knows my views on nutrition and hydration."

- *Identify the duties involved and explain how they relate to the case*: The team identified the duty to provide care based on need as well as the duty to respect the patient's autonomy. They saw upholding the standard of care as required. Providing standard-of-care treatment would include the residents and nurses making all of their regular visits to check on the patient's vital signs and condition so that they could respond with appropriate adjustments in her treatment. It would also involve preventing the sister from applying her unsanitary dressing changes. The team also recognized that because the patient could no longer communicate, respecting her autonomy would be shown by honoring her previous wishes.

- *Identify the duties that conflict in the situation*: The team members recognized that, in this case, the duty to provide needed care conflicted with respecting Mrs. H. T.'s previous wishes. Given her previous identification of her sister as her healthcare proxy and her acceptance of her sister performing dressing changes her own way, there was no reason to believe that Mrs. H. T. would object to what her sister was doing.

- *Formulate a question of ethics that reflects the conflict*: The team formulated an ethics question that expressed the conflict in terms of the duties involved. "Should the medical team abide by the surrogate's decisions or override them and provide needed standard-of-care medicine for the patient?"

- *Decide which duty should have priority and support that choice with factors relevant to the case*: As the group started to weigh in with their considerations for going one way or another, it quickly became apparent that nothing was going to make much of a difference to the outcome. Mrs. H. T.'s death was imminent, she was expected to survive for no more than a few days. It was unlikely that she would develop a painful infection related to her sister's dressing changes during that period, and if one developed and hastened her death, it could be considered a benefit under the circumstances.

When Mrs. H. T. had been able to communicate, she had no objections to what her sister did. She never asked her to stop, even when nurses or residents voiced their concern. She actually seemed comforted by having her sister close by.

Taking these factors into account, the team conceded that because there was no benefit to be had from interfering with the sister's actions, she should be allowed to continue in accordance with the apparent previous preferences of Mrs. H. T. Furthermore, they recognized that interfering with the sister when she was about to suffer a significant personal loss would be likely to cause her needless emotional distress.

- *Evaluate the decision by asking if it is what a consensus of exemplary doctors would agree is the resolution that would uphold the trustworthiness of the profession*: At that point, the team accepted that no physician who understood the facts of this case would fault them for not providing standard-of-care treatment for Mrs. H. T. When there were no foreseeable untoward consequences for the patient and the chosen path would avoid causing her sister anguish, they were able to imagine that exemplary and compassionate professionals would agree with their chosen course.
- *Plan the practical steps for implementing the decision, focusing on the details of the case and the foreseeable issues in the near future*: Communication was the needed step for moving forward. Because the ultimate solution had been so far from their original plan, the team members who participated in the discussion recognized that others would need to understand what was being done and why. To implement their decision, they needed to explain their rationale to the teams that would take over Mrs. H. T.'s care, the nurses, those on the night shift, and anyone else who would be involved.

In this case, working through the clinical moral reasoning process allowed the team to set aside their original discomforts and focus on the situation of their patient and her sister to arrive at a well-justified ethical conclusion. The conversation enabled the team to identify the right course of action and allowed them to support their patient and her sister with caring devotion. It also gave the team moral clarity and confidence in how to proceed.

Although I have presented this model of clinical moral reasoning as a template for resolving ethical dilemmas in medicine, it is only a guide, and sometimes improvisation may be in order. Case 1 fit the model rather well, and the process of clinical moral reasoning helped the team reach a conclusion that was very different from where they began. The next case illustrates how the model can be used in an unusual and complicated situation. Even though every step of the model was not quite a perfect fit with the case, following the template helped the team to distinguish relevant issues from those that were more tangential.

Case 2

A. R., a 16-year-old male, had recently become the patient of an adolescent psychologist, Dr. Orson, at a facility that provides a broad range of services for the youth of the community. A. R. was referred for treatment by his lawyer as part of a probation agreement. In Dr. Orson's third session with A. R., the teen disclosed that he was expelled from the private boarding school that he had attended on scholarship for his participation in the sexual abuse of another younger student at the school.

While discussing the situation with Dr. Samuels, a fellow psychologist at the facility, Dr. Samuels realized that his 14-year-old patient, L. S., was the boy who had been abused by A. R. Drs. Orson and Samuels recognized that they were involved in a messy situation that involved ethical issues, but they were at a loss for knowing how to proceed.

- *Collect all relevant data that could help with resolving the matter*: This is the starting point. Drs. Orson and Samuels shared what they know about their patients. Both boys lived relatively close to the facility and, by appearance and family names, both boys appear to be people of color but from different "racial" groups. Both boys are obviously bright and have been academically high performers.

L. S. had been Dr. Samuel's patient for 10 weeks. He is withdrawn and depressed, but he has started to attend a local high school that is north of the clinic. He attends school regularly, he has been keeping up with his schoolwork, and he hasn't missed any clinic appointments.

L. S. lives in a large extended family. He has three older brothers who know about the assault at the private school, and L. S. has reported that they say they would kill anyone who was a party to what happened to their kid brother. They are very protective of L. S., and for the first month or so the older brothers took turns bringing him to the facility for appointments. One brother has recently been released from prison, where he served time for assault.

A. R. lives with his maternal grandfather in the projects nearby. He has been supportive and nurturing and extremely proud of his grandson. He has remained supportive even after the termination of his scholarship and expulsion from the private school. Since the incident, he got his grandson a lawyer, and he has been taking him to church services to get him back on the right track. The lawyer has helped him arrange for a meeting with the principal of A. R.'s former high school so that he can restart classes after the Christmas break. A. R. has said that his parents are dead, but Dr. Orson believes that there is more to the story.

- *Identify the duties involved and explain how they relate to the case*: The group of medical professionals involved in this moral deliberation identified a number of duties that were relevant considerations: justice, provide care based on need, maintain nonjudgmental regard, maintain the confidentiality of patient information, promote patient interests. As their connection to the case was discussed, the understanding of what needed to be done started to become clear.

Those who thought that justice was at the heart of the matter focused on who should remain a patient at the facility and who should be turned away. Because L. S. had come to the facility for treatment first and had been a patient for a longer period of time, some thought that A. R. should be asked to find treatment elsewhere. Others also considered it relevant that L. S. was the victim. They thought that L. S. should therefore be given preference at the facility over the perpetrator, A. R.

As the discussion of justice continued, the group recognized that first come, first served was not a relevant conception of justice for the allocation of medical care in this situation. Furthermore, because Drs. Orson and Samuels agreed that both boys needed the care of a psychologist, and because no other facility in the area would provide the treatment without charge, justice and the duty to provide care based on need required that services be provided for both boys. In addition, the group noted that not enough was known about the circumstances to assume that one boy was the victim while the other had victimized him. Someone suggested that the sexual abuse may have been a pattern at the school, and that A. R. might have previously been abused in the same way. This line of argument led to the conclusion that the team was committed to nonjudgmental regard toward both patients regardless of what had been done by whom.

- *Identify the duties that conflict in the situation*: The duty to maintain the confidentiality of patient information and the duty to benefit patients seemed to be at the crux of the situation, but the direction for action was still elusive. It was not obvious whether the confidentiality of A. R. or L. S. should be violated and information divulged about either boy. It was also hard to say that confidentiality could be ensured when their identity could be revealed to each other inadvertently if one showed up for treatment of an unanticipated illness when the other was present at the facility.
- *Formulate a question of ethics that reflects the conflict*: The question that captured the team's dilemma therefore became, "Should we focus on protecting the boys' confidentiality, or should we try to benefit the boys by providing mental health care?"
- *Decide which duty should have priority and support that choice with factors relevant to the case OR find an alternative that avoids the dilemma*: Once the question was formulated, the answer started to emerge. In the long run, it seemed that an encounter between the boys was inevitable. The team had to try to take whatever measures they could to forestall a meeting at the facility, but boys who were close in age and living in the same geographic area were likely to run into one another at some point. To avert the potential serious harm of a violent confrontation, it was in the interest of everyone involved to try to prepare the boys and their families for that unavoidable event.
- *Evaluate the decision by asking if it is what a consensus of exemplary doctors would agree is the resolution that would uphold the trustworthiness of the profession*: The team recognized that divulging the identity of one boy to the other would be a betrayal of trust. They also realized that they would be negligent if they failed to address the potential dangers inherent in the situation. Leaving L. S. vulnerable to a potentially explosive attack by A. R.'s brothers would be irresponsible. A trustworthy response required proactive measures.
- *Plan the practical steps for implementing the decision, focusing on the details of the case and the foreseeable issues in the near*

future: Fortunately, the facility has two floors with separate entrances on opposite sides of the building. To minimize the possibility of a chance encounter at the facility, arrangements were put in place for the boys to have their regularly scheduled psychologist visits on different days and on different floors of the building. In addition, chart notes were placed for those who scheduled appointments to notify both Drs. Orson and Samuels when additional appointments were made.

Both psychologists recognized the need for coordinating strategies and preparing their patients for a possible encounter anywhere in the neighborhood. They also accepted that they needed to work with L. S.'s family, particularly his older brothers, to defuse the situation. They planned to hold family meetings on the main campus, which was a distance from the youth facility, in order to help them appreciate that a vengeful response was likely to harm L. S. and to encourage them to provide support and love for their little brother in more productive ways.

This was an extraordinarily difficult case to untangle. Going through the steps one by one allowed the team to address the thoughts of all of those involved. It also allowed them to reach a solution that directed them toward what needed to be done and provided them with an explanation of why that was required. In sum, going through the process enabled the team to reach a consensus on how to proceed. It also assured them that they had made the right decision and gave them confidence as they proceeded to implement their plan.

Conclusion

This systematic approach to resolving clinical ethical dilemmas serves dual purposes. It allows doctors to rely on a standardized model to prompt their thinking. This increases the likelihood that they will consider all of the relevant information and put it together in a way that leads to an ethically justified resolution. Following a structured thought process for addressing ethical dilemmas in medicine also ensures that physicians act for reasons that are consistent with the ethics of medicine and uphold duties that are clear to them and others.

Promoting a systematic thought processes is demanded in other areas of clinical decision-making because following a decision template helps to ensure that key issues are identified and receive necessary attention. Following a systematic thought process should also be the standard for addressing medical ethics issues. Doing so would enable doctors to develop skill in clinical moral reasoning so that they learn to reliably reason and act in accordance with medical professionalism.

12

Problems with Doctors Invoking the Best Interest Standard

As I explained in Chapter 2, the second duty of medical ethics is *serve the interests of patients and society*. It requires that doctors relinquish their liberty to pursue only self-interest and commits them to using their medical knowledge, skills, powers, privileges, and immunities in the service of patients and society. This is the core of medicine's *fiduciary responsibility*, and it requires doctors to put their patients' interests before their own.

In the 1977 first edition of *Principles of Biomedical Ethics*, Beauchamp and Childress presented their account of bioethics, which has since become widely accepted. There, and in all subsequent editions of the work, they referred to this primary commitment as the principle of beneficence.[1] If acting for the benefit of a child or a patient is good, then doing what is in their "best interest" sounds even better. From there, it was easy for bioethics theorists and clinicians to slide into speaking of "the best interest" as a principle of medical ethics and canonizing it as a moral imperative in clinical practice and biomedical research. Today, many prominent bioethicists vigorously defend its use.[2,3] The "best interest standard" has been widely accepted as a benchmark for decisions made on behalf of others, both patients and loved ones. It is employed to guide decisions in both law and medicine. It just seems like common sense, so relying on the best interest is widely accepted. It is taken to be as pleasing as apple pie, as wholesome as mother's milk, and as salutary as chicken soup.

The best interest standard is employed in a variety of contexts that seem to be reasonable and appropriate. It has been invoked in court proceedings primarily to indicate that the welfare of children should be at the forefront of

[1] Beauchamp TL and Childress JF, *Principles of Biomedical Ethics*, 7th edition (New York: Oxford University Press, 2012).
[2] Kopelman LM, "The Best-Interests Standard as Threshold, Ideal, and Standard of Reasonableness," *The Journal of Medicine and Philosophy* 22, 3 (1997): 271–289.
[3] Pope TM, "The Best Interest Standard: Both Guide and Limit to Medical Decision Making on Behalf of Incapacitated Patients," *Journal of Clinical Ethics* 22, 2 (2011): 134–138.

The Trusted Doctor. Rosamond Rhodes, Oxford University Press (2020). © Oxford University Press.
DOI: 10.1093/oso/9780190859909.001.0001

concern when legal decisions involving children have to be made, often in divorce proceedings or as a result of complicated family circumstances. In such a situation, a judge's decision may involve a choice between two parents who each seek custody, and the judge has to determine which of the two available options serves the child's best interests. Governmental and social service agencies also rely on best interest when formulating policies that are designed to regulate services for vulnerable individuals in their charge. In the medical domain, patients often have to consider which of several treatment options will serve their own best interests, and surrogates who are called upon to make decisions on behalf of patients who lack decisional capacity may try to sort out which of the available options serves the best interests of their loved one.

The issues that have to be decided by medical professionals are, however, very different from those decided by surrogates, courts, and agencies that provide or oversee care for vulnerable individuals who lack decisional capacity. Furthermore, the duty of medical professionals to care for patients and promote their interests is markedly different from doing what is in the patient's **best** interest. Doctors must be careful to distinguish their professional fiduciary responsibilities from the concept of best interest because confusing the two can lead to conceptual errors and serious blunders with unfortunate consequences. I expect that a number of readers will be surprised by my claim, so I will explain my several concerns.[4]

In what follows, I begin by briefly reviewing what is said in defense of the best interest standard and what is said in criticism of it. Because children are the paradigm example for best interest arguments,[5] I follow the example of other authors who discussed the best interest standard by employing cases from pediatrics to illustrate medical decision-making.

As others have noted, the best interest standard is both subjective and vague, making it less useful than supporters presume that it is. The larger problem is that its use leads to behavior that is intolerant and polarizing. Also, using it as a point of reference can be misleading, egocentric, irrelevant, and unjust. None of this should be taken to suggest that standards for

---

[4] Diekema has taken a position that in some respects is similar to the one presented here. Diekema argued against infringements on parental liberty and that the harm principle, rather than the best interest standard, should be the criterion for overruling parental decisions. Diekema DS, "Parental Refusals of Medical Treatment: The Harm Principle as Threshold for State Intervention," *Theoretical Medicine and Bioethics* 25 (2004): 243–264; Diekema DS, "Revisiting the Best Interest Standard: Uses and Misuses," *Journal of Clinical Ethics* 22, 2 (2011): 128–133.

[5] Kopelman, "Best-Interests Standard."

assessing surrogate appropriateness or surrogate decisions should be abandoned. Because of their fiduciary responsibility to their patients, doctors must accept responsibility for monitoring the decisions that others make on behalf of patients. It also suggests that the standards for assessing surrogate appropriateness and surrogate decisions require refinement.

Insight into this issue begins with understanding the duties of physicians when a surrogate is the decision-maker on behalf of a patient and recognizing that making judgments about best interest exceeds their authority.

The Best Interest Standard in the Bioethics Literature

Loretta M. Kopelman is well known for her defense of the best interest standard. As she pointed out, it is the "prevailing standard . . . in pediatrics as well as other professions,"[6] and it has been widely embraced in the literature.[7-15] Ideally, adhering to the best interest standard involves selecting "the option that maximizes the person's overall good and minimizes the person's overall risks of harm."[16] Kopelman has argued that upholding the best interest standard is required by the public's trust in medicine as a profession. She maintained "that it is generally clear how this standard should be applied . . . and that it is a useful standard for making professional

---

[6] Kopelman LM, "Using the Best Interests Standard to Generate Actual Duties," *AJOB Primary Research* 4, 2 (2013): 11–14, 11.

[7] Beauchamp and Childress, "*Principles*," 138–140.

[8] Buchanan AE and Brock DW, *Deciding for Others: The Ethics of Surrogate Decision Making* (Cambridge: Cambridge University Press, 1990: 122–134.

[9] Kopelman LM, "A New Analysis of the Best Interests Standard and Its Crucial Role in Pediatric Practice," *The Journal of Law, Medicine and Ethics* 35, 1 (2007): 187–196; Kopelman LM, "Using the Best Interests Standard to Decide Whether to Test Children for Untreatable, Late-Onset Genetic Diseases," *Journal of Medicine and Philosophy* 32, 4 (2007): 375–394.

[10] Shah S, "Does Research With Children Violate the Best Interests Standard? An Empirical and Conceptual Analysis," *Northwestern Journal of Law and Social Philosophy* 8, 2 (2013): 121–173.

[11]. Ahronheim JC, Moreno JD, and Zuckerman C, *Ethics in Clinical Practice* (Sudbury, MA: Jones & Bartlett Learning, 2005: 39–45, 95–96, 138–139).

[12] Arras JD, "The Severely Demented, Minimally Functional Patient: An Ethical Analysis," in Steinbock B, Arras JD, and London AJ, editors, *Ethical Issues in Modern Medicine* (New York: McGraw-Hill, 2003: 333–341).

[13] Kuczewski MG, *Fragmentation and Consensus: Communitarian and Casuist Bioethics* (Washington, DC: Georgetown University Press, 1997: 151–153).

[14] Tress DM, "Classical and Modern Reflections on Medical Ethics and the Best Interests of the Sick Child," in Kuczewski MG and Polansky R, editors, *Bioethics: Ancient Themes in Contemporary Issues* (Cambridge, MA: MIT Press, 2002: 197–202).

[15] Garrett TM, Ballie HM, Garrett RM, and McGeehan, *Healthcare Ethics: Principles and Problems*, 4th edition, (Upper Saddle River, NJ: Pearson, 2009).

[16] Kopelman, "Using the Best Interests Standard," 12.

recommendations and decisions for those unable to decide for themselves about what is in their best interest."[17] Kopelman sees best interest as an ideal, a threshold, and a constraint that most often produces consensus on what should be done. In her experience, disputes over what is in a patient's best interest are rare, and when they arise, "disputes . . . are often solved by better communication."[18] In sum, Kopelman took the best interest standard to be the unproblematic touchstone for medical professionals and family members who are making medical decisions on behalf of those who cannot decide for themselves.

Robert M. Veatch, one of the most prominent critics of the best interest standard,[19] has raised many of the more common objections that are found in the literature.[20-24] He noted that the best interest standard has "achieved the status on an unquestioned platitude," and he found it to be "terribly implausible."[25] In great detail he explicated the source of ambiguity and disagreement in the determination of what is in the patient's best interest. He noted the possibility of conflicts between those who focus exclusively on health concerns and those who factor in other interests and goals. He elucidated different theories of the good, in his terms, hedonistic theories, desire-fulfillment theories, and objective list theories that could provide radically different conclusions about what is actually in a patient's best interest. The possibility of differences that arise from people having different perspectives on what makes something good led Veatch to conclude "that physicians are no better than the rest of us at guessing what counts as the medical good, how the medical good relates to the total good, and whether the patient's total good should be promoted."[26] In the end, he suggested that "to know what is good for this particular person," decisions should be made by someone who shares "deep values" with the patient because that would allow the patient's beliefs and values to govern the decision. In contrast with the best interest standard, Veatch called his alternative the "reasonable interest standard"

---

[17] Kopelman, "Using the Best Interests Standard," 11.
[18] Kopelman, "Using the Best Interests Standard," 12.
[19] Veatch R, "Abandoning Informed Consent," *Hastings Center Report* 25, 2 (1995): 5–12.
[20] Loewy EH, *Textbook of Healthcare Ethics* (New York: Plenum Press, 1996: 88–89).
[21] Elliot C, "Patients Doubtfully Capable or Incapable of Consent," in Kuhse H and Singer P, editors, *A Companion to Bioethics* (Hoboken, NJ: Wiley-Blackwell, 1998: 454–459).
[22] Lo B, *Resolving Ethical Dilemmas: A Guide for Clinicians*, 2nd edition (Philadelphia: Lippincott, Williams & Watkins, 2000: 113–115).
[23] Diekema, "Parental Refusals."
[24] Diekema, "Revisiting the Best Interest Standard."
[25] Veatch 1995, 6.
[26] Veatch 1995, 9.

and allowed that it will tolerate any choice that is consonant with a patient's values. Obviously, we don't consider young children or individuals with profound mental impairment to be capable of having deep values, so Veatch is willing to accept any choice that is consistent with the parents' or surrogate's values and beliefs.

Veatch's approach would require doctors to accept surrogates' decisions as long as the surrogates themselves had decisional capacity. It amounts to equating a surrogate's decisions with the decisions of a competent patient. Yet, the difference between a patient's and a surrogate's decision are significant.

What About the Best Interest Standard
Is Problematic?

When we identify something as the best, we are picking out one thing. There is only one best apple pie at the state fair, one best student in the class, and one best picture of the year. But there can be disagreement about which one in each category is the best. Different people value different things. Some like large chunks of apple in their pie; others prefer the apples to be sliced thinly. Some prefer thin crust, and others prefer a crumb topping. Some prefer their pie to be sweet with hints of cinnamon and nutmeg; others prefer an unadulterated tart apple taste. In other words, what we call "best" is subjective. Even when people agree on a list of specific factors that are most relevant to a specific judgment, they can prioritize them differently and therefore reach different conclusions about what is best.

Today we live in a pluralistic society. Inherent in that reality is the fact that people have radically different views about what counts as good and widely divergent perspectives on what is best. When medical professionals adopt the view that they are the arbiters of what is best for a patient, it is certainly possible that other parties with an interest in the decision see the situation differently. When doctors maintain that their professional responsibility requires them to advocate for what is in the best interest of the patient, they trap themselves in a position that is ethically and socially untenable. When doctors regard their duty as doing what is best for the patient, accepting any different decision would be a violation of duty and totally unacceptable. Clinicians who allow themselves to believe that they are acting in their patient's best interest are inclined to feel justified in pressing their view on others and trying to ensure that their view wins out. In many instances, the imposition of the doctors' will exceeds their legitimate clinical authority because it requires a personal ranking of priorities and personal judgment.

Seeing a doctor's responsibility as a commitment to the patient's best interest can also put health professionals at odds with each other or set the stage for an irresolvable conflict with the patient's family. In other words, regarding doctors as being committed to doing what is in the best interest of the patient is intolerant of other people's values and perspectives. It polarizes the parties involved and leaves those with opposing views standing their ground and having no room to compromise.

A doctor's imposition of personal values on surrogates should be recognized as an abuse of authority. For example, a doctor who regards a peaceful natural death that doesn't prolong the dying process to be in a patient's best interest may employ language and fervor to advocate for "liberating" the patient from machines. A phrase like "liberate the patient from the machines"[27] is loaded language used to manipulate the hearers to a point of view. Using the term *liberate* is likely to ignite waves of guilt in any surrogate who had agreed to impose the original bondage to machines on the captive patient. If repairing that injustice requires liberation, it is hard for those who hear the charge to escape the conclusion that whoever imposed the ventilator did something really bad. I suggest that the bad actors are physicians who overstep their role to impose personal values on surrogates who may not share them.

---

[27] The use of the term *liberate* in the context of discontinuing ventilator treatment has a history going back to 1987. In a *JAMA* article, "Liberation of the Patient From Mechanical Ventilation" by Hall and Wood, the authors suggested that a process of slowly weaning patients from mechanical ventilation before discontinuing the intervention was unnecessary. Instead, they proposed a simple pathophysiologic approach to discontinuing mechanical ventilation. In their discussion, they used the term *liberation*. That term was then embraced, first by intensivists and then by palliative care practitioners. See, for example, the following references: Carson SS, Garrett J, Hanson LC, et al., "A Prognostic Model for 1-Year Mortality in Patients Requiring Prolonged Mechanical Ventilation," *Critical Care Medicine* 36, 7 (2008): 2061–2069; Hall JB and Wood LDH, "Liberation of the Patient From Mechanical Ventilation," *JAMA* 257, 12 (1987): 1621–1628; Hess DR, MacIntyre NR, Mishoe SC, and Galvin WF, *Respiratory Care: Principles and Practice,* 3rd edition (Sudbury, MA: Jones and Bartlett Learning, 2016); Manthous CA, Schmidt GA, and Hall JB, "Liberation From Mechanical Ventilation: A Decade of Progress," *Chest* 114, 3 (1998): 886–901; Nelson JE, Tandon N, Mercado AF, Camhi SL, Ely EW, and Morrison RS, "Brain Dysfunction: Another Burden for the Chronically Critically Ill," *Archives of Internal Medicine* 166 (2006):1993–1999; Nelson JE, Mercado AF, Camhi SL, et al. "Communication About Chronic Critical Illness," *Archives of Internal Medicine* 67, 22 (2007): 2509–15; Nelson JE, Cox CE, Hope AA, and Carson SS, "Chronic Critical Illness," *American Journal of Respiratory and Critical Care Medicine* 182, 4 (2010): 446–454; Unroe M, Kahn JM, Carson SS, et al., "One Year Trajectories of Care and Resource Utilization for Recipients of Prolonged Mechanical Ventilation," *Annals of Internal Medicine* 153, 3 (2010): 167–175; Vincent J-L, *Intensive Care Medicine: Annual Update* (New York: Springer, 2007).

Aside from this structural problem of intolerance, the best interest standard doesn't work as well as people imagine it does. Consider some cases that illustrate a variety of ways in which the best interest standard may be found wanting. Even though these cases share some similarity, each distinct problem is instructive.

Case 1: Misleading

When Mrs. J. L. was pregnant with her sixth child, the fetus was found to have trisomy 18 with no significant life-threatening anomalies. Mrs. J. L. was determined to have the child and bring him up at home. She requested resuscitation if needed at delivery. She had been in touch with other parents of children with trisomy 18, and she was very optimistic about her son's future.

When the child was born, he did not require resuscitation. He clearly had many of the features of trisomy 18, including diminished neurological functioning and an inability to handle secretions, necessitating frequent suctioning. He required feeding by nasogastric tube and a nasal cannula with oxygen and increased airway pressure to keep him comfortable.

After many weeks the neonatal team concluded that the child would not be able to go home any time in the near future, and informed the mother that he needed a tracheotomy and gastrostomy. She was told that these procedures were in his best interest. Mrs. J. L. was reluctant to agree to have these measures implemented. She was worried that something would go wrong.

It was never entirely clear that the recommendation was actually in the best interest of the child because he may not have needed the intervention if he stayed in the acute care setting for another month or two. The statement may have been motivated by the team's interest in having the infant transferred to a long-term care facility. Such institutions typically would not accept a child with a nasogastric tube and nasal cannula.

Often enough, medical professionals employ best interest language to move family members to accept their decisions. Psychologically and socially, it is extremely difficult for loving family members to refuse to accept interventions that are described as being in their loved one's best interest.

Yet, when an intervention is described in those terms, it may be only one of several acceptable options or a course that actually is not best for the patient, but best for others. In such circumstances, it is misleading and dishonest to frame a treatment option as being in the patient's best interest.

In this case, it was not at all obvious which course would be best for the patient and if any of the alternative decisions would be unacceptable. When the child was evaluated shortly after birth, the team may have accepted a decision to withhold aggressive treatment and allow him to die. In such circumstances, when choosing to allow a patient to die is acceptable and choosing to treat aggressively is also acceptable, it is hard to justify a position that would rule out a course that falls somewhere in between those extremes.

Case 2: Irrelevant

P. D. was a 3-month-old boy who was brought to the hospital after frequent vomiting and failure to thrive. He was found to have a rare genetic anomaly that made it impossible for him to digest certain proteins. During his hospitalization, one particular formula was found to be tolerated somewhat.

The parents, a young couple from a rural Mexican village, had accepted all of the recommended treatments and tests. When they were finally given a fatal prognosis and offered palliative care, they wanted to take P. D. home, feed him a regular baby formula, and treat him with Mexican medicine and prayer.

The pediatricians involved in P. D.'s care were appalled by what the parents wanted to do. As they saw it, restricting P. D.'s feeding to the special formula was in his best interest.

At an interdisciplinary conference called to discuss the situation, everyone agreed that P. D.'s condition was incompatible with life. The different approaches would not make much of a difference in what PD experienced, and he was expected to die soon regardless of what was done. Even if the parents' choice of how to proceed might be slightly worse than the medically recommended alternative, there was no appreciable difference in expectations for the course of PD's short life or the ultimate outcome. In this case, trying to distinguish what was in PD's best interest from his parents' chosen course was irrelevant. There were no good options, and there was no significant difference between the alternative courses because all of the options were bad.

This was not a case of a family refusing highly beneficial treatment: The parents wanted to take their son home and try another means to save their baby. Permitting them to do so could allow them some measure of satisfaction from trying what was accepted as best in their culture. All things considered, the ultimate recommendation was to support the parents in their decision while also offering them the option of returning PD to the hospital if his management at home became problematic.

Case 3: Irrelevant (to choosing a better option)

D. T. is an infant at 35 weeks of gestation born to an 18-year-old single mother. D. T. has an amniotic band syndrome involving the placental membranes becoming entangled with the fetus early in development. He has a huge facial cleft that looks like an axe split his face into two parts. (Actually, the umbilical cord was responsible.) There is no skull bone covering the brain over the top half of his head, only attached placenta. One eye is missing. He also has limb anomalies, amputations from fusions with the placental membranes. His brain is malformed, but he breathes normally and can tolerate tube feeding. Based on the extent of his brain anomalies, his doctors predict that D. T. will have seriously impaired cognitive and physical function, if any at all. To prevent life-threatening infections, D. T. has had multiple surgeries to cover and protect his brain.

The craniofacial service is willing to try and reconstruct his face. His mother wants everything done to make him look closer to "normal." The father is supportive of that goal, as is the maternal grandmother.

There is no clear and obvious answer regarding whether cosmetic surgery would be in D. T.'s best interest. Aside from his brain and his face, all of his other vital organs work well; his body from the neck down is healthy. D. T. currently has no life-threatening medical needs, but there is no evidence that he has any sentience: Without sentience, he can have no interests. We could project interests on him, but that would be mere imagination.

Is D. T.'s mother's desire to improve his appearance and make him look more normal in his best interest? It could make it easier for others to manage his care, which, in some metaphorical sense, may be in his long-term best interest. Because surgery and all of its attendant risks are involved, some might think that doing less would be better. The surgical procedures would involve discomfort if he were sentient, but there is no evidence that he can experience anything in any way. In this case, trying to distinguish what is in D. T.'s best interest from what is not seems irrelevant because there is no way of saying what would even count as being good or bad for him. This makes the best interest standard irrelevant in deciding whether to proceed with surgery and irrelevant in deciding whether to refuse to act on his mother's desire for improving her son's appearance.

Case 4: Egocentric

E. B. is a 2-month-old infant with several serious congenital anomalies. After an extensive workup, the treating team of pediatricians concludes that features of her brain make it clear that if she survives she will have very poor mental function. Furthermore, her only chance for survival is a small-bowel transplant. The team explains to the parents that because of the low chance of success and the high risk of complications, the parents may either opt for palliative care or have their baby listed for a transplant.

The parents do not want E. B. to have a transplant. They explain that they will pray, and God will heal her.

The pediatric team was uncomfortable with the parents' choice to pray rather than move ahead with the transplant. Prayer alone would not save E. B. The transplant team was willing to perform a small-bowel transplant because it was the only treatment that might prolong E. B.'s life. Because the best interest standard requires attention to only the patient's interests, they counted transplantation as her best interest.

The procedure was relatively new and often involved serious complications, so no one was prepared to go to court for a judge's order to perform the transplant. It was hard to imagine that a judge would order the transplant under the circumstance. Nevertheless, the team's reluctance to deviate from the best interest standard left them frustrated with the parents' choice.

In this case, the parents had very much wanted to have a child. The decision to forgo a small-bowel transplantation and allow their child to die was unspeakably difficult for them. Rather than having to say that they were choosing to let their daughter die, it was easier for them to live with their choice as a decision to pray rather than proceed with a transplant.

Forgoing transplantation was not an unreasonable decision under the circumstances. Also, the parents were the ones who would have to live with the pain of any decision that they made. They would remember their daughter E. B., what they had chosen to do, and how she died. Caring medical professionals should appreciate that the interests of the parents are legitimate factors that deserve attention. Compassion required the team to allow the parents to express their choice in their own terms. Pressuring the parents to accept the team's choice or demanding that the parents express their decision in terms that the team found acceptable, by declaring that they were choosing to allow their daughter to die, imposed demands that were simply cruel. A medical team that showed compassion for the difficult choice that the parents confronted should be willing to take the parents' pain into account, accept their language, and allow them to find some peace with their decision.

Typically, egoists are decried as selfish and reviled for failing to take others into account in their decisions. It is therefore peculiar to regard medical decisions on behalf of those who cannot make decisions for themselves to be made from the egoist perspective. There is no obvious justification for ascribing the immorality of a selfish egoist to incapacitated patients. We should at least acknowledge the oddness of that perspective. This case suggests that a different approach may be more ethically appropriate, one that acknowledges that sometimes the interests of others may be legitimate considerations, even in medical decisions. It also suggests that in such situations, adherence to the best interest standard could be the wrong thing to do.

Case 5: Justice (Avoiding the Worst Outcome)

At 3:00 AM on a Saturday, the nurses in the newborn intensive care unit (NICU) began to smell smoke. It seemed to be coming from the labor and delivery unit, one floor below. The fire alarm was activated. In accordance with institutional emergency planning guidelines, the neonatal attending announced that he was putting the full evacuation plan into effect. The attending directed that the least ill babies (those without respiratory support who were in the NICU) would be evacuated first. They would be followed by the babies requiring oxygen, and then the critically ill babies.

As the smoke became thicker, it became obvious that the evacuation must occur quickly.

One nurse demanded that her patient, a very sick 24-week premature infant who was being maintained on the jet ventilator, nitric oxide, and vasopressors, be evacuated with the first group. The team had previously devoted incredible resources to save him. The nurse argued that it was in her patient's best interest for him to be evacuated immediately.

The nurse was certainly correct in claiming that evacuating her fragile patient in the first wave was in his best interest. Disaster evacuation plans, however, typically reflect the well-accepted principles of medical triage. In drastic circumstances when it is presumed that not all can be saved, avoiding the worst outcome is taken to be the right course. We set aside all of those who have the least likelihood of surviving while requiring a great deal of medical attention so that more lives can be saved. In disasters, we consider a greater number of deaths to be the worst outcome, and we consider policies that reflect the commitment to avoiding the worst outcome to be just.

In less drastic circumstances, when it is expected that everyone will be saved—the circumstance of the intensive care unit and the emergency department on ordinary days, for instance—we treat those with urgent needs first in the expectation that those who can wait longer will not be permanently harmed by the wait. This approach is also accepted as being in accord with justice even though it is not in the best interest of those whose care is delayed. Neither disaster (wartime) triage nor emergency room (peacetime) triage reflects the best interest standard, but both policies are just because they reflect significant differences in the circumstances of the patients involved and the priorities that a consensus of experienced and thoughtful medical professionals endorse as the most appropriate response to those sorts of circumstance. Following the triage plan accords with justice because it treats all similarly situated patients in the same way.[28] And even Kopelman accepted that achieving the ideal of acting in the patient's best interest "would not be an actual duty if . . . [it] was unfair or dangerous to others."[29]

---

[28] The broad issue of what makes a medical policy or action just is discussed in detail in Chapter 9.
[29] Kopelman, "Using the Best Interests Standard," 11.

In sum, there are serious problems with employing the best interest standard in clinical medicine. It is subjective and, at the same time, intolerant and polarizing. It is also far less useful than people imagine it to be because its directions can be vague, insensitive to complexity, misleading, irrelevant, egocentric, and unjust. Fortunately, there is another option.

The Not Unreasonable Standard for Surrogate Decisions: The Three-Box Model

Physicians who frequently treat patients who lack decisional capacity need guidance on what to advocate on behalf of their patients and how to respond to surrogate decisions. Medical professionals are neither required to decide what an ideal choice for promoting the patient's best interest would be, as Kopelman suggested, nor required to accept any surrogate choice, as Veatch suggested. But if both of those options are rejected, doctors need a different model for navigating the complex normative terrain of surrogate decisions. Physicians' fiduciary responsibility as trusted guardians of their patients' well-being gives them important responsibilities for assessing the appropriateness of surrogates and for determining when to allow a surrogate's choice to rule.[30] They need a tool that will help them answer questions about whether a surrogate's decision should be accepted or refused and a way to explain those decisions.

T. M. Scanlon distinguished three kinds of reasons that people use in making their decisions.[31] Imagine a series of three concentric circles containing different kinds of reasons that people draw on to justify their actions. Reasons from the central core are the kinds of considerations that people everywhere find reasonable; for example, the choice would be likely to avoid death, pain, disability, loss of pleasure, and loss of freedom.[32] Reasons from the middle ring reflect decisions based on core reasons that reasonable people may order differently in the same situation. Reasons in

---

[30] Faden and Beauchamp discussed the "gatekeeping concept," the role of physicians in determining when a patient lacks the capacity for making decisions about his medical care. In what follows, I recognize a "gatekeeping" role with respect to the assessment of surrogate's decisional capacity and surrogates' decisions. Faden R and Beauchamp TL, *A History and Theory of Informed Consent,* (New York: Oxford University Press, 1986: 287–288).

[31] Scanlon TM, *What We Owe to Each Other* (Cambridge, MA: Belknap Press, Harvard University Press, 1998: 348–349).

[32] Gert B, Clouser KD, and Charles C, *Bioethics: A Return to Fundamentals* (New York: Oxford University Press, 1997).

the outermost ring are reasons that others may reject without being unreasonable. This third domain is significantly different from the other two because those reasons reflect an individual's personal commitments, moral standards, aesthetic values, or religious views. These are reasons that other reasonable people may not share and do not have inherent reasons to accept for themselves.

An adult patient who accepts a treatment because it is likely to preserve life invokes a reason from the central core to support her decision. But if more than one core reason could be relevant to the decision, different people could prioritize those core reasons differently and therefore reach different decisions. A patient who accepts a treatment because it offers some small chance of prolonging life, although a significant likelihood of causing pain and disability, invokes core reasons and prioritizes avoiding death. Another patient in a similar situation could share the same core values but prioritize them differently. He might refuse the life-extending treatment in order to avoid disability. These judgments would reflect the second ring of reasons.

An adult's personal commitments can also support a medical choice and determine whether or not she should accept or refuse a recommended intervention. A person who chooses to accept the intervention may do so because her son wants her to, and he would be distressed if his mother refused it. Someone who chooses to forgo treatment may also reach that decision for personal reasons from the outer ring, such as a religious commitment that prohibits use of that particular sort of intervention (e.g., blood transfusion).

Physicians accept patient choices that are justified by reasons from the first two domains because the supporting reasons are widely shared and recognized as being important to everyone. They are often uncomfortable about accepting patient choices that are justified by reasons from the third domain precisely because those supporting reasons are not broadly shared. Nevertheless, the duty to respect patient autonomy directs physicians to accept the refusals of patients with decisional capacity even when dire consequences are foreseen and when the justification comes from personal commitments or religious convictions.

Yet, it is hard to imagine a rationale from the outer ring of idiosyncratic reasons that would justify a surrogate's decision to withhold treatment that offered a good chance of averting a catastrophe. If a previously competent adult had expressed her own views on refusing treatment under the prevailing circumstances, withholding it would be consonant with her values or her advance directive. Doctors should not, however, accept a surrogate's refusal of treatment that offers significant and likely benefit without a central core justifying reason because, by definition, that rationale would not be reasonable for anyone who didn't share those values.

A surrogate's refusal of treatment that entailed significant risks and low likelihood of achieving benefits would be an entirely different matter. In such cases, surrogates should be given wide berth and allowed to decide either way precisely because neither choice would be unreasonable.

In previous articles, Dr. Ian Holzman and I explained this difference in authority to make surrogate decisions by using our three-box model (Figure 12.1). At one extreme is a box representing cases that are likely to have very poor outcomes regardless of the interventions that are tried. In such cases, medical interventions prolong an agonizing dying process or create greater burdens than benefits. Physicians in such situations should and do encourage surrogates to withhold or discontinue treatment and adopt a palliative mode of care because that approach would be humane and reasonable. At the opposite extreme is a box representing cases in which treatment promises a likely and significant medical benefit, whereas refusal of treatment is likely to result in significant harm or death. In such cases, surrogates should not be

THE **NOT UNREASONABLE STANDARD** FOR
SURROGATE DECISIONS:
THE THREE BOX APPROACH

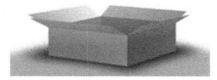

Unreasonable to Refuse/Highly Beneficial & Low Risk	Reasonable Options	Unreasonable to Request/ Harmful & Minimal Benefit

Figure 12.1 The Not Unreasonable Standard for Surrogate Decision-Making: The Three-Box Approach.

In this illustration, the middle box is largest because I assume that the circumstances where forgoing treatment is unreasonable are rare. In some specialties, however (e.g., emergency medicine), such circumstances may be more common.

allowed to refuse medical intervention because doing so would be unreasonable. Although patients with decisional capacity may refuse such treatment for themselves on the grounds of some personal commitment, surrogates should not be allowed the authority to impose their own personal values on another who will suffer a devastating result. Refusals of likely and beneficial interventions in that extreme box are paradigmatically unreasonable. Such decisions can only be justified by reasons from the outer ring of personal reasons that other reasonable people may refuse to endorse. Although personal reasons are sufficient for guiding one's own life, they should not be accepted in surrogate decisions.

Because physicians have a fiduciary responsibility to their patients, when a surrogate's choice would clearly subvert a treatment goal that is supported by core reasons, the choice must be rejected. Doctors should not accept a surrogate's personal reasons for refusing a significantly beneficial treatment when the choice violates core values, and they must refuse to honor decisions to withhold treatment that is likely to provide significant benefit.

Medical decisions involving a choice among acceptable alternative treatment options or a discretionary matter without significant consequences or decisions about treatments with uncertain outcomes should be sorted into the middle box. When nothing crucial turns on the decision or when reasonable people could accept or refuse the treatment option, medical teams should accept the decisions of surrogates. In these cases, where core reasons can be prioritized in different ways, there is neither an obvious reasonable choice nor an obvious unreasonable choice and no unique and clear way to prioritize the various considerations.

Three further considerations support the acceptance of surrogate discretion for decisions sorted into the middle box. First, because the surrogate is far more likely to bear at least some part of the physical, psychological, and financial burdens of the decision than the medical professionals, who can be expected to have no more than limited interaction with the patient who leaves the hospital, it is appropriate to leave the choices to those who will have the responsibility. Second, because people derive some of their priorities from their own family or culture, decisions by surrogates on behalf of patients who previously had decisional capacity are more likely to reflect the patient's values than people who do not belong to the patient's (biological or social) family and culture. Third, a vast majority of patients want their surrogates to make decisions on their behalf in circumstances when they are unable to decide for themselves.

Once physicians determine that the decision may be sorted into the middle box, acceptable surrogates should be allowed to make decisions that reflect their reasons and values without physicians delving into their priorities. In other words, if a surrogate's decision is **not unreasonable**, it should be allowed to govern what is done.

Conversations with surrogates who refuse recommended treatment should focus on eliciting the kinds of special considerations that might be relevant for reclassification of the case. For example, a surrogate might draw attention to how the patient's other medical problems make it likely that a proposed surgery will have serious complications. Or, perhaps a patient's fear of unfamiliar environments would make the anguish of hospitalization significant. Such reasons might justify a different conclusion and be sufficient for moving the case from a box at the extreme of required treatment to the more optional middle box.

Scanlon argued for determining the rightness of an action by looking to the specifics of the situation and the reasons for making one's choice. He maintained that the moral importance of choosing actions in this way "is adequately explained by the fact that people have reasons to want to act in ways that can be justified to others."[33] Doctors who have to manage a patient's care with direction from a surrogate should consider whether the reason(s) for their acceptance or rejection of the surrogate's choice can be justified to other experienced medical professionals who understood the details of the case at hand. The three-box model provides a template for assessing such decisions based on reasons that can be justified to other physicians.[34]

---

[33] Scanlon, *What We Owe*, 154.

[34] The 1983 report from the President's Commission for the Study of Ethical Problems in Medicine and Biomedical and Behavioral Research repeatedly endorsed the best interest standard for making decisions on behalf of others. At the same time, the report distinguished three categories that resemble the three box model. The commission also made recommendations comparable to ours. Based on the physician's assessment of treatment options, the commissioners distinguished (1) clearly beneficial therapies from (2) ambiguous or uncertain ones and (3) futile ones. The commissioners would require treatment when it is clearly beneficial, but leave the decision to surrogates when it is not. The commission also acknowledged the role of physicians in assessing the decisions of parents and interrogating or resisting those that are not justified. The not unreasonable standard that is characterized in the three boxes model goes beyond the report by explaining the shortcomings of the best interest standard and providing a rationale for treating these different kinds of circumstances differently. President's Commission for the Study of Ethical Problems in Medicine and Biomedical and Behavioral Research, *Deciding to Forego Life-Sustaining Treatment: A Report on the Ethical, Medical, and Legal Issues in Treatment Decisions* (Washington, DC: Georgetown University, 1983: 215–223). https://bioethicsarchive.georgetown.edu/pcbe/reports/past_commissions/deciding_to_forego_tx.pdf

Surrogates

Case 6

L. V. is a 3-year-old child. She has short-gut syndrome, and her doctors recommend a small-bowel transplant. L. V. has spent her entire life in hospitals. For the past 6 months, she has been in a tertiary care pediatric facility to be evaluated for transplantation. During this entire stay, no one from her family has visited. The parents do not respond to requests from the transplant team for a meeting to discuss transplantation and post-transplant care for L. V. They have not responded to phone messages or registered letters asking them to contact the transplant team.

L. V.'s family consistently failed to be involved with her or even to communicate with the medical team about her treatment. This sort of situation raises a different sort of question. If they should eventually come to a meeting about whether or not to proceed with small-bowel transplantation, should the transplant team accept their decision? Although a decision about small-bowel transplantation would usually be sorted into the middle optional box because it is still a relatively new procedure with a high risk of complications or failure, we should be reluctant to leave the decision in the hands of her parents. Their absence and lack of involvement, effectively abandoning their daughter, raises questions about whether they have appropriate concern for her well-being.

Because physicians have a fiduciary responsibility to their patients, they have to take a skeptical and cautious stance toward surrogates, and they are obliged to assess those who might be entrusted to make decisions on their patients' behalf. It is certainly legitimate for physicians to informally evaluate surrogates' decisional capacity even though it may not be feasible to subject them to a standard clinical capacity assessment. It is also necessary for physicians to gauge surrogates' attitude toward the patient.

Although a surrogate's full-blown commitment to the patient's best interest may be admirable, a more circumscribed commitment to the patient's well-being and a minimally appropriate level of concern are indispensable. In this vein, it is useful to keep in mind that most states allow friends to serve as surrogates for patients who lack decisional capacity and have no one closer to make decisions on their behalf. This suggests that the surrogate must have some concern for the patient's well-being, but it needn't be an overwhelming or a primary interest. That said, a surrogate's display of disinterest or opposing interests should disqualify a surrogate from making any significant decisions on the patient's behalf.

For these reasons, the team should seek the legal appointment of a surrogate other than L. V.'s parents to make all decisions about her future medical treatment. L. V. needs a concerned and caring decision maker to choose the course for her future medical treatment. If no family member is able to provide that direction, someone else must be designated to take on that responsibility. Once it becomes apparent that her parents do not provide the appropriate involvement or concern for her well-being, the medical professionals have to take steps to ensure that she will have a responsible and responsive surrogate decision-maker available for the numerous treatment decisions that her future will involve. When time permits, the need for an appropriate surrogate involves taking the matter to the courts for a resolution.

Conclusions

In cases involving patients who lack decisional capacity, physicians have important responsibilities in assessing surrogates and surrogate decisions, and they have to make unusual and weighty decisions. I have argued that the decision they should avoid making is one that would determine the best interest of the patient. I caution doctors to avoid thinking in terms of what is in a patient's best interest: Doing so is counterproductive and a fool's errand. This chapter provides arguments for rejecting the best interest standard even though it continues to be widely supported in the bioethics literature and it is frequently invoked as the basis for making choices on behalf of patients who are unable to make their own decisions.

Instead, doctors need to be aware that decisions made by patients and surrogates are different from the choices that they are required to make. Doctors have to make judgments about the range of acceptable surrogate decisions and the appropriateness of both the surrogate and the surrogate's decision. They have to assess both the surrogate's decisional capacity and determine whether the surrogate has a caring attitude toward the patient. Doctors also have to evaluate surrogates' reasons for their refusals of recommended treatment. Only decisions based on widely shared reasons should be accepted for surrogate refusal of highly beneficial treatment.

The not unreasonable standard, coupled with the three-box model, provides a framework and rationale for navigating this complicated moral terrain and justifying the treatment decisions that have to be made. They can guide doctors in identifying acceptable surrogate decisions and blocking inappropriate surrogate decisions. When physicians determine that a surrogate's chosen course is not unreasonable, the decisions should rest with the surrogate, and the physician should support the surrogate's choice. Doctors need to understand that they have an obligation to ensure that surrogate decisions do not compromise their patient's interests and understand that they have no right to identify the best of several reasonable options. Doctors who can distinguish their duty and its limits are prepared to interact with surrogate decision-makers. Understanding the scope of their responsibility, as well as the limits of their authority, makes doctors trustworthy in managing patient care that is directed by surrogates.

Although it is admirable for surrogates to think in terms of what is best for their loved one, unnecessary problems are created when medical professionals employ the phrase *best interest* in considering or discussing the clinical options for a patient. Medical professionals should eschew the phrase *best interest* and avoid taking it as the standard for guiding their clinical decisions because using that language invites intolerance. In many circumstances, asserting that a particular treatment choice is "in the patient's best interest" can be polarizing, misleading, egocentric, irrelevant, or unjust.

Instead, by omitting the word *best*, doctors can simply speak about how particular options will serve the patient's interests. Equipped with conceptual clarity about both the scope of physician obligations and the limits of their authority, doctors can be trusted to steer a path through their surrogate decision maker interactions with medical professionalism.

13

Professional Responsibility and Conscientious Objection

This chapter has a place in this book because conscience and conscientious objection have become prominent and controversial topics in our society. The most prominent conscience issues in medical ethics concern abortion and the provision of aid in dying, but individuals also register objections to providing services based on gender, sexual identity, withholding and withdrawing treatment, contraception, assisted reproduction, and more. Matters of conscience may also involve doctors' decisions on cooperating with orders to report patients who might be undocumented to immigration authorities, refusing to accept pediatric patients whose parents refuse to have them vaccinated, assisting patients in avoiding military service in an unjust war, refusing to provide needed medical care for injured terrorists, and so on. In addition, recent versions of the Australian Medical Association Code of Ethics[1] and the Canadian Medical Association Code of Ethics[2] have added items that appear to sanction physicians claiming conscientious objection as grounds for refusing services to patients.

Because the concept of conscience has a long and controversial history in moral philosophy, because the fundamental concepts involved are not adequately understood, and because the controversies have become tangled and obscured by politics, discussing the concepts and issues is relevant, important, and timely. The central issues in today's disputes over conscience in medicine are, first, whether claims of conscientious objection should allow medical professionals to refuse to perform tasks that would otherwise

---

[1] Australian Medical Association, *AMA Code of Ethics, Editorially Revised 2006, Revised 2016* (2016), item 2.1.13. Accessed October 28, 2018, at https://ama.com.au/system/tdf/documents/ AMA%20Code%20of%20Ethics%202004.%20Editorially%20Revised%202006.%20Revised%20 2016.pdf?file=1&type=node&id=46014

[2] Canadian Medical Association. *CMA Code of Ethics (Update 2004)* (2004), responsibility 12. Accessed October 28, 2018, at http://www.cpsa.ca/wp-content/uploads/2019/01/CMA_Policy_ Code_of_ethics_of_the_Canadian_Medical_Association_Update_2004_PD04-06-e.pdf

The Trusted Doctor. Rosamond Rhodes, Oxford University Press (2020). © Oxford University Press.
DOI: 10.1093/oso/9780190859909.001.0001

be regarded as part of their professional responsibility and whether denial of service counts as a failure of duty, abandonment, or negligence and, second, whether claims of conscience give medical professionals license to do things that are prohibited by civil law. These issues can leave doctors uncertain about what a trustworthy physician should do and uncertain about when and why medical professionals should act according to the dictates of conscience.

In the United States today, it may be that peoples' understanding of the concept of conscience has been influenced more by Jiminy Cricket than by the authors who have wrestled with the concept over the centuries. Jiminy was the insect in a blue hat who served as the conscience for the puppet who wanted to be a real boy in Walt Disney's 1940 film *Pinocchio*. The concept of conscience expressed in that cartoon presents conscience bathed in the Blue Fairy's ethereal light as a supernaturally bestowed authoritative voice that enables us to tell right from wrong. People who have absorbed that view are inclined to assign privilege to actions done in obedience to the voice of conscience. At the same time, however, our ordinary understanding of ethics also privileges moral laws, such as don't break a promise, which most influential moral philosophers have regarded as the dictates of conscience.

The inherent conflict between these unexamined ideas about what conscience is needs to be recognized and explored in order to develop a defensible stand on today's issues. Because so much can turn on that understanding, it is irresponsible to continue with merely a cartoon characterization of the matter. The competing conceptions of conscience and claims of conscientious objection require examination with the critical tools of moral analysis. I therefore begin with a brief digression into the historical literature to review some of the canonical ideas that have played an important role in the theological and philosophical debates related to conscience.

Conscience: Some Historical Background

Most of the positions on conscience fall into one of two camps. As is the case in most of the long-standing arguments in philosophy, one camp is rooted in the philosophy of Plato while the other is rooted in Aristotle's philosophy. The discussions of conscience bear all of the traditional marks of these two philosophers' positions on the source of knowledge.

Conscience as the Innate, Moral Sense of Right and Wrong

The concept of conscience that is most consonant with today's use and the cartoon representation can be traced back to platonic roots. In most of its incarnations, the concept is closely tied to the idea that truth is absolute, unchanging, and closely associated with God, the Word of God, or the divine imprinted on our souls. We gain access to this source of moral knowledge by exploring what is within us. Since early Christianity, from the Christian Platonists to the Cambridge Platonists to twentieth-century authors such as C. S. Lewis, the concept is understood to express God's relation to individual humans and each person's deep, innate, and natural sense of right and wrong. Although there is some variation in the concept as it is employed by different authors, and even what it is called, it is typically taken to represent something short of innate knowledge and more of an ability "to receive the simple ideas of approbation and condemnation."[3,4] As Jean Jacques Rousseau (1712–1778) explained in his *Emile: Or, on Education* (1762), "Conscience is the voice of the soul. . . . Too often reason deceives us; . . . but conscience never deceives us; it is the true guide of man; it is to man what instinct is to the body; which follows it, obeys nature, and never is afraid of going astray."[5]

The concept has a long history in Christianity. St. Augustine's *Confessions* is commonly read as a search for understanding by searching within oneself to comprehend the Word of God. Although Augustine did not present a fully articulated conception of conscience, he did explain that, "But when a deep consideration had from the secret bottom of my soul drawn together and heaped up all my misery in the sight of my heart, there arose a mighty storm, bringing a mighty shower of tears."[6] Theologians of the early Latin Middle Ages expressed the Augustinian view that full understanding of the deepest truths is accessible to all through scriptural revelation, simple faith, and the spirit of grace.

The idea of conscience, as an authoritative inner voice or true heart, is associated with Reformation Protestant thinking dating back to Martin Luther (1483–1546) and John Calvin (1509–1564). Both of these reformers were

---

[3] Raphael DD, editor, *British Moralists 1650–1800*, Vols. 1 and 2 (London: Oxford at the Clarendon Press, 1969: vol. 1, 269).
[4] Beauchamp and Childress present a similar take on the meaning of "conscience." Beauchamp and Childress, *Principles*, 2013, 407.
[5] Rousseau J, *Emile: Or, on Education*, translated by A Bloom (New York: Basic Books, 1979: 269).
[6] Augustine, *The Confessions of Augustine*, edited by J Gibb and W Montgomery (New York: Garland, 1980: 398).

inclined toward Augustinian ideas, both were opposed to the central authority of the pope and the Catholic Church, and both held the view that each person could be his own priest and read the Bible for himself.

Pierre Bayle (1647–1706) provided a fulsome account of the concept of conscience in French Protestantism of the early modern period in his *Historical and Critical Dictionary*. There he provided six principles related to conscience and concluded

> that the first and most indispensable of all our Obligations, is that of never acting against the Instincts of Conscience. . . . There is therefore an eternal and immutable Law, obliging Man, upon pain of incurring the Guilt of the most heinous mortal Sin that can be committed, never to do any thing in violation and in despite of Conscience.[7]

The Cambridge Platonists, a group of British moralists writing in England during the same period, held similar views on conscience, its divine origin, and its moral authority. Henry More (1614–1687), in his *An Antidote Against Atheism* (1652), maintained that the "natural remorse of conscience . . . intimate[s] that there is a God."[8] He wrote that, "Wherefore I conclude from natural conscience in a man that puts him upon hope and fear of good and evil from what he does or omits, . . . that there is an intelligent principle over universal nature that takes notice of the actions of men—that is, that there is a God; for else this natural faculty would be false and vain."[9] Benjamin Whichcote (1609–1683) expressed a comparable view in his *Moral and Religious Aphorisms*; he declared, "Both Heaven and Hell have their foundation within us. Heaven primarily lies in a refined temper, in an internal reconciliation to the nature of God and to the rule of righteousness. The guilt of conscience and the enmity to righteousness is the inward state of Hell. The guilt of conscience is the fuel of Hell."[10] In the same vein, Lord Shaftesbury (1671–1713), writing in *An Inquiry Concerning Virtue or Merit*, offered that

---

[7] Bayle P, Extracts from: *Philosophical Commentary on the Words of the Gospel, 'Compel Them to Come In'* (translator anonymous), London, 1708. https://www.constitution.org/primarysources/bayle.html

[8] Craig GR, editor, *The Cambridge Platonists* (New York: Oxford University Press, 1968: 184).

[9] Craig, *Cambridge Platonists*, 184.

[10] Craig, *Cambridge Platonists*, 424.

To have the reflection in his mind of any *unjust* action or behavior, which he knows to be naturally *odious* and *ill-deserving* . . . is alone properly called CONSCIENCE; . . . it has its force however from the apprehended moral deformity and odiousness of any act, with respect purely to the divine presence, and the natural veneration due to such a supposed being.[11]

In the seventeenth century, when the authority of conscience was an important issue in theology and political philosophy, both Samuel Clarke (1675–1729), an Anglican clergyman, and Bishop Joseph Butler (1692–1752) identified St. Paul's statement in Romans 2:14, 15, as biblical authority for the idea that conscience is imprinted in human hearts by God.[12]

For when the Gentiles which have not the law, do by nature the things contained in the law, these having not the law, are a law unto themselves; which shows the work of the law written in their hearts, their conscience also bearing witness, and their thoughts the mean while *accusing* or else *excusing* one another.

Sometimes, the word *conscience* was explicitly used in discussions, but other terms were employed as well, with the same author often employing different words to express roughly the same concept. For example, British moralist Francis Hutcheson (1694–1746) sometimes wrote about conscience and at other points referred to how "men must consult their own breast," "a superior sense," the "moral sense," "approbation," "perception of moral excellence," "opinion of natural goodness," and "some secret sense."[13] Another British moralist, Thomas Reid (1710–1796), sometimes referred to conscience and at other points called it "our constitution" or the "sense of duty."[14]

British moralist Joseph Butler (1692–1752) presented a more complex view of conscience in his *Fifteen Sermons Preached at the Rolls Chapel* and *A Dissertation Upon the Nature of Virtue*. Like the Cambridge Platonists, Butler conceived of conscience as a distinct faculty that, by nature, is the superior, supreme, chief, or highest faculty, and it carries moral authority. In his *Dissertation* (and similarly in *Sermon* II, 4, and *Sermon* III, 3 and 5) he stated,

---

[11] Raphael, *British Moralists*, vol. 1, 185 (220).
[12] Raphael, *British Moralists*, vol. 1, 194, 346.
[13] Raphael, *British Moralists*, vol. 1, 261–266.
[14] Raphael, *British Moralists*, vol. 2, 268.

> Conscience does not only offer itself to shew us the way we should walk in, but it likewise carries its own authority with it, that it is our natural guide; the guide assigned us by the Author of our nature: it therefore belongs to our condition of being, it is our duty to walk in that path, and follow this guide . . . as it is absolutely the whole business of a moral agent, to conform ourselves to it.[15,16]

The inner voice idea of conscience is vulnerable to serious lines of criticism. There is no way to determine just what the source of the inner voice is. When we notice people from different cultures performing vengeance or shame killings as acts dictated by conscience, it is reasonable to doubt the authenticity of conscience claims and to regard them as social artifacts or the products of cultural influence. There is also no way to discern whether the inner voice is spoken by a demon rather than a deity, or even if the person who claims to have heard an inner voice actually did.

Suspicion about the origin of the alleged moral sense, and hence its message, becomes more pronounced when we notice that different people who sincerely claim to act from conscience passionately disagree with each other. It's hard to imagine that people who regard conscience as the voice of God would also accept that God speaks with a forked tongue or issues conflicting messages. Yet even today we witness people who claim that they are acting on the dictates of conscience when they provide abortions and others who are at least as passionate in following the dictates of conscience in their opposition to abortion.

---

[15] Butler J, *Fifteen Sermons Preached at the Rolls Chapel and a Dissertation Upon the Nature of Virtue* (London: Bell, 1964: 195).

[16] Although Butler was clear on the authority of conscience, he was somewhat unclear on what he took conscience to be, leading to controversy in the ethics literature of the mid-twentieth century over just how to read Butler's position on conscience. For example, T. McPherson held that "this then is Butler's idea of human nature: a hierarchy of principles, with conscience or reflection at the top." The key issue in arguments over Butler's understanding of conscience concerns whether conscience is primarily intuitive (McPherson), primarily rational (Broad), both (Baumrin) or deliberately ambiguous (Selby-Bigge). Baumrin BH, new introduction in Selby-Bigge LA, *British Moralists*, edited and introduction by L.A. Selby-Bigge (Indianapolis: The Bobbs-Merril Company, 1964).

Broad CD, *Five Types of Ethical Theory* (New York: Harcourt, Brace and Company, 1934): 175–179. McPherson T, "The Development of Butler's Ethics," *Philosophy*, 23 (1948): 320.

Selby-Bigge LA, *British Moralists*, edited and introduction by L.A. Selby-Bigge, and new introduction by Bernard H. Baumrin (Indianapolis: The Bobbs-Merril Company, 1964).

Conscience as Right Reason

These sorts of concerns led at least three of the most prominent authors in the history of ethics to expound a radically different understanding of what conscience is. They held similar positions on conscience as a rational, cognitive, and propositional element of morality rather than an intuitive, noncognitive, and nonpropositional inner sense. These authors are Saint Thomas Aquinas (1225–1274) in his *Summa Theologica*, Thomas Hobbes (1588–1679) in his *Leviathan*, and Immanuel Kant (1724–1804) in his *Metaphysical Principles of Virtue*. Each of them considered the rules reached by right reason based on their observations and experience of the world to be morally authoritative. They counted those dictates of reason to be conscience properly understood. They also regarded the inner voices or feelings that people claimed to experience, as well as reflections that were not formulated and grounded in terms of moral law that should govern the actions of everyone, to be mistakenly called "conscience." They were especially suspicious of claims based on a moral sense and inner voice and considered them to be erroneous when they deviated from right reason. Aquinas explained that,

> Since conscience is a kind of dictate of the reason (for it is an application of knowledge to action), to inquire whether the will is evil when it is at variance with erring reason, is the same as to inquire "whether an erring conscience binds." . . . If a man's reason or conscience tells him that he is bound by precept to do what is evil in itself; or that what is good in itself, is forbidden, then his reason or conscience errs. . . . We must therefore conclude that, absolutely speaking, every will at variance with reason, whether right or erring, is always evil.[17]

Aquinas explained that because the nonpropositional moral sense experiences that are taken to be dictates of conscience can be in error, following them does not excuse evil action. For Aquinas, right reason was conscience; it was the highest authority and therefore the ultimate arbitrator.

For Hobbes the moral authority of conscience wasn't a side issue, but a central question that his moral and political philosophy aimed to resolve.

[17] Aquinas, *Summa Theologica*, translated by Fathers of the English Dominican Province (Cincinnati, OH: Benziger, 1947: First Part of the Second Part, Article 5). http://www.ccel.org/ccel/aquinas/summa.FS_Q19_A5.html

Hobbes's views are especially important because for one hundred years they were the target of many of the British authors mentioned previously, particularly the Cambridge Platonists. Hobbes regarded the careful use of language and correcting misuses of language as critical for right reason, and linguistic precision was a critical element of Hobbes's argument in *Leviathan*. Although Hobbes's position on conscience was repeated throughout the work, it was most clearly and directly addressed toward the end of Part 2, in Chapter 29, "Of those things that Weaken or tend to the Dissolution of a Common-wealth." There Hobbes listed as the first "poyson of seditious doctrines. . . . That every private man is Judge of Good and Evill actions." His second listed seditious doctrine "is that *whatsoever a man does against his Conscience, is Sinne.*" He went on to explain that, "For a mans Conscience, and his Judgement is the same thing; and as the Judgement, so also the Conscience may be erroneous."[18]

Like Aquinas, Hobbes was deeply suspicious of conscience as an inner sense or voice because there is no way of telling whether or not the sense or voice belongs to God or the devil. He saw the God-given ability of "naturall Reason" to be "the undoubted Word of God . . . and therefore not to be folded up in the Napkin of an Implicite Faith, but to be employed in the purchase of Justice, Peace, and true Religion."[19]

In Part 1, Chapter 8, Hobbes identified "Inspiration, called commonly, Private Spirit," as a defect in intellectual virtue, apparently to distinguish reason-based, law-giving "conscience" from what others erroneously called conscience. As defects in intellect, Inspiration or Private Spirit are anything but reliable guides for action.[20] In Part 3 of *Leviathan*, Hobbes explicated the Bible to show how his moral and political views were consonant with Christianity and the obligations of Christians. There he cautioned that in trying to understand biblical texts, "we are not to renounce our Senses, and Experience; nor (that which is the undoubted Word of God) our natural Reason."[21] Hobbes's general view was that we can deduce the immutable and

---

[18] Hobbes T, *Hobbes's Leviathan* (Oxford: Oxford at the Clarendon Press, 1965: 249;29/168233).

[19] Hobbes, *Hobbes's Leviathan*, 286; 32/195.

[20] Hobbes accounted for this sort of defect of intellect and for why conscience is mistakenly accepted as authoritative, explaining that it

> begins very often, from some lucky finding of an Errour generally held by others; and not knowing, or not remembering, by what conduct of reason, they came to so singular a truth (as they think it, though it be many times an untruth they light on,) they presently admire themselves; as being in the speciall grace of God Almighty, who hath revealed the same to them supernaturally, by his Spirit. (Hobbes, Hobbes, *Hobbes's Leviathan*, 58–59)

[21] Hobbes, *Hobbes's Leviathan*, 286; 32/186.

eternal Laws of Nature from our experience by using right reason.[22] With a long list of examples, he cautioned readers to be wary of being taken in by false prophets, concluding that, "If one Prophet deceive another, what certainty is there of knowing the will of God, by other way than that of Reason?"[23]

Immanuel Kant's position on conscience can be grouped along with that of Aquinas and Hobbes. For him, conscience was an inner moral court of judgment that determines whether a maxim, a description of a proposed action, can be willed as a law to govern everyone who is similarly situated. "Conscience is practical reason holding up before a man his duty for acquittal or condemnation in every case under a law."[24] He went on to explain that

> Every concept of duty contains objective constraint through the law (a moral imperative limiting our freedom) and belongs to practical understanding, which gives the rule. . . . All of this takes place before a tribunal called a court of justice, as though before a moral person who gives effect to the law. The consciousness of an inner court of justice within man ("before which his thoughts accuse or excuse one another") is *conscience*.[25]

These views, which equate conscience with the God-given faculty of reason, lack the emotional appeal of conscience as an inner moral sense. They also lack the personal and self-aggrandizing status of being directly informed by God's voice. Reasoning and developing principles to guide one's actions are hard intellectual work that smacks of elitism. It is, therefore, no surprise that the right reason perspective on conscience is less popular with the masses than the view of conscience as a moral sense or an inner voice of God.

---

[22] Hobbes's Laws of Nature direct people to obey their civil sovereign, who has the authority to make civil law and dictate limits on religious practices. He therefore maintained that the civil laws,

> As far as they differ not from the Laws of Nature, there is no doubt, but that they are the Law of God, and carry their Authority with them, legible to all men that have the use of naturall reason: but this is no other Authority, then that of all other Morall Doctrine consonant to Reason; the Dictates whereof are Laws, not *made*, but *Eternall*. (Hobbes, *Hobbes's Leviathan*, 300; 33/200)

[23] Hobbes, *Hobbes's Leviathan*, 288; 32/197.

[24] Kant I, *Immanuel Kant: Ethical Philosophy*, translated by JW Ellington (Indianapolis, Indiana: Hackett, 1983). See "The Metaphysics of Morals, Part II, The Metaphysical Principles of Virtue, Introduction, XII. Sensitive Basic Concepts of the Susceptibility of the Mind to Concepts of Duty Generally, B. Concerning Conscience," 59/400.

[25] Kant, *Immanuel Kant*, "The Metaphysics of Morals, Part II, The Metaphysical Principles of Virtue, §13 Concerning Man's Duty to Himself Insofar as He Is the Innate Judge of Himself," 100/438.

The Link: How Conscience Binds

The nature of conscience and its authority in directing action were especially important topics in the ethics literature of the seventeenth and eighteenth centuries and continued to be important to numerous later authors. For example, the early twentieth century author C. S. Lewis (1898–1963) identified conscience as the "internal witness,"[26] and with similar import, people recently have defended their acts of civil disobedience as inspired by conscientious objection. Even some late twentieth-century bioethicists who experienced revulsion in contemplating possible future applications of biomedical technology identified their reactions with the inner sense of conscience, what they called "the yuk factor."[27]

Conscientious objection remains a controversial issue in society, and today's moral dilemma is whether a person who believes she acts from conscience can be doing something wrong when the action violates a moral law. The question is whether a person should follow the dictates of private conscience, obey the civil law, or abide by professional ethics. The inner voice, moral sense advocates' position, has been that conscience should determine assent, and one should always act in accordance with one's moral sense.

Aquinas, Hobbes, and Kant viewed conscience more as setting moral limits on action, so that it was never acceptable for a person to violate the moral law. According to those moral theorists, people are free to act as they see fit as long as their actions do not transgress the moral law, and they each expressed that conclusion in their own terms. For Aquinas, the moral law is what the Bible commands that we must not do. For Hobbes, the Laws of Nature tell us what we must not do. And for Kant, we must not act on maxims that cannot be categorically willed as moral laws that should bind everyone.[28]

Thus, even though the two groups of theorists had very different views on what conscience is and how we can recognize what conscience requires of us, they all agreed that the dictates of conscience must be accepted as either directing or limiting action, and people who regard themselves as being bound by conscience must conform their action with what conscience requires of them. In other words, a person who commits herself to following

[26] Lewis CS, *Studies in Words*, 2nd edition (Cambridge: Cambridge University Press, 1967: 187).

[27] Kass L, "The Wisdom of Repugnance: Why We Should Ban the Cloning of Humans," *The New Republic* 216, 22 (1997): 17–26.

[28] Kant, *Immanuel Kant*, "The Metaphysics of Morals, Part II, The Metaphysical Principles of Virtue, Introduction, VI. Ethics Does Not Give Laws for Actions but Only for the Maxims of Actions," 47/389.

the dictates of conscience regards herself as committed to fulfilling her commitment to follow the dictates of conscience. This approach to morality, in essence, derives moral authority from binding oneself. It is both an overarching perspective on ethics as arising from a personal acceptance of the responsibility to conform one's actions to morality and an instance of the view that we should uphold the commitments that we make. Stated in simple terms, it means that that we should keep the promises that we make to ourselves and keep the promises that we make to others.

Thus, someone who regards certain actions as being contrary to the dictates of conscience should not commit herself to performing them. Said another way, someone who undertakes an obligation commits herself to fulfilling that obligation. And said in Kantian terms, a person should not make a promise that she does not intend to keep.[29]

Putting this digression aside for a few pages, let's return to the issue of conscientious objectors.

Conscientious Objectors

Disgusted by slavery and the war that would spread slavery into Mexico's territory, American intellectual Henry David Thoreau (1817–1862) published an essay, "Civil Disobedience," in 1849. There he argued that people should not permit government to overrule their conscience, and that they had a duty not to acquiesce and thereby enable government to make them agents of injustice. Thoreau demonstrated his conscience-directed nonviolent resistance to the Mexican-American War by refusing to pay his taxes and choosing to be jailed instead. Taking a stand that is compatible with the inner sense view of conscience, Thoreau asked,

> Must the citizen ever for a moment, or in the least degree, resign his conscience to the legislator? Why has every man a conscience, then? I think that we should be men first, and subjects afterward. It is not desirable to cultivate a respect for the law, so much as for the right. The only obligation which I have a right to assume is to do at any time what I think right. It is truly enough said that a corporation has no conscience; but a corporation

---

[29] Kant, *Immanuel Kant*, "The Grounding for the Metaphysics of Morals, Part I, Second Section," 31/423. Kant regarded this as a perfect duty.

of conscientious men is a corporation *with* a conscience. Law never made men a whit more just; and, by means of their respect for it, even the well-disposed are daily made the agents of injustice.[30,31]

Mohandas Gandhi (1869–1948) was influenced by Thoreau's view of nonviolent civil disobedience, and he held a similar view on conscience. He maintained, "In matters of conscience, the law of the majority has no place."[32] Gandhi employed nonviolent resistance in his struggles to overcome oppression, first on behalf of Indians living in South Africa and later in India. In India he initiated a noncooperation movement involving marches and fasts and called on his fellow Indians to withdraw from British institutions, return honors conferred by the British, and learn self-reliance. His conscientious objection and nonviolent activism culminated in his call for Indian independence from British rule in 1942. In response, the British government held Gandhi under arrest until after the end of World War II.

Martin Luther King Jr. (1929–1968) was a Baptist minister who became a US civil rights activist early in his career largely because his view of Christianity committed him to follow his conscience. Gandhi's achievements inspired him to adopt nonviolent civil disobedience. With a call for a coalition of conscience, King led nonviolent marches and massive protests to end racial segregation and discrimination and promote justice and human dignity, declaring, "There comes a time when we must take a position that is neither safe, nor politic, nor popular, but one must take it because it is right."[33] In the course of his civil rights activism, Dr. King had his house bombed, was arrested upward of twenty times, was assaulted at least four times, and was ultimately assassinated.

In June 2018, some US Immigration Department Employees became conscientious objectors when they refused to participate in President Trump's and Attorney General Jeff Sessions's policy and orders to separate children from their asylum-seeking parents. When they recognized that what they were being ordered to do was immoral and unlawful and chose to abide by

---

[30] Thoreau HD, "Civil Disobedience" [Originally published as "Resistance to Civil Government"] (1849). Accessed June 23, 2018, at http://sniggle.net/Experiment/index5.php?entry=rtcg

[31] Thoreau's position is clearly at odds with Hobbes's view on the substance of what conscience dictates for subjects of a civil society.

[32] Gandhi M, Accessed August 5, 2019, at https://wealthygorilla.com/78-mahatma-gandhi-quotes/.

[33] King, M. Accessed August 5, 2019, at http://www.famous-quote.net/comes-time-one-must-take-position-neither-safe-politic-popular.html

the limitations that their consciences imposed, they risked their jobs, prosecution, and other unknown penalties. Nevertheless, they refused to participate in wrongdoing and were willing to bear the burdens of their decisions.

Conscientious Objectors in Medicine Today

Most recently, defending rights of conscientious objection has become a cause, primarily for people concerned with what they regard as infringements on religious freedom and political right-wing moral conservatives. In the medical arena, these advocates invoke conscientious objection to exempt healthcare workers from participating in the provision of legal abortion services and life-ending refusal of treatment or aid in dying, and they champion state and federal legislation to protect healthcare provider conscience rights.[34] The Church Amendments, 42 U.S.C. § 300a-7 Section 245 of the Public Health Service Act, and the Weldon Amendment, collectively known as the "federal health care provider conscience protection statutes," were first enacted in the 1970s.[35] They prohibit recipients of certain federal funds from discriminating against healthcare professionals who base their refusal to participate in abortion or sterilization procedures, training, performance, or arrangements on religious or moral objections. Since 2005, the Weldon Amendment has been incorporated into each subsequent Health and Human Services appropriations act. Its protections extend to "an individual physician or other health care professional, a hospital, a provider-sponsored organization, a health maintenance organization, a health insurance plan, or any other kind of health care facility, organization, or plan." Even the 2010 Affordable Care Act includes conscience protections within the health insurance exchange program.[36] Section 1303(b)(4) of the act provides that "no qualified health plan offered through an Exchange may discriminate against

---

[34] Among those who defend significant discretionary space for medical professionals' conscientious objection are the following: Lynch H, *Conflicts of Conscience in Health Care* (Cambridge, MA: MIT Press, 2008); Wicclair MR, *Conscientious Objection in Healthcare* (Cambridge: Cambridge University Press, 2011); Weinstock D, "Conscientious Refusal and Healthcare Professionals: Does Religion Make a Difference?" *Bioethics* 28, 1 (2014): 8–15; Sulmasy DP, "Tolerance, Professional Judgment, and the Discretionary Space of the Physician," *Cambridge Quarterly of Healthcare Ethics* 26, 1 (2017): 18–31.

[35] US Department of Health and Human Services. *Federal Statutory Health Care Provider Conscience Protections*. Accessed June 27, 2018, at https://www.hhs.gov/conscience/conscience-protections/index.html

[36] HealthCare.gov. *Patient Protection and Affordable Care Act*. Accessed June 27, 2018, at https://www.healthcare.gov/glossary/patient-protection-and-affordable-care-act/

any individual health care provider or health care facility because of its un-willingness to provide, pay for, provide coverage of, or refer for abortions."

There are two straightforward reasons for challenging these claims of con-scientious objection and allowing them legal protections.[37] (1) A person who makes a choice for self-serving reasons and imposes burdens on others is not a conscientious objector. (2) A conscience-based refusal to provide a lawful and medically beneficial service is not an acceptable option for a medical professional. Allow me to explain each of these objections.

(1) Traditionally, as the examples illustrate, people who invoke conscience as their reason for refusing to abide by a civil law or the commands of someone with authority are willing to bear the burdens of their moral commitments. Pacifists in World War I who refused to take violent action against others ac-cepted particularly dangerous service as medics on the battlefield rather than violate their beliefs. Thoreau, Gandhi, and King accepted their incarcerations because that was the price for the civil disobedience that their consciences compelled them to perform. The US Immigration Department employees who refused to participate in separating children from their parents at the border accepted the unknown penalties of their conscientious objection.

Today's medical professionals who assert a conscience-based refusal ask to be protected from bearing the burdens of their inner discomfort. In doing so, they are willing to impose burdens of compromised liberty and health or possible death on patients. They show no compunction over causing patients affront with their judgmental refusal, no empathy for the inconveniences

[37] Several articles in the bioethics literature have offered arguments opposing rights of con-scientious objection in medicine. Some authors argued forcefully against claims of conscien-tious objection in medicine. Others provided compelling reasons for accommodating objectors and drawing a line between acceptable and unacceptable refusals to provide medical services. Here, I am not responding directly to those positions, but engaging in the debate by taking a dif-ferent approach to the issue. This literature includes the following: Cantor J and Baum K, "The Limits of Conscientious Objection—May Pharmacists Refuse to Fill Prescriptions for Emergency Contraception?" *New England Journal of Medicine* 351, 19 (2004): 2008–2012; Charo RA, "The Celestial Fire of Conscience: Refusing to Deliver Medical Care," *New England Journal of Medicine* 352, 24 (2005): 2471–2473; Swarz MS, "'Conscience Clauses' or 'Unconscionable Clauses': Personal Beliefs Versus Professional Responsibilities," *Yale Journal of Health Policy, Law & Ethics*, 6, 2 (2006): 269–350; Savulescu J, "Conscientious Objection in Medicine," *British Medical Journal*, 332, 7536 (2006): 294–297; Savulescu J and Schuklenk U, "Doctors Have No Right to Refuse Medical Assistance in Dying, Abortion or Contraception," *Bioethics* 31, 3 (2016): 162–170; West-Oram P and Buyx A, "Conscientious Objection in Health Care Provision: A New Dimension," *Bioethics* 30, 5 (2016): 336–343; Giubilini A, "Objection to Conscience. An Argument Against Conscience Exemptions in Healthcare," *Bioethics* 31, 5 (2017): 400–408; Schuklenk U and Smalling R, "Why Medical Professionals Have No Moral Claim to Conscientious Objection Accommodation in Liberal Democracies," *Journal of Medical Ethics* 43, 4 (2017): 234–240; McConnell D, "Conscientious Objection in Healthcare: How Much Discretionary Space Best Supports Good Medicine?" *Bioethics* 33, 1 (2019): 154–161.

that they impose of having to find another doctor, and no compassion for the financial costs related to missed work, child care, and transportation expenses that their patients then have to bear.

For the sake of their own comfort, they are also willing to burden the shrinking number of medical professionals who continue to put the interests of patients before their own with increasing risks to their safety and their lives. In sum, today's medical professionals who make claims of conscientious objection to refuse patients services are unwilling to sacrifice anything for their beliefs. They are, therefore, not entitled to be counted conscientious objectors. In any other context, they instead would be fittingly described as selfish egoists. They misappropriate the term and abuse the language to claim the moral high ground when their behavior is at odds with the historical use of the term.

(2) There are some duties that everyone has: to be truthful, to be kind, to avoid harming others, to keep promises, and so forth. Other duties are distinctive obligations that only those who voluntarily undertake them have to fulfill. The duties of parenthood, of repaying a debt, of hosting a guest, and the like are responsibilities that we have only when we choose to accept them. These are special duties that arise from personal commitments, and they bind only those who assume them. People who take on special responsibilities may be granted special powers, privileges, and immunities, but the essence of assuming a special obligation is giving up freedoms that they had before. People who choose to become parents, for example, are allowed the powers to discipline their offspring and require them to complete household chores without pay, the privileges of naming them and choosing whether they are to be raised with or without a religion and which one, and the immunity from prosecution for kidnapping when they move their reluctant brood away from their friends to another state. At the same time, in their act of choosing to become parents people give up the freedoms of sleeping through the night, spending all of their money on themselves, and all of their afterwork hours alone and doing as they please. By freely accepting the role of parents, people who might otherwise have preferred to avoid messes and unpleasant odors become obliged to change their infants' dirty diapers and clean up these offspring when they vomit.

Individuals who voluntarily take on special duties that involve interactions with others give people good reason to rely on them to carry out their obligations and fulfill the responsibilities of the jobs that they have freely accepted. The person who agrees to water your plants or look after your pet assumes those obligations and ethically must, therefore, fulfill them even when the tasks turn out to be inconvenient or when they find the chores obnoxious or repulsive.

Choosing to become a professional is promising to take on the special responsibilities of that profession. Thus, someone who loves uniforms, medals, military parades, and big war machines and chooses to become a soldier is not free to assert a pacifist conscientious objection to killing or using force. Taking on professional obligations entails giving those duties at least prima facie priority over other commitments. We would find it outrageous for firefighters or police who had moral convictions in opposition to Nazis or political right-wingers to refuse them the aid or protections that they were otherwise due. This is because the firefighters and police had taken on their professional responsibilities to fulfill their obligations to all of the people in their society.

As the American Board of Internal Medicine (ABIM), the American College of Physicians (ACP) Foundation, and the European Federation of Internal Medicine declared in their 2005 statement, "Medical Professionalism in the New Millennium: A Physician Charter," medical professionalism "demands placing the interests of patients above those of the physician."[38] Every ethical code, each oath of medical professionals, and all of the discussions of medical professionalism that I have encountered similarly assert the primacy of medicine's commitment to its fiduciary responsibility and putting the welfare of patients before the doctor's own.[39-46] Furthermore,

[38] Brennan T, et al., "Medical Professionalism in the New Millennium: A Physician Charter," *Lancet* 359, 9305 (2002): 520–522, and *Annals of Internal Medicine* 136, 3 (2002): 243–246. It is interesting to note that this joint statement by US and European physicians lists 10 professional responsibilities which are consistent with the 16 duties on my list.

[39] Cruess RL and Cruess SR, "Expectations and Obligations: Professionalism and Medicine's Social Contract With Society," *Perspectives in Biology and Medicine* 51, 4 (2008): 579–598.

[40] Miles SH, *The Hippocratic Oath and the Ethics of Medicine* (New York: Oxford University Press, 2005).

[41] Liaison Committee on Medical Education, *Functions and Structure of a Medical School Standards for Accreditation of Medical Education Programs Leading to the MD Degree*, Association of American Medical Colleges and the American Medical Association, March 2014. Accessed June 27, 2018, at https://med.virginia.edu/ume-curriculum/wp-content/uploads/sites/216/2016/07/2017-18_Functions-and-Structure_2016-03-24.pdf

[42] Brody H and Doukas D, "Professionalism: A Framework to Guide Medical Education," *Medical Education* 48, 10 (2014): 980–987.

[43] Carrese JA, Malek J, Watson K, et al., "The Essential Role of Medical Ethics Education in Achieving Professionalism: The Romanell Report," *Academic Medicine* 90, 6 (2015): 744–752.

[44] DeAngelis CD, "Medical Professionalism in the Twenty-First Century," in DeAngelis CD, editor, *Patient Care and Professionalism* (New York: Oxford University Press, 2014): 61–76.

[45] Byyny RL, "Reflections on Best Practices for Medical Professionalism in the Modern Era," in Byyny RL, Paauw DS, Papadakis M, and Pfeil S, editors, *Professionalism Best Practices: Professionalism in the Modern Era* (Aurora, CO: Alpha Omega Alpha Honor Medical Society, 2017: 129–143).

[46] Humphrey H and Levinser D, "Becoming a Doctor: The Learner and the Learning Environment: A Complex Interaction," in Byyny RL, Paauw DS, Papadakis M, Pfeil S, editors, *Professionalism Best Practices: Professionalism in the Modern Era* (Aurora, Colorado: Alpha Omega Alpha Honor Medical Society, 2017: 97–116).

only members of the medical profession are allowed the powers, privileges, and immunities required for the performance of pregnancy termination and sterilization procedures, and in the states that allow aid in dying, only physicians may provide the prescriptions. Because they have chosen to be doctors, and because they uniquely have the knowledge, skills, tools, powers, privileges and immunities to perform these tasks, they are obliged to use that license in serving their patients. There is no obvious reason why soldiers, police, firefighters, teachers, priests, judges, and members of other professions should be regarded as duty bound to fulfill their responsibilities when they might prefer not to, while medical professionals are allowed to invoke conscience and opt out at the expense of others.

In his *A Letter Concerning Toleration* [hereafter, *Letter*], philosopher and physician John Locke (1632–1704) asserted that, "Promises, covenants, and oaths, . . . are the bonds of human society."[47] Thomas Hobbes had also noted the moral importance of promise keeping when he set it down as the Third Law of Nature, "that men perform covenants made" (XV, 1). And in his *Grounding for the Metaphysics of Morals,* Immanuel Kant argued that making a promise with the intention of breaking it would be a violation of the moral law.[48] The list of like-minded moral theorists, theologians, and others on both sides of the conscientious objection debate who share that basic view on promise keeping goes on and on.

Becoming a physician is making a commitment to patients and society and taking on the medical profession's special obligations. As physician Edmund Pellegrino noted in his article, "Professionalism, Profession and the Virtues of the Good Physician," " 'Profession' is to declare aloud, . . . publicly. . . . Professionals commit themselves when the 'Oath' is taken." "It is . . . a binding commitment [of] enter[ing] a moral community whose defining purpose is to respond to and to advance the welfare of patients." Pellegrino recognized that "the doctor voluntarily promises that he can be trusted and incurs the moral obligations of that promise." He continued to explain that, "The profession is 'declared' in the daily encounter with patients. Every time a physician sees a patient and asks 'What can I do for you?' . . . he or she is professing to use . . . competence in the best interests of the patient."[49]

---

[47] Locke J, *Toleration 1689* [Conventionally known as *A Letter About Toleration*], Section 10,4:21. Accessed June 23, 2018, at http://www.earlymoderntexts.com/assets/pdfs/locke1689b.pdf. Copyright Jonathan Bennett 2017.

[48] Kant, *Immanuel Kant,* "The Grounding for the Metaphysics of Morals, Part I, Second Section," 31/423.

[49] Pellegrino ED, "Professionalism, Profession and the Virtues of the Good Physician," *The Mount Sinai Journal of Medicine* 69, 6 (2002): 378–384; 379.

Although this view is widely endorsed by physicians and the public in most contexts, some people appear to forget this insight when they approach the issues of abortion and aid in dying. For example, Dr. Pellegrino clearly understood what a physician's professional commitment entailed when he considered the obligations of physicians broadly and even when he focused on specific challenges like the duty to provide medical care for patients living with HIV. In his article, "Physician's Duty to Treat: Altruism, Self-Interest and Medical Ethics," Pellegrino argued that individual physicians are not entitled to make individual, personal judgments about the dangerousness of treating HIV-positive patients.[50] Instead, he asserted that each individual physician must provide treatment because, according to the judgment of the profession, the risk of infection is not significant enough to defeat the professional duty to provide treatment. Pellegrino's conclusion, that personal values and personal assessment of risk have no place in the response of the medical professional, amounts to a general principle of medical ethics.

Unfortunately, the clarity of his discernment became clouded when he considered abortion and took a stand that was inconsistent with his other writing on the subject to defend the supremacy of personal morality over professional responsibility. In a 1987 article, "Toward a Reconstruction of Medical Morality," Pellegrino fell back on the view that other physicians put forward when they refuse to provide medical services based on a claim of conscientious objection. There he maintained that each of the parties in a doctor-patient relationship "must respect the dignity and values of the other," and that physicians should not be expected to sacrifice their own values in the service of their patients as long as they announce their positions in advance.[51]

That stand strikes me as having your cake and eating it, too. Yes, each party in a relationship should respect the values of the other. That means parties should not disparage one another based on their private values and continue to treat each other with respect. But nothing in that truth suggests that either party should be freed from fulfilling her obligations to the other. A person who acts with dignity honors her commitments and fulfills her obligations. So, as I see it, respectful interactions require all parties to uphold their commitments and abstain from shirking the duties that they have

---

[50] Pellegrino ED, "Physician's Duty to Treat: Altruism, Self-Interest and Medical Ethics," *Journal of the American Medical Association* 258, 14 (1987): 1939–1940.

[51] Pellegrino ED, "Toward a Reconstruction of Medical Morality," *The Journal of Medical Humanities* 8, 1 (1987): 7–18.

accepted. Priests who come to realize that they cannot uphold their commitment to celibacy recognize that they must resign from the priesthood regardless of how much they enjoy other aspects of that role. Similarly, people who choose to become doctors need to consider whether or not the commitments of medical professionals are consistent with their own values. If not, they should pursue another career, and we "must respect the dignity and values" that lead them to make their choice.

A similar confusion to Pelligrino's is evidenced in a recent article, "Tolerance, Professional Judgment, and the Discretionary Space of the Physician," by philosopher physician Daniel Sulmasy where he drew on John Locke's *A Letter Concerning Toleration*. Sulmasy rightly highlighted Locke's claim that we should tolerate the "practical principles or opinions by which men think themselves obliged to regulate their actions with one another." He correctly pointed out that Locke argued for tolerating different religious views as long as they were not "apparently destructive to society . . . because the conscience, or persuasion of the subject, cannot possibly be a measure by which the magistrate can, or ought to frame his laws, which ought to be suited to the good of all his subjects, not the persuasions of a part."[52,p.21]

It seems to me, however, that Sulmasy may have overlooked a distinction that Locke made. Although Locke supported religious tolerance of "private persons," he also drew a distinction between them and the professional duties of magistrates. In Locke's day, the term *magistrate* included judges, legislators, and monarchs.[53] Locke was pointedly focused on distinguishing magistrates' professional duty created by their "promises, covenants, and oaths" from the responsibilities of other people when he remarked, "In the last place, let us now consider what is the **magistrate's duty** in the business of toleration, which certainly is very considerable" [emphasis added].[54] He then asserted, "The public good is the rule and measure of all law-making."[55]

Locke went on to make a statement about conscientious objection by posing the following question:

[52] Sulmasy D, "Tolerance, Professional Judgment, and the Discretionary Space of the Physician," *Cambridge Quarterly of Healthcare Ethics* 28, 1 (2017): 18–31.
[53] Locke, "Toleration 1689," note by J Bennett, 1.
[54] Locke J, "A Letter Concerning Toleration," The Federalist Papers Project, 13. Accessed June 23, 2018, at https://www.thefederalistpapers.org/wp-content/uploads/2012/12/John-Locke-A-Letter-Concerning-Toleration.pdf
[55] Locke, "A Letter," 17.

What if the **magistrate** should enjoin anything by his authority that appears unlawful to the conscience of a **private person**? . . . Such a **private person** is to abstain from the action that he judges unlawful, and he is to undergo the punishment which it is not unlawful for him to bear. . . . For the private judgement of any person concerning a law enacted in political matters, for the public good, does not take away the obligation of that law, nor deserve a dispensation. [emphasis added][56]

In other words, Locke took the position that a conscientious objector should be willing to bear the burdens of personal commitments.

Whereas Locke defended toleration of private beliefs, he argued that those who take on professional obligations as the magistrate did must uphold them all, that they should not be exempt from any responsibilities by invoking conscience, and that those who claim exemption from duty have no right to toleration. His statements show that Locke's position on tolerance was at odds with the claims that Sulmasy made in his name. In addition to maintaining that people with a conscientious objection should bear the burdens of their commitment themselves, Locke held that people who impose their private value-based restrictions on others overstep and abuse their authority and thereby act with intolerance.

Hospital Claims of Conscientious Objector Status

Taking the argument a step further, it is important to note that we rely on hospitals as well as physicians to fulfill the full range of medical obligations to the extent that their resources allow.[57] Thus, people who are brought to an emergency department by ambulance and people who follow a blue and white road sign with a large H to deliver an ill passenger to a hospital have reason to expect medical care that is consistent with medical standards regardless of hospital ownership. Hospitals that have the wherewithal but refuse to provide emergency contraception to rape victims or abortion to patients with a medical need for the procedure are failing to meet their responsibilities, and they are not functioning as we reasonably expect hospitals to respond

---

[56] Locke, "A Letter," 23–24.
[57] Nelson L, "Provider Conscientious Refusal of Abortion, Obstetrical Emergency, and Criminal Homicide Law," *American Journal of Bioethics*, 18, 4 (2018): 87. Nelson made the point that arguments against conscientious objection claims also apply to hospitals.

to medical needs. We would not allow an institution that chose to withhold blood from patients who required transfusions to use the title *hospital*, even if it were owned by a Jehovah's Witness, precisely because withholding the service would be inconsistent with good medical practice.

Limiting hospital services to accord with religious beliefs is especially egregious and intolerant when patients are not aware of the institution's deliberate deviations from standard practice and not informed of the unwanted constraints that are imposed by the religiously affiliated owners. It is also intolerant of the physicians working at those institutions who are directed by conscience to serve their patients and provide the medical services that they need. Today, at least 14.5% of hospitals are owned by the Catholic Church.[58] Investigative reporters have found that one in six hospital beds in the United States is in a Catholic hospital. In some States, such as Washington, more than 40 percent of hospital beds are in Catholic hospitals and entire regions of the country have no other option for hospital care. Catholic hospitals also receive billions in taxpayer dollars.[59] Very few of the Catholic hospitals are transparent about the services that they refuse to provide, and some have recently changed their names, apparently to conceal their affiliation and their chosen limitations on services.[60]

It is ethically untenable for any hospital to impose religious doctrines to limit the care of patients who need it. Society grants hospitals numerous privileges (financial and legal) because of the valuable services that we rely on them to provide. It is therefore fair to expect them to meet their responsibilities to society and its members. Hospital ownership is not an essential function of religions, and it is not an inherent element of religious practice. Operating a hospital is, however, a voluntarily undertaken obligation to provide essential services. Therefore, prohibiting hospital owners from imposing religious restrictions on the services they provide would not be a violation of religious freedom.

If any religious group finds the performance of legal and professionally accepted medical procedures to be in opposition to their core religious beliefs,

[58] I am grateful to Udo Schuklenk for bringing these facts to my attention.

[59] Kaye J, Amiri B, Melling L, and Dalven J, *Health Care Denied: Patients and Physicians Speak Out About Catholic Hospitals and the Threat to Women's Health and Lives*, American Civil Liberties Union (2016, May). Accessed May 1, 2018, at https://www.aclu.org/sites/default/files/field_document/healthcaredenied.pdf

[60] Hafner K, "As Catholic Hospitals Expand, So Do Limits on Some Procedures," *The New York Times*, August 10, 2018. Accessed September 3, 2018, at https://www.nytimes.com/2018/08/10/health/catholic-hospitals-procedures.html

they can avoid entanglements with medical facilities and get out of the hospital business. It is unacceptable for them, or any group that will not live up to its voluntarily assumed obligations, to operate a hospital. Operating a hospital that refuses to fulfill its legal and social obligations is unethical because it is making a promise without the intention to keep it.

The Conscience of a Trustworthy Physician

Medical professionals bind themselves to fulfilling all of their professional obligations when they take public oaths and sign public documents that indicate their acceptance of those duties. The act of assuming their professional role entails undertaking the full range of moral responsibilities associated with that position. Medical professionals voluntarily don the white coat and the trappings of their professional role and attach their titles to their names (e.g., MD). These public marks identify individuals as members of their chosen medical profession and allow other members of their societies to rely on them.

The conscience of a trustworthy physician should therefore be determined by the broadly shared views of medical ethics. When a person chooses to join the profession, she makes the duties of medical ethics and professionalism the dictates of her conscience. Whenever she acts in her professional role, she should therefore uphold the duties that she committed herself to fulfill. The well-developed conscience of a physician will direct her practice toward upholding the obligations that she accepted, the most obvious one being the primacy of acting for the good of patients and society. Thus, when a civil authority or institution demands actions that would violate the standard of the profession, a trustworthy doctor should follow the dictates of her conscience to abide by the promises she made and refuse. And when a civil authority or institution refuses to allow doctors to respond to the needs of their patients as medical ethics demands, physicians should follow their conscience and fulfill their professional promises and fiduciary responsibilities.

Because both the sense of conscience as an inner voice and the sense of conscience as the rules of reason provide physicians with clear direction to abide by their commitments, physicians are ethically bound to uphold the duties of medical ethics. A trustworthy psychiatrist will rightly claim conscientious objection to safeguard a patient's confidentiality and accept the penalties that law enforcement agents or institutions might impose. And any other trustworthy doctor's conscience will direct her to provide medical care to patients who may be undocumented or prevent her from reporting her suspicion to immigration officials. The doctor's fiduciary duty to her patients and the duty to uphold confidentiality provide that direction from conscience.[61] When different professional duties conflict in a particular situation, there may not be a set rule for resolving the conflict. Deliberating with colleagues, as doctors do in their rounds and conferences by offering reasons for upholding one professional duty or sacrificing another that happens to conflict in some specific circumstances, is the medical equivalent of the Kantian court of conscience that should guide a physician through a complex dilemma of medical ethics.

Conclusions

Neither the moral sense/inner voice conception of conscience nor the right reason sense of conscience can defend today's obfuscating claims of conscientious objection by members of medical professions or medical institutions. Because the claimants are unwilling to bear the burdens of their choices and are instead quite willing to impose burdens on patients and colleagues so that they may be excused from their responsibilities, their misappropriation of the term should be recognized as employing what Locke termed "deceitful words" to manipulate public opinion and promote their self-advantage.

Most people who hold the moral sense/inner voice conception of conscience regard being true to your word as a conscience-given moral truth that must be followed. People who regard honoring promises and fulfilling commitments to be required by moral laws produced by right reason also conclude that they must abide by their conscience and not violate the moral law. In sum, both perspectives recognize the immorality of undertaking commitments without intending to fulfill them.

When an individual recognizes that the performance of certain professional role responsibilities would conflict with his conscience, he has a moral decision to make. He may either accept the full responsibilities of the profession or bear the burdens of his own conviction and choose another

[61] Sconyers J and Tate T, "How Should Clinicians Treat Patients Who Might Be Undocumented?" *AMA Journal of Ethics* 18, 3 (2016): 229–236. Accessed June 29, 2018, at http://journalofethics.ama-assn.org/2016/03/ecas4-1603.html

path in which his personal beliefs would be compatible with the roles that he voluntarily assumes. A true conscientious objector does not ask others to suffer the burdens of his commitments, but accepts the consequences of the principles that he values. Some people's career choices are limited by financial resources or life circumstances. Other people's career options are restricted by their aptitudes and faculties, and some people's selections are limited by their tastes and aversions. No injustice is involved in recognizing that some people's alternatives may also be limited by their personal values, commitments, or religious affiliation.

People who freely choose to become doctors bind their conscience to the rules and principles of medical ethics. They are no longer free to act on private conscience when they serve in their professional role. When acting as doctors, their conscience should direct them to conform to the duties of medicine. Thus doctors who expect to withhold legal and professionally accepted medical procedures from patients for their own sense of inner comfort violate their professional obligations and the fundamental standard of morality by making a promise that they do not intend to keep. That is an obvious violation of the trust that society invests in doctors.

In sum, because the people in our society trust doctors and hospitals to fulfill all of their obligations to us and rely on them to put the interests of patients before their own, individuals and institution choosing not to fulfill the duties of their station should recognize that what they do is immoral. They should not take on roles that are incompatible with their personal values when they intend not to satisfy some of their voluntarily undertaken duties. Instead, they should limit their choices to commitments that they are willing to honor.

14

Concluding Thoughts

Reprise

The image of doctors that I have evoked throughout this book represents the popular view that medicine is a higher calling and that the medical professional is committed to behavior on a higher standard than what is acceptable in other areas of society. We think that the behavior of soldiers is deplorable when we learn that they were involved in the torture of prisoners, but it seems worse when we learn that *doctors* were involved. We may oppose the death penalty, but it seems especially bad for *doctors* to be involved in its administration. We were dismayed to learn that *doctors* had abandoned patients in the aftermath of Hurricane Katrina. And people were revolted and outraged when they learned that *doctors* were involved in Nazi genocide.

These widely shared sentiments are evidence that common morality is not equivalent to the ethics of medicine. This implies that we need reasons from medical ethics, rather than everyday ethics, to justify the actions and decisions of medical professionals. This was the starting point of my exploration of medicine's distinctive ethical domain, and it ultimately led to the theory of medical ethics that I have presented.

This perspective on medical ethics leads to the further conclusion that because medical ethics is not something that good people already know, and because the duties of physicians are distinctive and different from the duties of common morality, medical ethics must be taught. Doctors need to learn about their professional duties and develop the supporting doctorly virtues so that their actions are consistent with medical professionalism.

Even though I have presented a novel way of describing the obligations that medical ethics requires doctors to fulfill, the duties that I listed capture the well-understood, profession-endorsed responsibilities of physicians and the associated virtues that facilitate the medical behavior that we admire. Because the ethics of medicine is internal to the profession, meaning that the profession's distinguishing morality has been constructed by medical professionals for medical professionals, this fact should not be surprising.

The Trusted Doctor. Rosamond Rhodes, Oxford University Press (2020). © Oxford University Press.
DOI: 10.1093/oso/9780190859909.001.0001

Thoughtful and experienced doctors have recognized the necessity of similar sets of rules since the practice of medicine began.

For the most part, this book's primary contribution is explaining why the ethics of medicine must be as it is and providing an overview and structure that makes sense of the distinct morality of the profession. In this sense, the book is not primarily a criticism of the profession, but an effort to organize the insights of the field into a consistent and reasoned theory of medical ethics. My aim has been to provide a coherent and useful framework that arranges the various aspects of medical professionalism into a structure that makes the requirements of professionalism easy to comprehend and appreciate.

Providing this broad overview of the moral commitments of medicine fills in some serious gaps by explaining broadly acknowledged professional responsibilities that have somehow been omitted from codes of medical ethics promulgated by medical societies. The book also provides a basis for criticizing some elements of medical practice that have been incorporated into today's professional statements and clinical practice. In addition, the book explains important concepts that may have been misunderstood or oversimplified and clarifies confusions that have been created by incorporating concepts and terminology from other domains (e.g., law) or common morality into the ethics of medicine.

Throughout this book I argued that the ethics of medicine is different and distinct from the ethics of everyday life.[1] In making my case, I challenged the common view of medical ethics as merely an extrapolation of the principles of common morality.[2] Instead, I offered a contractarian constructivist account of the distinctive ethical commitments of the medical profession and the basic moral duties that should guide physicians in the practice of medicine. In sum, this adds up to a theory of medical ethics.

Beauchamp and Childress appreciated that a theory of ethics should address a "limited range of morality" and also meet the goals of a moral theory, namely, "to locate and justify general norms." As my explanations and numerous examples illustrate, this theory of medical ethics satisfies all of Beauchamp and Childress's eight criteria for a theory: clarity, coherence,

---

[1] Gert B, Culver CM, and Clouser KD, *Bioethics: A Systematic Approach* (New York: Oxford University Press, 2006).
[2] Beauchamp TL and Childress JF, *Principles of Biomedical Ethics*, 7th edition (New York: Oxford University Press, 2012), 352.

comprehensiveness, simplicity, explanatory power, justificatory power, output power, and practicability.[3]

Regarding medical ethics as the profession's commitment to society, as I do, has two important consequences. First, it implies that physicians' actions must be informed by professional judgment, not personal judgment. Although peer judgment is largely irrelevant in personal morality, peer judgment is a crucial feature of medical ethics. Patients and society rely on physicians to provide treatment according to profession-wide technical and moral standards. This requires doctors to justify the ethical dimension of their actions with reasons from professional ethics and the commitments and values that they share with their peers. The second implication is that becoming a doctor is a moral commitment that involves ceding authority to professional judgment over personal preference.

Medical Ethics and the Structure of Clinical Practice

In presenting a clear theory of medical ethics and explaining why each of the specific duties is a necessary element of professionalism, I avoided discussion of how structural elements of today's medicine impact clinical practice. This omission may have created the impression that I expect doctors to be superheroes and overcome all of the real-life obstacles that they encounter in clinical practice. To try to correct that false impression, I need to say a bit about healthcare structure and how it both eases some physician burdens and creates others. Today's healthcare structure affects clinical practice in at least three different ways: (1) clinical practice arrangements, (2) healthcare financing arrangements, and (3) institutional arrangements.

Clinical Practice Arrangements

In describing a doctor's duties, it may have seemed as if I expect each physician to be superhuman and meet all of the medical needs of each patient. In previous ages, when medicine had little to offer, and before the dramatic growth of cities, the rise of hospitals, and the commitment of many

---

[3] Beauchamp and Childress, *Principles*, 334–336. In Chapter 1, I explain what I take those requirements to be and how they may be satisfied.

societies to make medical care available to all of their people, independent practitioners largely acted alone and did what they could to meet the needs of their relatively small communities. Today, particularly in our urban centers, a variety of practice arrangements have developed to meet the medical needs of large patient populations and provide patients with the specialty care that medical science can offer.

Now, physicians often work in group practices where individual doctors see patients for regularly scheduled office visits and take turns covering emergent patient needs at night and on weekends. A number of different variations on this sort of arrangement work well. They allow doctors to sleep through many nights; have some time for family, friends, and other interests; and even take vacations from time to time. These practice arrangements allow patient needs to be met and medical duties to be fulfilled.

In addition, now that there is so much to know, today's doctors are trained to call on the expertise of colleagues to better serve their patients. Primary care doctors and clinicians of every specialty develop referral networks of various specialties to meet the particular needs of their patients. For example, an oncologist may need to refer a patient to a dermatologist, an oral surgeon, or a psychiatrist so that the patient's needs may be met. No single physician is expected to have expertise in all medical specialties and subspecialties.

And in today's medicine, when a patient has serious and complex medical needs that require round-the-clock attention, patient needs are met in hospitals. There rotating teams of medical professionals provide the care that patients require and call on additional teams with different skills and areas of expertise.

Any of these arrangements that can be trusted to meet patient needs for medical care and provide needed care in a way that promotes the trust of patients and society fulfills the ethical obligations of the profession.

Healthcare Financing Arrangements

Some societies provide their people with healthcare or health insurance; some leave their people to arrange for their own healthcare through employer-provided services or insurance or privately purchased insurance;[4]

---

[4] By leaving its members to make their own arrangements for healthcare, some societies leave many people without access to the care that they may need. Such arrangements are ethically unacceptable

some allot care on a fee-for-service basis; and some operate with a combination of these different financing arrangements. Each comes with its own
advantages and disadvantages, and each mechanism provides incentives and
disincentives for different physician behaviors.

Fee-for-service insurance systems provide payment based on the numbers
and kinds of test and treatments. Such arrangements encourage doctors to
perform many tests and offer many procedures. This is especially the case in
societies where medical malpractice legislation encourages doctors to practice defensive medicine.

To counter the tendencies that increase spending on medical services, various measures have been implemented to control medical inflation and keep
programs from insolvency. Some systems impose limitations on the kinds of
treatments that are offered, eligibility for particular treatments, the number
of people who may receive a particular level of care, the amount of time for
office visits, and the like. Others employ payment mechanisms to control
costs, such as diagnosis-related group (DRG) classifications, which limit
payment for services based on medically relevant patient characteristics
and the patient's diagnosis. This approach imposes financial consequences
to limit tests and treatments and encourages discharging patients from
hospitals as soon as possible. Other approaches that impose penalties for patient readmissions for the same sort of problem aim to encourage adequate
treatment and discharge planning. And some less scrupulous insurers simply
reject claims for expensive treatments, expecting that many who they insure
will simply accept their claim denials without a fight.

By design, these cost containment structures have a significant impact on what individual medical professionals choose to do in the service
of their patients. In addition, many hospitals respond to financial pressures
with staffing cuts (sometimes while also increasing management staff and
salaries).

To some extent, doctors should attend to the costs of the services that they
offer. They should prescribe inexpensive measures rather than expensive
ones when the less costly ones will do the job, and avoid needless spending
so that the available resources can be spread across the population to meet
the needs of more individuals. Doctors also need to muster the courage to resist system-imposed limitations on the treatment of patients who need it and

and they leave physicians with intolerable burdens. They require discussion and action as matters of
urgent public policy.

support extra treatment for patients who are likely to benefit significantly from more than what is standardly allowed and who would suffer for the lack of extra measures. Physicians who are attuned to their duties are often left in the time-consuming, frustrating position of having to battle healthcare financing structures that impose limits on clinical tests and care and the relentless stress of more patient care demands than they can reasonably handled.[5]

Institutional Arrangements

Whereas medicine is a profession and a livelihood for each physician, independent doctors can make their own decisions about how much time to work, how much time to spend with each patient, what treatments to prescribe, and what to charge. We expect that their choices will be guided by their insight into the situations they encounter, their doctorly character, and their commitment to medical professionalism.

A good deal of today's healthcare, however, is provided under the umbrella of some institution. Care is often delivered at an institution or within some sort of relationship with an institution. Medical professionals who provide the care are either employees of institutions or have some financial and practice relationships with institutions. These complex relationships mean that in most cases doctors are no longer fully independent actors who can fully decide what to do or not do, when, where, how, and to whom and what to charge for their services. Instead, administrators at different levels make many decisions that impose limits on what individual physicians may do and encourage physicians to do more or less than they might otherwise decide to do.

Ideal institutional administrators are concerned with delivering quality care and also with the financial viability of their institution. Administrators have to pay attention to the bottom line of their expenditures and accounts receivable because an institution that cannot balance its books will not be able to continue providing patient services. At the same time, administrators have to pay attention to the structural decisions involving healthcare regulations and financing made at higher levels and at greater remove from clinical encounters. To achieve their goals, which may include profits for

---

[5] Ofri D, "The Business of Health Care Depends on Exploiting Doctors and Nurses," *New York Times* Opinion, June 8, 2019.

stockholders of for-profit institutions or obscenely large executive salaries, institutions create their own incentives to encourage cost-conscious behavior from doctors.

Like any other life endeavor, medical practice becomes complicated, and often it is hard to tell whether the practices that are implemented with the aim of meeting lofty goals actually conform to ethical standards or violate them. Thus, the structural arrangements that are adopted to help the profession fulfill its commitments need to be examined and reexamined periodically to determine whether the structures and practices can be trusted to meet the needs of patients and society and whether their implementation is trustworthy. In some respects, each of these kinds of structural arrangements is necessary. The demands for medical care are huge, and as biomedical science and technology advance, the demands for demonstrably effective care keep growing.[6] Yet, the amount of money that any society provides for medical care is limited, the time and energy of medical professionals is limited, and these scare resources have to be rationed.[7] To the extent that different structural arrangements enable the profession to meet the needs of a population, they should be embraced but they also have to be held up to the standards of medical ethics.

Doctors who confront the needs of actual patients need to be alert to the structural influences that institutions impose on them. The institution's interests may encourage the use of only the drugs in the formulary; limit referrals to the institution's staff; and require more or fewer admissions, more or fewer tests, longer or shorter hospital stays, more or fewer procedures, and different approaches at different times. Doctors in these situations need to employ judgment, first to discern the influences at play and then to recognize whether and when the influences need to be resisted. And when resistance is in order, doctors need to marshal their doctorly virtues to confront what needs to be done. Caring is critical for keeping the focus on the patient's good rather than one's own. Courage is needed to stand up to the challenge. Skills in social engagement are needed for managing the conversations that may be involved. Anger over being put in a difficult position will have to

[6] Baumrin B, "Why There Is No Right to Health Care," in Rhodes R, Battin MP, and Silvers A, editors, *Medicine and Social Justice: Essays on the Distribution of Health Care,* 2nd edition (New York: Oxford University Press, 2012: 91–96).
[7] Sreenivasan G, "Why Justice Requires Rationing in Health Care," in Rhodes R, Battin MP, and Silvers A, editors, *Medicine and Social Justice: Essays on the Distribution of Health Care,* 2nd edition (New York: Oxford University Press, 2012: 143–154).

be contained. When financial incentives are provided for conforming to a policy, sometimes the temptation of money must be resisted.

How Medical Ethics Is Good

Coming to the end of this book, I want it to be apparent that medical ethics is good. In presenting this theory of medical ethics, I have been arguing that the goodness of medical ethics lies in its defining medical professionalism and explaining why it is important. I presented arguments to show that physicians must understand their distinctive duties and commit themselves to becoming doctors who can fulfill them. Inherent in my presentation is the view that the ability to identify ethical issues, distinguish relevant duties, employ skill in moral reasoning, and having a doctorly character are essential elements of medical professionalism. These features of medical ethics are critical tools for guiding clinical practice.

In clinical contexts, medical ethics is useful in resolving ethical dilemmas. Physicians need to understand medical ethics and develop their moral as well as clinical judgment to facilitate trustworthy medical treatment decisions. When the decision is less medical and more about the patient's goals and values or sorting out what duty requires, doctors need to be prepared to meet the moral challenges that we expect them to handle with professionalism.

Recognizing the importance of medical ethics leads to the conclusion that a focus on nurturing these elements of physician professionalism should be incorporated as robust features of medical education. Doing so would advance clinicians' thinking about the ethical issues that arise in their practice, inform biomedical research, and give direction to healthcare policy. Unfortunately, clinicians typically receive limited training for addressing the decisions that have to be made. They often experience the situations that they find themselves confronting as some sort of a mess and feel ill prepared for resolving the ethical matters.[8] In such circumstances, facility in medical ethics can be useful in clarifying the issues, providing a road map for navigating the ethical dilemma, and helping clinicians to sort out relevant issues from those that are more tangential.

---

[8] Leitman M, Yim C, and Rhodes R, *Centering Housestaff Ethics Education*, presentation at American Society for Bioethics and Humanities (ASBH), Kansas City, October 19, 2017.

In medical education, medical ethics should play a significant role in preparing trainees to navigate the ethical dilemmas that arise frequently in clinical practice. A medical ethics curriculum that is integrated into all years of training should focus on developing the core competencies that all medical professionals need to have. A good program will aim at fostering understanding of physician duties, developing skills in clinical moral reasoning, nurturing the attitudes and virtues that incline medical professionals to do their duty and become models of medical professionalism, and providing sufficient opportunities to practice those skills over the course of medical training. That training should involve different activities unified by a theory that explains each element and why it is important. Without the explanatory rationale, the enterprise doesn't make sense, and learners may not appreciate why their attention is necessary.

What Is Good Medical Ethics?

From the beginning of this book, I have been arguing that some of what has been called medical ethics is not so good, and my explorations of the field have led me to offer an approach to medical ethics that is radically different from the view that has been dominant for many decades. I have reached the conclusion that the ethics of medicine is different from common morality, and I have laid out what I've identified as its essential duties and virtues. I turn now to trying to show why I take my approach to be good and better than the popular alternatives.

Academic contributions to medical ethics are good when they advance the field. They provide insights, clarify issues, challenge accepted views, provide useful guidance for clinicians and researchers, and spur further discussions. They are well argued, well organized, and well written. Good medical ethics makes valuable contributions to the development of healthcare policy with input that is informed by moral and political philosophy and informed about the relevant medical facts and health systems concerns that are at issue. Good medical ethics offers arguments that are measured, fair, and presented in the interest of the appropriate stakeholders.

That said, I recognize that my attempt to accurately express what comprises good medical ethics is vague, and, therein, somewhat jejune, and I acknowledge that more precision is in order. For me to be more informative and do a better job of explaining what good medical ethics is requires explaining what bad medical ethics is. In this case, bad medical ethics wears the trousers. Here's what I mean: In *Sense and Sensibilia*, when trying to distinguish what is real from what is not, philosopher J. L. Austin identified the kind of difficulty that I am confronting and offered a solution.[9] He noted that sometimes saying what something is not can be more informative than trying to explain what it is. So, while my description of good medical ethics may not be adequately edifying, I am better able to identify and illustrate some of the ways that medical ethics goes wrong. In doing so I identify behaviors, pronouncements, decisions, and policies that wrap themselves in the banner of medical ethics or bioethics that may not be salubrious.

Not So Good Medical Ethics

I consider a good theory of medical ethics to be coherent, illuminating, accurate, reasonable, consistent, and informed and one that is not so good to be lacking in those qualities.

Incoherent

Sometimes an important role of medical ethics is to point out features of medical practice that require some measure of reform or adjustment. Whereas I certainly see room for improvement, for the most part and in many respects, I regard medical practice to be quite admirable. For that reason, good medical ethics should cohere with what we regard as good medical practice.

Regrettably, most approaches to medical ethics view the field as an application of the ethics of everyday life to medicine. Even though authors who take that approach do teach us a great deal and offer numerous valuable insights, I find their overall theoretical approach to medical ethics wanting. As I have tried to show throughout this book, that approach to medical ethics is incoherent. Its principles and rules sometimes direct physicians to act in opposition to their professional duties and they do not explain why doctors have the distinctive duties that we expect them to uphold.

[9] Austin JL, *Sense and Sensibilia*, edited by GJ Warnock GJ (New York: Oxford University Press, 1964).

Not Illuminating

Frequently, the cases that trouble clinicians involve ethical dilemmas. A dilemma can be framed as a question about which of two important principles should be upheld in the particular circumstances or which of two irreconcilable paths is more consistent with professional responsibility. In trying to sort out dilemmas that arise in clinical practice, many people rely on a simplistic version of Beauchamp and Childress's four principles approach for adjudicating and reaching a decision. Typically, they list the ways in which each principle is related to the decision at hand. As Clouser and Gert pointed out in their insightful article, "A Critique of Principlism," the four principles do not provide a mechanism for resolving dilemmas.[10] Similarly, the four topics approach advocated by Albert Jonsen, Mark Siegler, and William Winslade offers no guidance for how to use the information collected into four boxes to adjudicate a problem.[11] And neither does the Gert, Culver, and Clouser approach, which never explains how or why ideals become duties in professions. Yet, Beauchamp and Childress as well as Gert, Culver, and Clouser appeared to take pride in tolerating disagreement. That attitude strikes me as especially inappropriate because doctors need to resolve their disagreements and arrive at a particular course of action that can be endorsed by the entire medical team. Thus, none of these popular approaches to medical ethics provides illuminating guidance for resolving ethical dilemmas.

At the same time, insisting that physicians attend to all four principles, all four topics, or all ten rules diverts attention from key issues and introduces needless confusion by focusing attention on tangential matters, namely principles, topics, or rules that are not at issue. Rote ticking off principles, topics, or rules can be unproductive and distracting without clarifying the issue or helping to resolve the problem.

Furthermore, I am aware that most accounts of medical ethics include discussions of the principles of beneficence and nonmaleficence[12] or moral rules that require doctors to avoid causing death, pain, disability, loss of pleasure, or loss of freedom.[13] In medicine, doctors frequently speak of the

[10] Clouser KD and Gert B, "A Critique of Principlism," *Journal of Medicine and Philosophy* 15, 2 (1990): 219–236.
[11] Jonsen AR, Siegler M, and Winslade WJ, *Clinical Ethics: A Practical Approach to Ethical Decisions in Clinical Medicine*, 7th edition (New York: McGraw-Hill Medical, 2010).
[12] Beauchamp and Childress, *Principles*.
[13] Gert, Culver, and Clouser, *Bioethics*.

"do no harm" principle, which is taken as a gloss of the Hippocratic standard of medical ethics, and amounts to much the same.

My omission of this standard exposition is not an oversight. I chose not to include a separate discussion of these concepts for two reasons. In one sense, they merely express the negative content of ordinary morality, namely, *That which is hateful to you, do not do to your fellow*. Hence, they are not specific features of the ethics of medicine. In another sense, they are redundant expressions of medicine's fiduciary responsibility. Some consequences of medical interventions are beneficial; others are harmful. It is always important for physicians to assess and compare the beneficial and harmful consequences of alternative interventions and their likelihood in determining the course of treatment that serves their patient's interests. Performing that basic analysis is a core duty of medicine and not a dilemma that arises from unusual circumstances. In that sense, discussion of beneficence and nonmaleficence is not illuminating because it adds nothing to our understanding of medical ethics while distorting the view of this constant feature of medical analysis.

Inaccurate

Medical ethics is supposed to serve as a moral compass that provides useful guidance. Instead, medical ethics frequently muddies the waters and points people in the wrong direction. Often, confusion is introduced by conflating issues of personal morality with political issues and issues of professional responsibility, or importing concepts from another domain (e.g., law) into medicine. The "best interest standard" is a case in point. As I have explained, this concept is used in adjudicating legal decisions and it has been widely invoked in medical ethics as the criterion for clinical decisions and clinical behavior. Best interest sounds like mother's milk, and without attending to the problems it introduces, it has become an accepted standard for making medical decisions. Nevertheless, clinicians who have more than one patient and more than one responsibility are frequently not acting in their patient's best interest. When a physician attends to a bleeding accident victim's urgent needs before seeing the patient who arrived earlier with less urgent needs, the physician does the right thing although she is not acting in the best interest of the patient who is left to wait longer. When multiple patients require medical resources or attention, some patient's best interest may have to be sacrificed for the good of others. And when achieving educational goals requires an extra examination of a patient or practice by someone low down on the learning curve, again, the patient's best interest is sacrificed. And when research goals require extra tests or extra time, again, the patient's best interest is sacrificed. Although the patient's interests must always be considered, and clinicians must always strive to achieve optimal outcomes for each patient, often good clinical practice does not actually reflect every patient's best interest. Using best interest language is inaccurate, and it presents a distorted picture of what medicine is and should be.[14]

Seeing significant moral differences between acts and omissions, killing and letting die, or accepting the doctrine of double effect are additional glaring examples of misdirection that has infected medical ethics thinking. Simplistic understanding of these concepts has encouraged some to accept fallacies as truths and led some clinicians to negligent practice, which in any other setting would be identified as blameworthy. As a guide to medical professionalism, medical ethics must be accurate.

Unreasonable

Simplicity is appealing. People like simple principles and rules because knowing them seems to make it easy to avoid wrongdoing. Yet, every simple rule has exceptions. Morality requires making difficult judgments, taking responsibility for them, and living with the uncertainty of not knowing if you made the right call.

In medical ethics, simplicity has its usual appeal. When a doctor fails to distinguish circumstances that require following the principle or rule from those that require a deviation, the result is not good. Consider privacy and informed consent, two key factors that should be carefully assessed in clinical practice and biomedical research. When those factors are taken to be absolute standards, policymakers can make unreasonable demands and sacrifice other important responsibilities (e.g., safety, advancing science) for the sake of protecting privacy or defending the primacy of informed consent.

To make this problem vivid, imagine a bike-riding policy for children that someone committed to preventing harm would advocate. Bike riding would be prohibited because there is no way to allow the activity and absolutely

---

[14] An extended argument against using best interest language is provided in Chapter 12.

guarantee that no child would suffer harm. It's obvious that a "no bike riding" policy would be unreasonable because it would also obstruct the development of important learning and skills. Yet, policymakers in medicine who are absolutely committed to ensuring privacy and informed consent frequently advocate policies that are similarly unreasonable. Whereas privacy and informed consent must be considered, in contexts including public health, clinical practice, education, and research, ensuring absolute privacy and prohibiting any interaction for which informed consent cannot be elicited introduces unreasonable risks and imposes unreasonable burdens. Regarding these protections as "absolutely essential" fails to appreciate that ethics always requires discernment and mindfulness.[15]

Similar problems are created when policymakers regard any risk to a "vulnerable" research participant as a violation of an inviolable moral rule. Risks should always be considered in context. Often enough, risks that are unlikely and harms that are small and fleeting can be justified, even when those who are at risk can be regarded as vulnerable.

Inconsistent

Although Ralph Waldo Emerson chided that "a foolish consistency is the hobgoblin of little minds,"[16] when a point is incisive it should be applied consistently even though some exclusions may be justified. Unfortunately, a lot of inconsistency is incorporated into today's bioethics discussion. For instance, one valuable insight of contemporary medical ethics is the importance of respect for patient autonomy. Yet, in the medical ethics literature we find people employing this concept with meanings from opposite ends of the interpretation spectrum, and sometimes the very same individuals take opposing and inconsistent views in different contexts. In clinical ethics we find clinicians who presume that every patient, including children, the demented, and those who are minimally conscious, has autonomy that must be respected. At the same time, we find authors, policymakers, investigators, and research review board members paternalistically protecting research subjects by advocating that research participants must demonstrate near-perfect understanding of a

---

[15] *The Nuremberg Code*. Accessed August 22, 2018, at https://history.nih.gov/research/downloads/nuremberg.pdf. The first principle states, "1. The voluntary consent of the human subject is absolutely essential."

[16] Emerson RW, *Self-Reliance: A Classic Essay by Emerson* (Rockville, MD: Arc Manor, 2007).

research study before they can be accepted as autonomous participants. On the one hand, as the term is used in clinical medicine it is overly inclusive suggesting that anyone who indicates a preference has autonomy and those preferences must be respected. On the other hand, it is understood too narrowly in biomedical research to suggest that anyone without complete and perfect comprehension of a study lacks the autonomy to make an enrollment decision. At the very least people need to acknowledge that the two contrasting positions on respect for autonomy are inconsistent, and that the difference is rarely noticed.

To belabor the point, consider a few additional common inconsistencies that arise in bioethics discussions:

- Some geneticists who staunchly demand genetic privacy in research also assert the "duty to warn" in clinical genetics. That would require violating the privacy of individual patients who have relied on medical confidentiality and expressed their opposition to sharing personal information.
- In the context of human subject research, bioethicists often insist that the focus must be on the research participants only, regardless of the impact that an inefficient and wasteful study design might have on the broader affected community. Frequently enough, these same bioethicists advocate for considering the welfare of all humanity in public health and environmental matters.
- Many are quick to debunk duties to future generations in arguments for participating in research while they vigorously endorse duties to future generations again when they discuss environmental concerns.

I am not supporting any of these positions but drawing attention to the inconsistencies that abound among bioethicists. Although there may be circumstances that justify shifting one's focus of concern, the change in perspective should be noted and explained. Conceptual sloppiness of this magnitude is not good.

Uninformed

Medical ethics decisions affect the lives of others. People in clinical settings, within institutions, and in the broader society rely on the counsel of physicians, and their reliance entails responsibilities to get the recommendations right. The easiest way to get things wrong in medical ethics is to offer a recommendation that is uninformed. Sometimes it's hard to know what you don't know, but the more novel the issue is, the greater the responsibility to delve into the facts. This point is important both in offering recommendations and in voicing criticism. Without pointing fingers, suffice it to say that offering ethical recommendations without first educating oneself about the facts and the issues and without hearing from key medical and scientific personnel can amount to culpable ignorance rather than good medical ethics.

Ineffectual babble is not advice, and responding by merely reciting vapid platitudes of medical or research ethics without an adequate appreciation of the issues fails to fulfill one's obligations. At the very least, physicians who face ethical issues should make a sincere effort to gather the facts, digest the material, and offer reasoned recommendations or at least a framework for sorting through the problem.

In sum, I trust that the theory of medical ethics that I have provided succeeds by being coherent, illuminating, accurate, reasonable, consistent, and informed while avoiding the pitfalls of being incoherent, not illuminating, inaccurate, unreasonable, inconsistent, and uninformed. My aim was to make my explication of the duties of medical ethics clear and compelling and demonstrate their relevance with informative examples. My intention was to make the approach useful for clinicians and a valuable resource for medical educators.

Final Thoughts

More often than I can recall, after sorting through the ethical issues in a difficult case and reaching a resolution that everyone agrees is what should be done, a doctor who has been part of the discussion will exclaim, "That's not ethics, it's just good medicine." In a way, that statement is wrong, and in a way, it is exactly right. It is wrong because the doctor who makes the remark is failing to appreciate that medicine is through and through about ethics. Medicine is biomedical science applied to promoting the interests of patients and society. That core commitment makes all of medical practice a matter of applied ethics. The doctor's claim that "it's just good medicine" is also correct because good medicine exemplifies medical professionalism by according with the ethics of medicine. In other words, good medicine is inseparable from good medical ethics.

The goal of this book has been to explain that a good doctor is someone who identifies herself with the standards of medical professionalism, is committed to fulfilling the duties of the profession, and seeks the trust of patients and society in her every action. These are demanding requirements that doctors must meet, but doctors expect no less from the physicians who they ask to treat their loved ones and themselves. And because of the extraordinary license that society allows to the profession and our reliance on doctors to measure up to our expectations, it should now be clear that physicians are obliged to uphold the ethics of medicine.

Appendix

The documents that are provided below are intended for the reader's convenient reference. Different versions of the historical documents can be found, and the contemporary documents are revised and updated periodically.

The Hippocratic Oath

I swear by Apollo the Physician, by Asclepius, by Hygeia, by Panacea and by all the gods and goddesses, making them witnesses, to bring the following oath and written covenant to fulfillment, in accordance with my power and my judgment:

To regard him who has taught me this art as equal to my parents, and to share, in partnership, my livelihood with him and to give him a share when he is in need of necessities, and to judge the offspring coming from him equal to my male siblings, and to teach them this art, should they desire to learn it, without fee and written covenant, and to give a share both of rules and of lectures, and of all the rest of learning, to my sons and to the sons of him who has taught me and to the pupils who have both made a written contract and sworn by a medical convention but by no other.

And I will use regimens for the benefit of the ill in accordance with my ability and my judgment, but from what is to their harm or injustice I will keep them. And I will not give a drug that is deadly to anyone if asked for it, nor will I suggest the way to such a counsel. And likewise I will not give a woman a destructive pessary. And in a pure and holy way I will guard my life and my art. I will not cut, and certainly not those suffering from stone, but I will cede this to men who are practitioners of this activity. Into as many houses as I may enter, I will go for the benefit of the ill, while being far from all voluntary and destructive injustice, especially from sexual acts both upon women's bodies and upon men's, both of the free and of the slaves. And about whatever I may see or hear in treatment, or even without treatment, in the life of human beings—things that should not ever be blurted out outside— I will remain silent, holding such things to be unutterable sacred, not to be divulged.

If I render this oath fulfilled, and if I do not blur and confound it making it to no effect, may it be granted to me to enjoy the benefits both of life and of art, being held in good repute among all human beings for time eternal. If, however, I transgress and perjure myself, the opposite of these.

English translation by Heinrich von Staden, "'In a Pure and Holy Way': Personal and Professional Conduct in the Hippocratic Oath?" *Journal of the History of Medicine and Allied Sciences* 51 (1996): 404–437, at 406–408, modified.

Oath of Maimonides

The eternal providence has appointed me to watch over the life and health of Thy creatures.

May the love for my art actuate me all time; may neither avarice nor miserliness, nor thirst for glory or for a great reputation engage my mind; for the enemies of truth and philanthropy could easily deceive me and make me forgetful of my lofty aim of doing good to Thy children.

May I never see in the patient anything but a fellow creature in pain.

Grant me the strength, time and opportunity always to correct what I have acquired, always to extend its domain; for knowledge is immense and the spirit of man can extend indefinitely to enrich itself daily with new requirements.

Today he can discover his errors of yesterday and tomorrow he can obtain a new light on what he thinks himself sure of today.

Oh, God, Thou has appointed me to watch over the life and death of Thy creatures; here am I ready for my vocation and now I turn unto my calling.

Accessed December 13 at https://www.einstein.yu.edu/uploadedFiles/education/md-program/diversity/March%202013%20Office%20of%20Diversity%20Enhancement%20Newsletter.pdf

American Medical Association Code of Medical Ethics

American Medical Association Principles of Medical Ethics (Revised June 2001)

Preamble

The medical profession has long subscribed to a body of ethical statements developed primarily for the benefit of the patient. As a member of this profession, a physician must recognize responsibility to patients first and foremost, as well as to society, to other health professionals, and to self. The following Principles adopted by the American Medical Association are not laws, but standards of conduct that define the essentials of honorable behavior for the physician.

Principles of medical ethics

I. A physician shall be dedicated to providing competent medical care, with compassion and respect for human dignity and rights.

II. A physician shall uphold the standards of professionalism, be honest in all professional interactions, and strive to report physicians deficient in character or competence, or engaging in fraud or deception, to appropriate entities.

III. A physician shall respect the law and also recognize a responsibility to seek changes in those requirements which are contrary to the best interests of the patient.

IV. A physician shall respect the rights of patients, colleagues, and other health professionals, and shall safeguard patient confidences and privacy within the constraints of the law.

V. A physician shall continue to study, apply, and advance scientific knowledge, maintain a commitment to medical education, make relevant information available to patients, colleagues, and the public, obtain consultation, and use the talents of other health professionals when indicated.

VI. A physician shall, in the provision of appropriate patient care, except in emergencies, be free to choose whom to serve, with whom to associate, and the environment in which to provide medical care.

VII. A physician shall recognize a responsibility to participate in activities contributing to the improvement of the community and the betterment of public health.

VIII. A physician shall, while caring for a patient, regard responsibility to the patient as paramount.

IX. A physician shall support access to medical care for all people.

https://www.ama-assn.org/sites/default/files/media-browser/principles-of-medical-ethics.pdf

Australian Medical Association Code of Ethics 2004.

Editorially Revised 2006. Revised 2016

Members are advised of the importance of seeking the advice of colleagues should they be facing difficult ethical situations.

1. PREAMBLE
   1.1 Medical professionalism embodies the values and skills that the profession and society expects of doctors (medical practitioners). A Code of Ethics is essential for setting and maintaining the expected standards of ethical behaviour within the medical profession.
   1.2 The AMA Code of Ethics articulates and promotes a body of ethical principles to guide doctors' conduct in their relationships with patients, colleagues and society.
   1.3 This Code has grown out of other similar ethical codes stretching back into history including the Hippocratic Oath and those from other cultures.
   1.4 Because of their particular knowledge and expertise, doctors have a responsibility to patients who entrust themselves to medical care.
   1.5 The doctor-patient relationship is a partnership based on mutual respect, collaboration and trust. Within the partnership, both the doctor and the patient have rights as well as responsibilities.
   1.6 While doctors have a primary duty to individual patients, they also have responsibilities to other patients and the wider community.
   1.7 The principles in the AMA Code of Ethics apply to all doctors regardless of their professional roles.
2. The Doctor and the Patient
   2.1 Patient care
      2.1.1 Consider first the well-being of the patient.
      2.1.2 Treat the patient as an individual, with respect, dignity and compassion in a culturally and linguistically appropriate manner.
      2.1.3 Respect the patient's right to choose their doctor freely.
      2.1.4 Communicate effectively with the patient and obtain their consent before undertaking any tests, treatments or procedures (there may be an exception in emergency circumstances) or involving them in research, teaching or disclosing their personal information to others.
      2.1.5 Respect the patient's right to make their own health care decisions. This includes the right to accept, or reject, advice regarding treatments and procedures including life-sustaining treatments.

2.1.6 Respect the patient's right to refuse consent or to withdraw their consent.

2.1.7 Encourage and support the patient to take an interest in managing their health.

2.1.8 Respect the patient's request for a support person.

2.1.9 Facilitate coordination and continuity of care.

2.1.10 Respect the fact that a patient may have more than one established doctor-patient relationship.

2.1.11 Recognise that you may decline to enter into a therapeutic relationship where an alternative health care provider is available and the situation is not an emergency one.

2.1.12 Recognise that you may decline to continue a therapeutic relationship if it becomes ineffective or compromised. Under such circumstances, you can discontinue the relationship if an alternative health care provider is available and the situation is not an emergency one. You must inform the patient so that they may seek care elsewhere and assist in facilitating arrangements for their continuing care.

2.1.13 If you refuse to provide or participate in some form of diagnosis or treatment based on a conscientious objection, inform the patient so that they may seek care elsewhere. Do not use your conscientious objection to impede patients' access to medical treatments including in an emergency situation.

2.1.14 Where a patient's death is deemed to be imminent and where curative or life-prolonging treatment appears to be of no medical benefit, try to ensure that death occurs with comfort and dignity.

2.1.15 Respect the right of a terminally ill patient to receive relief from pain and suffering, even where that may shorten their life.

2.1.16 Avoid providing care to anyone with whom you have a close personal relationship, where possible.

2.1.17 Facilitate the ongoing care of your patients, including the management of their medical records, if closing or relocating your practice.

2.1.18 Recognise the patient's right to make a complaint in relation to their health care. Ensure they are provided with information on the complaints process and do not let a complaint adversely affect the patient's care.

2.2 Protection of patient information

2.2.1 Respect the patient's right to know what information is held about them, their right to access their medical records and their right to have control over its use and disclosure, with limited exceptions.

2.2.2 Maintain the confidentiality of the patient's personal information including their medical records, disclosing their information to others only with the patient's express up-to-date consent or as required or authorised by law. This applies to both identified and de-identified patient data.

2.2.3 Maintain accurate, contemporaneous medical records.

2.2.4 Ensure patient information is kept secure.

2.2.5 Facilitate arrangements for accessing, transferring and storing medical records upon retirement.

2.3 Patients with limited, impaired or fluctuating decision-making capacity

2.3.1 Presume an adult patient has decision-making capacity, the ability to make and communicate a decision, unless there is evidence to the contrary.

2.3.2 Recognise that some patients may have limited, impaired or fluctuating decision-making capacity. As such, any assessment of capacity for health care decision-making is relevant to a specific decision at a specific point in time.

2.3.3 Respect the patient's ability to participate in decisions consistent with their level of capacity at the time a decision needs to be made. This includes decisions involving their health care as well as the use and disclosure of their personal information.

2.3.4 Recognise that some patients will have capacity to make a supported decision while others will require a substitute decision-maker.

2.3.5 Recognise that a competent minor may have the capacity to make a specific health care decision on their own behalf.

2.4 **Patients' family members, carers and significant others**

2.4.1 Treat the patient's family members, carers and significant others with respect.

2.4.2 Recognise that the patient's family members and carers may also need support, particularly where the patient's condition is serious or life-limiting. Provide them with information regarding respite care, bereavement care, carer's support and other relevant services, where appropriate.

2.5 **Clinical research**

2.5.1 Endeavour to participate in properly designed, ethically approved research involving human participants in order to advance medical progress.

2.5.2 Recognise that the rights and interests of the individual research participant takes precedence over the interests of others including the research team, affiliated institutions, funders and the broader community.

2.5.3 Make sure that all research participants are fully informed and have consented to participate in the study.

2.5.4 Seek patient consent to inform treating doctors of the involvement of patients under their care in any research project, the nature of the project and its ethical basis.

2.5.5 Respect the patient's right to withdraw from a study at any time without prejudice to medical treatment.

2.5.6 Make sure that the patient's decision not to participate in a study does not compromise the doctor-patient relationship or appropriate treatment and care.

2.5.7 Ensure that research results are reviewed by an appropriate peer group before public release.

2.6 **Clinical teaching**

2.6.1 Honour your obligation to pass on your professional knowledge and skills to colleagues and students, where appropriate.

2.6.2 Before conducting clinical teaching involving patients, ensure that the patient is fully informed and has consented to participate.

2.6.3 Respect the patient's right to refuse or withdraw from participating in clinical teaching at any time without compromising the doctor-patient relationship or appropriate treatment and care.

2.6.4 Avoid compromising patient care in any teaching exercise. Ensure that the patient is managed according to the best-proven diagnostic and therapeutic methods and that the patient's comfort and dignity are maintained at all times.

2.7 **Fees**

    2.7.1 Set a fair and reasonable fee having regard to the time, skill and experience involved in the performance of your services, the relevant practice costs and the particular circumstances of the case and the patient.

    2.7.2 Recognise the importance of informed financial consent, ensuring that the patient is informed of and consents to your fees prior to the medical service being provided, where possible. Where a service you provide is in conjunction with other doctors or hospitals who will charge separate fees, advise the patient of this and how they can obtain information on those separate fees.

    2.7.3 Encourage open discussion of health care costs with the patient.

3. **The Doctor and the Profession**

3.1 **Professional conduct**

    3.1.1 Practise medicine to the best of your ability, recognising and working within your ability and scope of practice.

    3.1.2 Build a professional reputation based on integrity and ability.

    3.1.3 Recognise that your personal conduct may affect your reputation and that of your profession.

    3.1.4 Take responsibility for your own health and well-being including having your own general practitioner.

    3.1.5 Continue lifelong professional development to keep your knowledge, skills and performance up-to-date and improve your standard of medical care.

    3.1.6 Keep up-to-date on relevant codes of practice and legal responsibilities.

    3.1.7 Accept responsibility for maintaining and improving the standards of the profession.

    3.1.8 Maintain appropriate professional boundaries with patients and their close family members, not entering into sexual, exploitative or other inappropriate relationships.

    3.1.9 Refrain from offering inducements to patients, accepting inducements from patients or encouraging patients to give, lend or bequeath you money or gifts.

    3.1.10 Report suspected unethical or unprofessional conduct by a colleague to the appropriate authority.

    3.1.11 Report any form of bullying or harassment of, or by, students, colleagues or other health care professionals.

3.2 **Working with colleagues**

    3.2.1 Treat your colleagues with respect and dignity.

    3.2.2 Recognise colleagues who are unwell or under stress. Know how and when to respond if you are concerned about a colleague's health and take action to minimise the risk to patients and the doctor's health.

    3.2.3 Refrain from undertaking actions such as making comments which may unfairly damage the reputation of a colleague.

    3.2.4 Treat those under your supervision with respect, care and patience.

3.3 **Referral to colleagues**

    3.3.1 Recognise your professional limitations and be prepared to refer as appropriate.

    3.3.2 Obtain the opinion of an appropriate colleague acceptable to the patient if diagnosis or treatment is difficult or in response to a reasonable request by the patient.

3.3.3 When referring a patient, make available to your colleague, with the patient's knowledge and consent, all relevant information and indicate whether or not they are to assume the continuing care of the patient during their illness.

3.3.4 When an opinion has been requested by a colleague, report in detail your findings and recommendations to that doctor.

3.3.5 Respect the central role of the general practitioner in patient care. Should a patient require a referral to another specialist, ideally the referral should be made following consultation with the patient's general practitioner— except in an emergency situation. Any decision should be communicated to the general practitioner in a timely fashion.

3.4 **Working with other health care professionals and as part of a health care team**

3.4.1 Treat other health care professionals with respect and dignity.

3.4.2 Ensure that doctors and other health care professionals upon whom you call to assist in the care of the patient are appropriately qualified.

3.4.3 Work collaboratively with other members of the patient's health care team.

3.4.4 Adhere to your responsibility in delegation and handover of care of the patient.

3.4.5 Recognise the role of other support services including translators, Indigenous community members, religious, spiritual and cultural advisers.

3.5 **Managing conflicts of interests**

3.5.1 Ensure your financial or other interests are secondary to your primary duty to serve patients' interests. Financial and other interests should not compromise, or be perceived to compromise, your professional judgement, capacity to serve patients' interests or the community's trust in the integrity of the medical profession.

3.5.2 Disclose your financial or other interests that may affect, or be perceived to affect, patient care.

3.5.3 If you refer a patient to a facility, or recommend a treatment or product in which you have a financial interest, inform them of that interest and provide the patient with other options, where possible.

3.5.4 If you work in a practice or institution, place your professional duties and responsibilities to patients above the commercial interests of the owners or others who work within these practices.

3.6 **Advertising**

3.6.1 Confine advertising of professional services to the presentation of information reasonably needed by patients or colleagues to make an informed decision about the availability and appropriateness of your medical services.

3.6.2 Ensure that any announcement or advertisement directed towards patients or colleagues is demonstrably true in all respects. Advertising should not bring the profession into disrepute.

3.6.3 Do not endorse therapeutic goods in public advertising.

3.6.4 Exercise caution in endorsing non-therapeutic goods in public advertising.

3.6.5 Do not have any public association with products that clearly affect health adversely.

4. The Doctor and Society

4.1 Responsibility to society

4.1.1 Participate in activities that contribute to the health of the community and the wider public health. These can include matters relating to health education, environmental protection, public health and legislation impacting on health.

4.2 Professional autonomy and clinical independence

4.2.1 Uphold professional autonomy and clinical independence and advocate for the freedom to exercise professional judgement in the care and treatment of patients without undue influence by individuals, governments or third parties.

4.2.2 Refrain from entering into any contract with a colleague or organisation which you consider may conflict with your professional autonomy, clinical independence or your primary obligation to the patient.

4.2.3 Recognise your right to refuse to carry out services which you consider to be professionally unethical, against your moral convictions, imposed on you for either administrative reasons or for financial gain or which you consider are not in the best interests of the patient.

4.2.4 Alert appropriate authorities when the health care service or environment within which you work is inadequate or poses a threat to health.

4.2.5 The doctor who reasonably believes that significant harm will occur to the public as a result of the delivery or non-delivery of health care, despite the process mentioned in paragraph 4.2.4, would be open to taking whistleblowing action. Contemporary protections for whistleblowers should be supported by doctors.

4.3 Health standards, quality and safety

4.3.1 Participate in risk management, quality assurance and improvement activities.

4.3.2 Accept a share of the profession's responsibility to society in matters relating to the health and safety of the public, health education and literacy and legislation affecting the health of the community.

4.3.3 When providing scientific information to the public, recognise a responsibility to give the generally held opinions of the profession in a form that is readily understood. When presenting any personal opinion which is contrary to the generally held opinion of the profession, indicate that this is the case.

4.4 Stewardship

4.4.1 Practise effective stewardship, the avoidance or elimination of wasteful expenditure in health care, in order to maximise quality of care and protect patients from harm while ensuring affordable care in the future. Remember, however, that your primary duty is to provide the patient(s) with the best available care.

4.4.2 Practise effective stewardship in any setting in which your work, whether clinical, research or administrative.

4.4.3 Use your knowledge and skills to assist those responsible for allocating health care resources, advocating for their transparent and equitable allocation.

4.5 Medico-legal responsibilities

4.5.1 Recognise your responsibility when preparing medico-legal documents such as medical certificates or independent medical assessments. The information you provide must be honest, accurate and not misleading.

4.5.2 Recognise your responsibility to assist the courts, tribunals (or similar forums) by providing informed, fair opinion based on impartial, expert evidence when reasonably called upon to do so.

4.5.3 Ensure the patient understands your medico-legal role and responsibilities as it relates to their care.

4.6 Health equity and human rights

4.6.1 Endeavour to improve the standards and quality of, and access to, medical services in the community.

4.6.2 Provide care impartially and without discrimination on the basis of age, disease or disability, creed, religion, ethnic origin, gender, nationality, political affiliation, race, sexual orientation, criminal history, social standing or any other similar criteria.

4.6.3 Do not countenance, condone or participate in the practice of torture or other forms of cruel, inhuman or degrading procedures.

https://ama.com.au/system/tdf/documents/AMA%20Code%20of%20Ethics%20 2004.%20Editorially%20Revised%202006.%20Revised%202016.pdf?file=1&type=node &id=46014

Canadian Medical Association Code of Ethics (Update 2004)

This Code has been prepared by the Canadian Medical Association as an ethical guide for Canadian physicians, including residents, and medical students. Its focus is the core activities of medicine—such as health promotion, advocacy, disease prevention, diagnosis, treatment, rehabilitation, palliation, education and research. It is based on the fundamental principles and values of medical ethics, especially compassion, beneficence, nonmaleficence, respect for persons, justice and accountability.

Fundamental Responsibilities

1. Consider first the well-being of the patient.
2. Practise the profession of medicine in a manner that treats the patient with dignity and as a person worthy of respect.
3. Provide for appropriate care for your patient, even when cure is no longer possible, including physical comfort and spiritual and psychosocial support.
4. Consider the well-being of society in matters affecting health.
5. Practise the art and science of medicine competently, with integrity and without impairment.
6. Engage in lifelong learning to maintain and improve your professional knowledge, skills and attitudes.
7. Resist any influence or interference that could undermine your professional integrity.

8. Contribute to the development of the medical profession, whether through clinical practice, research, teaching, administration or advocating on behalf of the profession or the public.
9. Refuse to participate in or support practices that violate basic human rights.
10. Promote and maintain your own health and well-being.

Responsibilities to the Patient

General Responsibilities

11. Recognize and disclose conflicts of interest that arise in the course of your professional duties and activities, and resolve them in the best interest of patients.
12. Inform your patient when your personal values would influence the recommendation or practice of any medical procedure that the patient needs or wants.
13. Do not exploit patients for personal advantage.
14. Take all reasonable steps to prevent harm to patients; should harm occur, disclose it to the patient.
15. Recognize your limitations and, when indicated, recommend or seek additional opinions and services.
16. In determining professional fees to patients for non-insured services, consider both the nature of the service provided and the ability of the patient to pay, and be prepared to discuss the fee with the patient.

Initiating and Dissolving a Patient-Physician Relationship

17. In providing medical service, do not discriminate against any patient on such grounds as age, gender, marital status, medical condition, national or ethnic origin, physical or mental disability, political affiliation, race, religion, sexual orientation, or socioeconomic status. This does not abrogate the physician's right to refuse to accept a patient for legitimate reasons.
18. Provide whatever appropriate assistance you can to any person with an urgent need for medical care.
19. Having accepted professional responsibility for a patient, continue to provide services until they are no longer required or wanted; until another suitable physician has assumed responsibility for the patient; or until the patient has been given reasonable notice that you intend to terminate the relationship.
20. Limit treatment of yourself or members of your immediate family to minor or emergency services and only when another physician is not readily available; there should be no fee for such treatment.

Communication, Decision Making and Consent

21. Provide your patients with the information they need to make informed decisions about their medical care, and answer their questions to the best of your ability.
22. Make every reasonable effort to communicate with your patients in such a way that information exchanged is understood.
23. Recommend only those diagnostic and therapeutic services that you consider to be beneficial to your patient or to others. If a service is recommended for the benefit of others, as for example in matters of public health, inform your patient of this fact and proceed only with explicit informed consent or where required by law.

24. Respect the right of a competent patient to accept or reject any medical care recommended.
25. Recognize the need to balance the developing competency of minors and the role of families in medical decision-making. Respect the autonomy of those minors who are authorized to consent to treatment.
26. Respect your patient's reasonable request for a second opinion from a physician of the patient's choice.
27. Ascertain wherever possible and recognize your patient's wishes about the initiation, continuation or cessation of life-sustaining treatment.
28. Respect the intentions of an incompetent patient as they were expressed (e.g., through a valid advance directive or proxy designation) before the patient became incompetent.
29. When the intentions of an incompetent patient are unknown and when no formal mechanism for making treatment decisions is in place, render such treatment as you believe to be in accordance with the patient's values or, if these are unknown, the patient's best interests.
30. Be considerate of the patient's family and significant others and cooperate with them in the patient's interest.

Privacy and Confidentiality

31. Protect the personal health information of your patients.
32. Provide information reasonable in the circumstances to patients about the reasons for the collection, use and disclosure of their personal health information.
33. Be aware of your patient's rights with respect to the collection, use, disclosure and access to their personal health information; ensure that such information is recorded accurately.
34. Avoid public discussions or comments about patients that could reasonably be seen as revealing confidential or identifying information.
35. Disclose your patients' personal health information to third parties only with their consent, or as provided for by law, such as when the maintenance of confidentiality would result in a significant risk of substantial harm to others or, in the case of incompetent patients, to the patients themselves. In such cases take all reasonable steps to inform the patients that the usual requirements for confidentiality will be breached.
36. When acting on behalf of a third party, take reasonable steps to ensure that the patient understands the nature and extent of your responsibility to the third party.
37. Upon a patient's request, provide the patient or a third party with a copy of his or her medical record, unless there is a compelling reason to believe that information contained in the record will result in substantial harm to the patient or others.

Research

38. Ensure that any research in which you participate is evaluated both scientifically and ethically and is approved by a research ethics board that meets current standards of practice.
39. Inform the potential research subject, or proxy, about the purpose of the study, its source of funding, the nature and relative probability of harms and benefits, and the nature of your participation including any compensation.
40. Before proceeding with the study, obtain the informed consent of the subject, or proxy, and advise prospective subjects that they have the right to decline or withdraw from the study at any time, without prejudice to their ongoing care.

Responsibilities to Society

41. Recognize that community, society and the environment are important factors in the health of individual patients.
42. Recognize the profession's responsibility to society in matters relating to public health, health education, environmental protection, legislation affecting the health or well-being of the community and the need for testimony at judicial proceedings.
43. Recognize the responsibility of physicians to promote equitable access to health care resources.
44. Use health care resources prudently.
45. Recognize a responsibility to give generally held opinions of the profession when interpreting scientific knowledge to the public; when presenting an opinion that is contrary to the generally held opinion of the profession, so indicate.

Responsibilities to the Profession

46. Recognize that the self-regulation of the profession is a privilege and that each physician has a continuing responsibility to merit this privilege and to support its institutions.
47. Be willing to teach and learn from medical students, residents, other colleagues and other health professionals.
48. Avoid impugning the reputation of colleagues for personal motives; however, report to the appropriate authority any unprofessional conduct by colleagues.
49. Be willing to participate in peer review of other physicians and to undergo review by your peers. Enter into associations, contracts and agreements only if you can maintain your professional integrity and safeguard the interests of your patients.
50. Avoid promoting, as a member of the medical profession, any service (except your own) or product for personal gain.
51. Do not keep secret from colleagues the diagnostic or therapeutic agents and procedures that you employ.
52. Collaborate with other physicians and health professionals in the care of patients and the functioning and improvement of health services. Treat your colleagues with dignity and as persons worthy of respect.

Responsibilities to Oneself

53. Seek help from colleagues and appropriately qualified professionals for personal problems that might adversely affect your service to patients, society or the profession.
54. Protect and enhance your own health and wellbeing by identifying those stress factors in your professional and personal lives that can be managed by developing and practising appropriate coping strategies.

http://www.cpsa.ca/wp-content/uploads/2019/01/CMA_Policy_Code_of_ethics_of_the_Canadian_Medical_Association_Update_2004_PD04-06-e.pdf

Indian Medical Council (Professional Conduct, Etiquette and Ethics) Regulations

Medical Council of India, Code of Medical Ethics (2002)

Chapter I. Code of Medical Ethics

1.1 Character of Physician

    1.1.1 A physician shall uphold the dignity and honour of his profession.

    1.1.2 The prime object of the medical profession is to render service to humanity; reward or financial gain is a subordinate consideration. Who-so-ever chooses his profession, assumes the obligation to conduct himself in accordance with its ideals. A physician should be an upright man, instructed in the art of healings. He shall keep himself pure in character and be diligent in caring for the sick; he should be modest, sober, patient, prompt in discharging his duty without anxiety; conducting himself with propriety in his profession and in all the actions of his life.

    1.1.3 No person other than a doctor having qualification recognised by Medical Council of India and registered with Medical Council of India/State Medical Council (s) is allowed to practice Modern system of Medicine or Surgery. A person obtaining qualification in any other system of Medicine is not allowed to practice Modern system of Medicine in any form.

1.2 Maintaining good medical practice:

    1.2.1 The Principal objective of the medical profession is to render service to humanity with full respect for the dignity of profession and man. Physicians should merit the confidence of patients entrusted to their care, rendering to each a full measure of service and devotion. Physicians should try continuously to improve medical knowledge and skills and should make available to their patients and colleagues the benefits of their professional attainments. The physician should practice methods of healing founded on scientific basis and should not associate professionally with anyone who violates this principle. The honoured ideals of the medical profession imply that the responsibilities of the physician extend not only to individuals but also to society.

    1.2.2 Membership in Medical Society: For the advancement of his profession, a physician should affiliate with associations and societies of allopathic medical professions and involve actively in the functioning of such bodies.

    1.2.3 A Physician should participate in professional meetings as part of Continuing Medical Education programmes, for at least 30 hours every five years, organized by reputed professional academic bodies or any other authorized organisations. The compliance of this requirement shall be informed regularly to Medical Council of India or the State Medical Councils as the case may be.

1.3 Maintenance of medical records:

    1.3.1 Every physician shall maintain the medical records pertaining to his / her indoor patients for a period of 3 years from the date of commencement of the treatment in a standard proforma laid down by the Medical Council of India.

    1.3.2 If any request is made for medical records either by the patients / authorised attendant or legal authorities involved, the same may be duly acknowledged and documents shall be issued within the period of 72 hours.

    1.3.3 A Registered medical practitioner shall maintain a Register of Medical Certificates giving full details of certificates issued. When issuing a medical certificate he / she shall always enter the identification marks of the patient and keep a copy of the certificate. He / She shall not omit to record the signature and/or thumb mark, address and at least one identification mark of the patient on the medical certificates or report.

    1.3.4 Efforts shall be made to computerize medical records for quick retrieval.

1.4 Display of registration numbers:

    1.4.1 Every physician shall display the registration number accorded to him by the State Medical Council / Medical Council of India in his clinic and in all his prescriptions, certificates, money receipts given to his patients.

    1.4.2 Physicians shall display as suffix to their names only recognized medical degrees or such certificates/diplomas and memberships/honours which confer professional knowledge or recognizes any exemplary qualification/achievements.

1.5 Use of Generic names of drugs: Every physician should, as far as possible, prescribe drugs with generic names and he / she shall ensure that there is a rational prescription and use of drugs.

1.6 Highest Quality Assurance in patient care: Every physician should aid in safeguarding the profession against admission to it of those who are deficient in moral character or education. Physician shall not employ in connection with his professional practice any attendant who is neither registered nor enlisted under the Medical Acts in force and shall not permit such persons to attend, treat or perform operations upon patients wherever professional discretion or skill is required.

1.7 Exposure of Unethical Conduct: A Physician should expose, without fear or favour, incompetent or corrupt, dishonest or unethical conduct on the part of members of the profession.

1.8 Payment of Professional Services: The physician, engaged in the practice of medicine shall give priority to the interests of patients. The personal financial interests of a physician should not conflict with the medical interests of patients. A physician should announce his fees before rendering service and not after the operation or treatment is under way. Remuneration received for such services should be in the form and amount specifically announced to the patient at the time the service is rendered. It is unethical to enter into a contract of "no cure no payment". Physician rendering service on behalf of the state shall refrain from anticipating or accepting any consideration.

1.9 vasion of Legal Restrictions: The physician shall observe the laws of the country in regulating the practice of medicine and shall also not assist others to evade such laws. He should be cooperative in observance and enforcement of sanitary laws and regulations in the interest of public health.

Chapter 2. Duties Of Physicians to their Patients

2.1 Obligations to the Sick

2.1.1 Though a physician is not bound to treat each and every person asking his services, he should not only be ever ready to respond to the calls of the sick and the injured, but should be mindful of the high character of his mission and the responsibility he discharges in the course of his professional duties. In his treatment, he should never forget that the health and the lives of those entrusted to his care depend on his skill and attention. A physician should endeavour to add to the comfort of the sick by making his visits at the hour indicated to the patients. A physician advising a patient to seek service of another physician is acceptable, however, in case of emergency a physician must treat the patient. No physician shall arbitrarily refuse treatment to a patient. However for good reason, when a patient is suffering from an ailment which is not within the range of experience of the treating physician, the physician may refuse treatment and refer the patient to another physician.

2.1.2 Medical practitioner having any incapacity detrimental to the patient or which can affect his performance vis-à-vis the patient is not permitted to practice his profession.

2.2 Patience, Delicacy and Secrecy: Patience and delicacy should characterize the physician. Confidences concerning individual or domestic life entrusted by patients to a physician and defects in the disposition or character of patients observed during medical attendance should never be revealed unless their revelation is required by the laws of the State. Sometimes, however, a physician must determine whether his duty to society requires him to employ knowledge, obtained through confidence as a physician, to protect a healthy person against a communicable disease to which he is about to be exposed. In such instance, the physician should act as he would wish another to act toward one of his own family in like circumstances.

2.3 Prognosis: The physician should neither exaggerate nor minimize the gravity of a patient's condition. He should ensure himself that the patient, his relatives or his responsible friends have such knowledge of the patient's condition as will serve the best interests of the patient and the family.

2.4 The Patient must not be neglected: A physician is free to choose whom he will serve. He should, however, respond to any request for his assistance in an emergency. Once having undertaken a case, the physician should not neglect the patient, nor should he withdraw from the case without giving adequate notice to the patient and his family. Provisionally or fully registered medical practitioner shall not willfully commit an act of negligence that may deprive his patient or patients from necessary medical care.

2.5 Engagement for an Obstetric case: When a physician who has been engaged to attend an obstetric case is absent and another is sent for and delivery accomplished, the acting physician is entitled to his professional fees, but should secure the patient's consent to resign on the arrival of the physician engaged.

Chapter 3. Duties of Physician in Consultation

3.1 Unnecessary consultations should be avoided:

    3.1.1 However in case of serious illness and in doubtful or difficult conditions, the physician should request consultation, but under any circumstances such consultation should be justifiable and in the interest of the patient only and not for any other consideration.

    3.1.2 Consulting pathologists / radiologists or asking for any other diagnostic Lab investigation should be done judiciously and not in a routine manner.

3.2 Consultation for Patient's Benefit: In every consultation, the benefit to the patient is of foremost importance. All physicians engaged in the case should be frank with the patient and his attendants.

3.3 Punctuality in Consultation: Utmost punctuality should be observed by a physician in making themselves available for consultations.

3.4 Statement to Patient after Consultation:

    3.4.1 All statements to the patient or his representatives should take place in the presence of the consulting physicians, except as otherwise agreed. The disclosure of the opinion to the patient or his relatives or friends shall rest with the medical attendant.

    3.4.2 Differences of opinion should not be divulged unnecessarily but when there is irreconcilable difference of opinion the circumstances should be frankly and impartially explained to the patient or his relatives or friends. It would be opened to them to seek further advice as they so desire.

3.5 Treatment after Consultation: No decision should restrain the attending physician from making such subsequent variations in the treatment if any unexpected change occurs, but at the next consultation, reasons for the variations should be discussed / explained. The same privilege, with its obligations, belongs to the consultant when sent for in an emergency during the absence of attending physician. The attending physician may prescribe medicine at any time for the patient, whereas the consultant may prescribe only in case of emergency or as an expert when called for.

3.6 Patients Referred to Specialists: When a patient is referred to a specialist by the attending physician, a case summary of the patient should be given to the specialist, who should communicate his opinion in writing to the attending physician.

3.7 Fees and other charges:

    3.7.1 A physician shall clearly display his fees and other charges on the board of his chamber and/or the hospitals he is visiting. Prescription should also make clear if the Physician himself dispensed any medicine.

    3.7.2 A physician shall write his name and designation in full along with registration particulars in his prescription letter head.

Chapter 4. Responsibilities of Physicians to Each Other

4.1 Dependence of Physicians on each other: A physician should consider it as a pleasure and privilege to render gratuitous service to all physicians and their immediate family dependants.

4.2 Conduct in consultation: In consultations, no insincerity, rivalry or envy should be indulged in. All due respect should be observed towards the physician in-charge of the case and no statement or remark be made, which would impair the confidence reposed in him. For this purpose no discussion should be carried on in the presence of the patient or his representatives.

4.3 Consultant not to take charge of the case: When a physician has been called for consultation, the Consultant should normally not take charge of the case, especially on the solicitation of the patient or friends. The Consultant shall not criticize the referring physician. He / she shall discuss the diagnosis treatment plan with the referring physician.

4.4 Appointment of Substitute: Whenever a physician requests another physician to attend his patients during his temporary absence from his practice, professional courtesy requires the acceptance of such appointment only when he has the capacity to discharge the additional responsibility along with his / her other duties. The physician acting under such an appointment should give the utmost consideration to the interests and reputation of the absent physician and all such patients should be restored to the care of the latter upon his/her return.

4.5 Visiting another Physician's Case: When it becomes the duty of a physician occupying an official position to see and report upon an illness or injury, he should communicate to the physician in attendance so as to give him an option of being present. The medical officer / physician occupying an official position should avoid remarks upon the diagnosis or the treatment that has been adopted.

Chapter 5. Duties of Physician to the Public and to the Paramedical Profession

5.1 Physicians as Citizens: Physicians, as good citizens, possessed of special training should disseminate advice on public health issues. They should play their part in enforcing the laws of the community and in sustaining the institutions that advance the interests of humanity. They should particularly co-operate with the authorities in the administration of sanitary/public health laws and regulations.

5.2 Public and Community Health: Physicians, especially those engaged in public health work, should enlighten the public concerning quarantine regulations and measures for the prevention of epidemic and communicable diseases. At all times the physician should notify the constituted public health authorities of every case of communicable disease under his care, in accordance with the laws, rules and regulations of the health authorities. When an epidemic occurs a physician should not abandon his duty for fear of contracting the disease himself.

5.3 Pharmacists / Nurses: Physicians should recognize and promote the practice of different paramedical services such as pharmacy and nursing as professions and should seek their cooperation wherever required.

Chapter 6. Unethical Acts: A physician shall not aid or abet or commit any of the following acts which shall be construed as unethical.

6.1 Advertising:

    6.1.1 Soliciting of patients directly or indirectly, by a physician, by a group of physicians or by institutions or organisations is unethical. A physician shall not make use of him / her (or his / her name) as subject of any form or manner of advertising or publicity through any mode either alone or in conjunction with others which is of such a character as to invite attention to him or to his professional position, skill, qualification, achievements, attainments, specialities, appointments, associations, affiliations or honours and/or of such character as would ordinarily result in his self aggrandizement. A physician shall not give to any person, whether for compensation or otherwise, any approval, recommendation, endorsement, certificate, report or statement with respect of any drug, medicine, nostrum remedy, surgical, or therapeutic article, apparatus or appliance or any commercial product or article with respect of any property, quality or use thereof or any test, demonstration or trial thereof, for use in connection with his name, signature, or photograph in any form or manner of advertising through any mode nor shall he boast of cases, operations, cures or remedies or permit the publication of report thereof through any mode. A medical practitioner is however permitted to make a formal announcement in press regarding the following: (1) On starting practice. (2) On change of type of practice. (3) On changing address. (4) On temporary absence from duty. (5) On resumption of another practice. (6) On succeeding to another practice. (7) Public declaration of charges.

    6.1.2 Printing of self photograph, or any such material of publicity in the letter head or on sign board of the consulting room or any such clinical establishment shall be regarded as acts of self advertisement and unethical conduct on the part of the physician. However, printing of sketches, diagrams, picture of human system shall not be treated as unethical.

6.2 Patent and Copy rights: A physician may patent surgical instruments, appliances and medicine or Copyright applications, methods and procedures. However, it shall be unethical if the benefits of such patents or copyrights are not made available in situations where the interest of large population is involved.

6.3 Running an open shop (Dispensing of Drugs and Appliances by Physicians): A physician should not run an open shop for sale of medicine for dispensing prescriptions prescribed by doctors other than himself or for sale of medical or surgical appliances. It is not unethical for a physician to prescribe or supply drugs, remedies or appliances as long as there is no exploitation of the patient. Drugs prescribed by a physician or brought from the market for a patient should explicitly state the proprietary formulae as well as generic name of the drug.

6.4 Rebates and Commission:

    6.4.1 A physician shall not give, solicit, or receive nor shall he offer to give solicit or receive, any gift, gratuity, commission or bonus in consideration of or return for the referring, recommending or procuring of any patient for medical, surgical or other treatment. A physician shall not directly or indirectly, participate in or be a party to act of division, transference, assignment, subordination, rebating, splitting or refunding of any fee for medical, surgical or other treatment.

6.4.2 Provisions of para 6.4.1 shall apply with equal force to the referring, recommending or procuring by a physician or any person, specimen or material for diagnostic purposes or other study / work. Nothing in this section, however, shall prohibit payment of salaries by a qualified physician to other duly qualified person rendering medical care under his supervision.

6.5 Secret Remedies: The prescribing or dispensing by a physician of secret remedial agents of which he does not know the composition, or the manufacture or promotion of their use is unethical and as such prohibited. All the drugs prescribed by a physician should always carry a proprietary formula and clear name.

6.6 Human Rights: The physician shall not aid or abet torture nor shall he be a party to either infliction of mental or physical trauma or concealment of torture inflicted by some other person or agency in clear violation of human rights.

6.7 Euthanasia: Practicing euthanasia shall constitute unethical conduct. However on specific occasion, the question of withdrawing supporting devices to sustain cardio-pulmonary function even after brain death, shall be decided only by a team of doctors and not merely by the treating physician alone. A team of doctors shall declare withdrawal of support system. Such team shall consist of the doctor in charge of the patient, Chief Medical Officer / Medical Officer in charge of the hospital and a doctor nominated by the in-charge of the hospital from the hospital staff or in accordance with the provisions of the Transplantation of Human Organ Act, 1994.

https://www.mciindia.org/documents/rulesAndRegulations/Ethics%20Regulations-2002.pdf

Code of Ethics for the New Zealand Medical Profession

New Zealand Medical Association Code of Ethics (2014)

All medical practitioners, including those who may not be engaged directly in clinical practice, will acknowledge and accept the following Principles of Ethical Behaviour:

1. Consider the health and well being of the patient to be your first priority.
2. Respect the rights, autonomy and freedom of choice of the patient.
3. Avoid exploiting the patient in any manner.
4. Practise the science and art of medicine to the best of your ability with moral integrity, compassion and respect for human dignity.
5. Protect the patient's private information throughout his/her lifetime, and following death, unless there are overriding considerations in terms of public interest or patient safety.
6. Strive to improve your knowledge and skills so that the best possible advice and treatment can be offered to the patient.
7. Adhere to the scientific basis for medical practice while acknowledging the limits of current kno-wledge and contributing responsibly to innovation and research.
8. Honour the profession, its values and its principles in the ways that best serve the interests of patients.

9. Recognise your own limitations and the special skills of others in the diagnosis, prevention and treatment of disease.
10. Accept a responsibility to assist in the protection and improvement of the health of the community.
11. Accept a responsibility to advocate for adequate resourcing of medical services and assist in maximising equitable access to them across the community.
12. Accept a responsibility for maintaining and improving the standards of the profession.

https://www.nzma.org.nz/publications/code-of-ethics

UK General Medical Council, Good Medical Practice (2014)

Patients must be able to trust doctors with their lives and health. To justify that trust you must show respect for human life and make sure your practice meets the standards expected of you in four domains.

Professionalism in action

1. Patients need good doctors. Good doctors make the care of their patients their first concern: they are competent, keep their knowledge and skills up to date, establish and maintain good relationships with patients and colleagues, are honest and trustworthy, and act with integrity and within the law.
2. Good doctors work in partnership with patients and respect their rights to privacy and dignity. They treat each patient as an individual. They do their best to make sure all patients receive good care and treatment that will support them to live as well as possible, whatever their illness or disability.
3. Good medical practice describes what is expected of all doctors registered with the General Medical Council (GMC). It is your responsibility to be familiar with *Good medical practice* and the explanatory guidance which supports it, and to follow the guidance they contain.
4. You must use your judgement in applying the principles to the various situations you will face as a doctor, whether or not you hold a licence to practise, whatever field of medicine you work in, and whether or not you routinely see patients. You must be prepared to explain and justify your decisions and actions.
5. In *Good medical practice*, we use the terms 'you must' and 'you should' in the following ways.
   - 'You must' is used for an overriding duty or principle.
   - 'You should' is used when we are providing an explanation of how you will meet the overriding duty.
   - 'You should' is also used where the duty or principle will not apply in all situations or circumstances, or where there are factors outside your control that affect whether or how you can follow the guidance.
6. To maintain your licence to practise, you must demonstrate, through the revalidation process, that you work in line with the principles and values set out in this guidance. Serious or persistent failure to follow this guidance will put your registration at risk.

Domain 1: Knowledge, skills and performance

Develop and maintain your professional performance

7. You must be competent in all aspects of your work, including management, research and teaching.
8. You must keep your professional knowledge and skills up to date.
9. You must regularly take part in activities that maintain and develop your competence and performance.
10. You should be willing to find and take part in structured support opportunities offered by your employer or contracting body (for example, mentoring). You should do this when you join an organisation and whenever your role changes significantly throughout your career.
11. You must be familiar with guidelines and developments that affect your work.
12. You must keep up to date with, and follow, the law, our guidance and other regulations relevant to your work.
13. You must take steps to monitor and improve the quality of your work.

Apply knowledge and experience to practice

14. You must recognise and work within the limits of your competence.
    14.1 You must have the necessary knowledge of the English language to provide a good standard of practice and care in the UK.
15. You must provide a good standard of practice and care. If you assess, diagnose or treat patients, you must:
    a. adequately assess the patient's conditions, taking account of their history (including the symptoms and psychological, spiritual, social and cultural factors), their views and values; where necessary, examine the patient
    b. promptly provide or arrange suitable advice, investigations or treatment where necessary
    c. refer a patient to another practitioner when this serves the patient's needs.
16. In providing clinical care you must:
    a. prescribe drugs or treatment, including repeat prescriptions, only when you have adequate knowledge of the patient's health and are satisfied that the drugs or treatment serve the patient's needs
    b. provide effective treatments based on the best available evidence
    c. take all possible steps to alleviate pain and distress whether or not a cure may be possible
    d. consult colleagues where appropriate
    e. respect the patient's right to seek a second opinion
    f. check that the care or treatment you provide for each patient is compatible with any other treatments the patient is receiving, including (where possible) self-prescribed over-the-counter medications.
17. You must be satisfied that you have consent or other valid authority before you carry out any examination or investigation, provide treatment or involve patients or volunteers in teaching or research.
18. You must make good use of the resources available to you.

Record your work clearly, accurately and legibly

19. Documents you make (including clinical records) to formally record your work must be clear, accurate and legible. You should make records at the same time as the events you are recording or as soon as possible afterwards.
20. You must keep records that contain personal information about patients, colleagues or others securely, and in line with any data protection law requirements.
21. Clinical records should include:
    a. relevant clinical findings
    b. the decisions made and actions agreed, and who is making the decisions and agreeing the actions
    c. the information given to patients
    d. any drugs prescribed or other investigation or treatment
    e. who is making the record and when.

Domain 2: Safety and quality

Contribute to and comply with systems to protect patients

22. You must take part in systems of quality assurance and quality improvement to promote patient safety. This includes:
    a. taking part in regular reviews and audits of your own work and that of your team, responding constructively to the outcomes, taking steps to address any problems and carrying out further training where necessary
    b. regularly reflecting on your standards of practice and the care you provide
    c. reviewing patient feedback where it is available.
23. To help keep patients safe you must:
    a. contribute to confidential inquiries
    b. contribute to adverse event recognition
    c. report adverse incidents involving medical devices that put or have the potential to put the safety of a patient, or another person, at risk
    d. report suspected adverse drug reactions
    e. respond to requests from organisations monitoring public health.
When providing information for these purposes you should still respect patients' confidentiality.

Respond to risks to safety

24. You must promote and encourage a culture that allows all staff to raise concerns openly and safely.
25. You must take prompt action if you think that patient safety, dignity or comfort is or may be seriously compromised.
    a. If a patient is not receiving basic care to meet their needs, you must immediately tell someone who is in a position to act straight away.
    b. If patients are at risk because of inadequate premises, equipment or other resources, policies or systems, you should put the matter right if that is possible. You must raise your concern in line with our guidance and your workplace policy. You should also make a record of the steps you have taken.

c. If you have concerns that a colleague may not be fit to practise and may be putting patients at risk, you must ask for advice from a colleague, your defence body or us. If you are still concerned you must report this, in line with our guidance and your workplace policy, and make a record of the steps you have taken.

26. You must offer help if emergencies arise in clinical settings or in the community, taking account of your own safety, your competence and the availability of other options for care.

27. Whether or not you have vulnerable adults or children and young people as patients, you should consider their needs and welfare and offer them help if you think their rights have been abused or denied.

Risks posed by your health

28. If you know or suspect that you have a serious condition that you could pass on to patients, or if your judgement or performance could be affected by a condition or its treatment, you must consult a suitably qualified colleague. You must follow their advice about any changes to your practice they consider necessary. You must not rely on your own assessment of the risk to patients.

29. You should be immunised against common serious communicable diseases (unless otherwise contraindicated).

30. You should be registered with a general practitioner outside your family.

Domain 3: Communication, partnership and teamwork
communicate effectively

31. You must listen to patients, take account of their views, and respond honestly to their questions.

32. You must give patients the information they want or need to know in a way they can understand. You should make sure that arrangements are made, wherever possible, to meet patients' language and communication needs.

33. You must be considerate to those close to the patient and be sensitive and responsive in giving them information and support.

34. When you are on duty you must be readily accessible to patients and colleagues seeking information, advice or support.

Working collaboratively with colleagues

35. You must work collaboratively with colleagues, respecting their skills and contributions.

36. You must treat colleagues fairly and with respect.

37. You must be aware of how your behaviour may influence others within and outside the team.

38. Patient safety may be affected if there is not enough medical cover. So you must take up any post you have formally accepted, and work your contractual notice period before leaving a job, unless the employer has reasonable time to make other arrangements.

Teaching, training, supporting and assessing

39. You should be prepared to contribute to teaching and training doctors and students.

40. You must make sure that all staff you manage have appropriate supervision.

41. You must be honest and objective when writing references, and when appraising or assessing the performance of colleagues, including locums and students. References must include all information relevant to your colleagues' competence, performance and conduct.

42. You should be willing to take on a mentoring role for more junior doctors and other healthcare professionals.

43. You must support colleagues who have problems with their performance or health. But you must put patient safety first at all times.

Continuity and coordination of care

44. You must contribute to the safe transfer of patients between healthcare providers and between health and social care providers. This means you must:
    a. share all relevant information with colleagues involved in your patients' care within and outside the team, including when you hand over care as you go off duty, and when you delegate care or refer patients to other health or social care providers.
    b. check, where practical, that a named clinician or team has taken over responsibility when your role in providing a patient's care has ended. This may be particularly important for patients with impaired capacity or who are vulnerable for other reasons.

45. When you do not provide your patients' care yourself, for example when you are off duty, or you delegate the care of a patient to a colleague, you must be satisfied that the person providing care has the appropriate qualifications, skills and experience to provide safe care for the patient.

Establish and maintain partnerships with patients

46. You must be polite and considerate.

47. You must treat patients as individuals and respect their dignity and privacy.

48. You must treat patients fairly and with respect whatever their life choices and beliefs.

49. You must work in partnership with patients, sharing with them the information they will need to make decisions about their care, including:
    a. their condition, its likely progression and the options for treatment, including associated risks and uncertainties
    b. the progress of their care, and your role and responsibilities in the team
    c. who is responsible for each aspect of patient care, and how information is shared within teams and among those who will be providing their care
    d. any other information patients need if they are asked to agree to be involved in teaching or research.

50. You must treat information about patients as confidential. This includes after a patient has died.

51. You must support patients in caring for themselves to empower them to improve and maintain their health. This may, for example, include:

a. advising patients on the effects of their life choices and lifestyle on their health and well-being

b. supporting patients to make lifestyle changes where appropriate.

52. You must explain to patients if you have a conscientious objection to a particular procedure. You must tell them about their right to see another doctor and make sure they have enough information to exercise that right. In providing this information you must not imply or express disapproval of the patient's lifestyle, choices or beliefs. If it is not practical for a patient to arrange to see another doctor, you must make sure that arrangements are made for another suitably qualified colleague to take over your role.

Domain 4: Maintaining trust

Show respect for patients

53. You must not use your professional position to pursue a sexual or improper emotional relationship with a patient or someone close to them.

54. You must not express your personal beliefs (including political, religious and moral beliefs) to patients in ways that exploit their vulnerability or are likely to cause them distress.

55. You must be open and honest with patients if things go wrong. If a patient under your care has suffered harm or distress, you should:

a. put matters right (if that is possible)

b. offer an apology

c. explain fully and promptly what has happened and the likely short-term and long-term effects.

Treat patients and colleagues fairly and without discrimination

56. You must give priority to patients on the basis of their clinical need if these decisions are within your power. If inadequate resources, policies or systems prevent you from doing this, and patient safety, dignity or comfort may be seriously compromised, you must follow the guidance in paragraph 25b.

57. The investigations or treatment you provide or arrange must be based on the assessment you and your patient make of their needs and priorities, and on your clinical judgement about the likely effectiveness of the treatment options. You must not refuse or delay treatment because you believe that a patient's actions or lifestyle have contributed to their condition.

58. You must not deny treatment to patients because their medical condition may put you at risk. If a patient poses a risk to your health or safety, you should take all available steps to minimise the risk before providing treatment or making other suitable alternative arrangements for providing treatment.

59. You must not unfairly discriminate against patients or colleagues by allowing your personal views to affect your professional relationships or the treatment you provide or arrange. You should challenge colleagues if their behaviour does not comply with this guidance, and follow the guidance in paragraph 25c if the behaviour amounts to abuse or denial of a patient's or colleague's rights.

60. You must consider and respond to the needs of disabled patients and should make reasonable adjustments to your practice so they can receive care to meet their needs.

61. You must respond promptly, fully and honestly to complaints and apologise when appropriate. You must not allow a patient's complaint to adversely affect the care or treatment you provide or arrange.

62. You should end a professional relationship with a patient only when the breakdown of trust between you and the patient means you cannot provide good clinical care to the patient.

63. You must make sure you have adequate insurance or indemnity cover so that your patients will not be disadvantaged if they make a claim about the clinical care you have provided in the UK.

64. If someone you have contact with in your professional role asks for your registered name and/or GMC reference number, you must give this information to them.

Act with honesty and integrity
Honesty

65. You must make sure that your conduct justifies your patients' trust in you and the public's trust in the profession.

66. You must always be honest about your experience, qualifications and current role.

67. You must act with honesty and integrity when designing, organising or carrying out research, and follow national research governance guidelines and our guidance.

Communicating information

68. You must be honest and trustworthy in all your communication with patients and colleagues. This means you must make clear the limits of your knowledge and make reasonable checks to make sure any information you give is accurate.

69. When communicating publicly, including speaking to or writing in the media, you must maintain patient confidentiality. You should remember when using social media that communications intended for friends or family may become more widely available.

70. When advertising your services, you must make sure the information you publish is factual and can be checked, and does not exploit patients' vulnerability or lack of medical knowledge.

71. You must be honest and trustworthy when writing reports, and when completing or signing forms, reports and other documents. You must make sure that any documents you write or sign are not false or misleading.
    a. You must take reasonable steps to check the information is correct.
    b. You must not deliberately leave out relevant information.

72. You must be honest and trustworthy when giving evidence to courts or tribunals. You must make sure that any evidence you give or documents you write or sign are not false or misleading.
    a. You must take reasonable steps to check the information.
    b. You must not deliberately leave out relevant information.

73. You must cooperate with formal inquiries and complaints procedures and must offer all relevant information while following the guidance in *Confidentiality*.
74. You must make clear the limits of your competence and knowledge when giving evidence or acting as a witness.
75. You must tell us without delay if, anywhere in the world:
    a. you have accepted a caution from the police or been criticised by an official inquiry
    b. you have been charged with or found guilty of a criminal offence
    c. another professional body has made a finding against your registration as a result of fitness to practise procedures.
76. If you are suspended by an organisation from a medical post, or have restrictions placed on your practice, you must, without delay, inform any other organisations you carry out medical work for and any patients you see independently.

Honesty in financial dealings

77. You must be honest in financial and commercial dealings with patients, employers, insurers and other organisations or individuals.
78. You must not allow any interests you have to affect the way you prescribe for, treat, refer or commission services for patients.
79. If you are faced with a conflict of interest, you must be open about the conflict, declaring your interest formally, and you should be prepared to exclude yourself from decision making.
80. You must not ask for or accept—from patients, colleagues or others—any inducement, gift or hospitality that may affect or be seen to affect the way you prescribe for, treat or refer patients or commission services for patients. You must not offer these inducements.

https://www.gmc-uk.org/-/media/documents/good-medical-practice---english-1215_pdf-51527435.pdf

World Medical Association Declaration of Geneva (2017)

Adopted by the 2nd General Assembly of the World Medical Association, Geneva, Switzerland, September 1948
and amended by the 22nd World Medical Assembly, Sydney, Australia, August 1968
and the 35th World Medical Assembly, Venice, Italy, October 1983
and the 46th WMA General Assembly, Stockholm, Sweden, September 1994
and editorially revised by the 170th WMA Council Session, Divonne-les-Bains, France, May 2005
and the 173rd WMA Council Session, Divonne-les-Bains, France, May 2006
and amended by the 68th WMA General Assembly, Chicago, United States, October 2017

The Physician's Pledge

AS A MEMBER OF THE MEDICAL PROFESSION:

I SOLEMNLY PLEDGE to dedicate my life to the service of humanity;

THE HEALTH AND WELL-BEING OF MY PATIENT will be my first consideration;

I WILL RESPECT the autonomy and dignity of my patient;

I WILL MAINTAIN the utmost respect for human life;

I WILL NOT PERMIT considerations of age, disease or disability, creed, ethnic origin, gender, nationality, political affiliation, race, sexual orientation, social standing or any other factor to intervene between my duty and my patient;

I WILL RESPECT the secrets that are confided in me, even after the patient has died;

I WILL PRACTISE my profession with conscience and dignity and in accordance with good medical practice;

I WILL FOSTER the honour and noble traditions of the medical profession;

I WILL GIVE to my teachers, colleagues, and students the respect and gratitude that is their due;

I WILL SHARE my medical knowledge for the benefit of the patient and the advancement of healthcare;

I WILL ATTEND TO my own health, well-being, and abilities in order to provide care of the highest standard;

I WILL NOT USE my medical knowledge to violate human rights and civil liberties, even under threat;

I MAKE THESE PROMISES solemnly, freely, and upon my honour.

https://www.wma.net/policies-post/wma-declaration-of-geneva/

World Medical Association International Code of Medical Ethics (2006)

Adopted by the 3rd General Assembly of the World Medical Association, London, England, October 1949
and amended by the 22nd World Medical Assembly, Sydney, Australia, August 1968
and the 35th World Medical Assembly, Venice, Italy, October 1983
and the 57th WMA General Assembly, Pilanesberg, South Africa, October 2006

DUTIES OF PHYSICIANS IN GENERAL

A PHYSICIAN SHALL	always exercise his/her independent professional judgment and maintain the highest standards of professional conduct.
A PHYSICIAN SHALL	respect a competent patient's right to accept or refuse treatment.
A PHYSICIAN SHALL	not allow his/her judgment to be influenced by personal profit or unfair discrimination.
A PHYSICIAN SHALL	be dedicated to providing competent medical service in full professional and moral independence, with compassion and respect for human dignity.

A PHYSICIAN SHALL	deal honestly with patients and colleagues, and report to the appropriate authorities those physicians who practice unethically or incompetently or who engage in fraud or deception.
A PHYSICIAN SHALL	not receive any financial benefits or other incentives solely for referring patients or prescribing specific products.
A PHYSICIAN SHALL	respect the rights and preferences of patients, colleagues, and other health professionals.
A PHYSICIAN SHALL	recognize his/her important role in educating the public but should use due caution in divulging discoveries or new techniques or treatment through non-professional channels.
A PHYSICIAN SHALL	certify only that which he/she has personally verified.
A PHYSICIAN SHALL	strive to use health care resources in the best way to benefit patients and their community.
A PHYSICIAN SHALL	seek appropriate care and attention if he/she suffers from mental or physical illness.
A PHYSICIAN SHALL	respect the local and national codes of ethics.

DUTIES OF PHYSICIANS TO PATIENTS

A PHYSICIAN SHALL	always bear in mind the obligation to respect human life.
A PHYSICIAN SHALL	act in the patient's best interest when providing medical care.
A PHYSICIAN SHALL	owe his/her patients complete loyalty and all the scientific resources available to him/her. Whenever an examination or treatment is beyond the physician's capacity, he/she should consult with or refer to another physician who has the necessary ability.
A PHYSICIAN SHALL	respect a patient's right to confidentiality. It is ethical to disclose confidential information when the patient consents to it or when there is a real and imminent threat of harm to the patient or to others and this threat can be only removed by a breach of confidentiality.
A PHYSICIAN SHALL	give emergency care as a humanitarian duty unless he/she is assured that others are willing and able to give such care.
A PHYSICIAN SHALL	in situations when he/she is acting for a third party, ensure that the patient has full knowledge of that situation.
A PHYSICIAN SHALL	not enter into a sexual relationship with his/her current patient or into any other abusive or exploitative relationship.

DUTIES OF PHYSICIANS TO COLLEAGUES

A PHYSICIAN SHALL	behave towards colleagues as he/she would have them behave towards him/her.
A PHYSICIAN SHALL	NOT undermine the patient-physician relationship of colleagues in order to attract patients.
A PHYSICIAN SHALL	when medically necessary, communicate with colleagues who are involved in the care of the same patient. This communication should respect patient confidentiality and be confined to necessary information.

https://www.wma.net/policies-post/wma-international-code-of-medical-ethics/

Index

For the benefit of digital users, indexed terms that span two pages (e.g., 52–53) may, on occasion, appear on only one of those pages.

Tables and figures are indicated by *t* and *f* following the page number

as inner voice (innate), 323–26, 342–43
as internal witness, 330
as moral sense, 323–26, 343
as right reason, 327–29, 342–43
of trustworthy physician, 342–43
conscientious objection, 321, 330, 331–33
arguments against, 334, 340–41n57
duty of, 343–44
Federal Statutory Health Care Provider
Conscience Protections (US), 333–34
by hospitals, 340–42
by medical professionals, 333–40
consensus, overlapping, 234, 234n34,
283–84n2
consent
informed, 101, 172–73, 357
voluntary, 101–2, 357–58n12
consequentialism, 225
constructivism, contractarian, 37
consults, 193–94, 195–96, 197
contraception, 31n59, 340–41
contractarian constructivism, 37
Council for International Organizations of
Medical Sciences (CIOMS), 112, 113
courage, 264–66, 351–52
covenants, 337
critically scarce resource allocation,
243–48, 257t
Cruess, R.L., 336–37n40
culture, 24, 180
Culver, Charles, 355
Bioethics: A Return to Fundamentals
(Gert, Clouser, and Culver),
9–10, 23–29
Bioethics: A Systematic Approach (Gert,
Clouser, and Culver), 9–10, 23–29,
128n14, 283–84, 355–56
Curzer, H.J., 67n55, 274n47

Daniels, Norman, 219–20, 238–39
data collection, 285
four topics approach to, 9–10n5,
285n5, 355
DeAngelis, C.D. 336–37n45
decisional capacity, 24–25, 141
assessment of, 25, 138–60, 146–47n18
cases to consider 151, 152, 154, 155, 156
impaired, 146–47n18, 149–50, 152

decision-making
best interest standard for, 90–92,
301–20, 356–57
surrogate decision making case
example, 318–19
ethical decisions, 9–10, 9–10n5
evaluating decisions, 291–92
evaluation of, 291–92
informed, 173, 359–60
moral dilemmas, 281n54, 283–300, 284t
not unreasonable standard for, 313–17,
315f, 320
parental, 302n4
shared, 171–72, 171–72n50 (*see also*
information sharing)
surrogate, 176, 176n53, 301–20
systematic approach to, 283–300, 284t
three-box approach to, 313–19,
315f, 320
decisions
planning the practical steps for
implementing, 292
Declaration of Geneva (WMA), 47n4, 55–
56, 85, 90–91, 192, 389–90
Declaration of Helsinki:
Recommendations Guiding Medical
Doctors in Biomedical Research
Involving Human Subjects (WMA),
90–91, 92, 113
deep values, 304–5
democratic deliberations, 233–34
Descartes, Rene, 115
deservingness, 124
de Snoo-Trimp, Janine, 171–72
diagnosis-related groups (DRGs), 349
Diekema, D.S., 302n4
difference principle, 219, 231, 232–33, 257t
in chronic care, 236–37, 257t
in preventive care, 241–42, 257t
dilemmas
case examples, 293, 296
systematic approach to, 283–300, 284t
disability-adjusted life expectations
(DALEs), 217
disability-adjusted life years (DALYs), 217
disaster preparedness, 229–30
disaster response, 84–85, 223–24
discipline, peer, 203

408 INDEX